PLURAL+PLUS

COMPANION WEBSITE

Purchase of *Cases in Head and Neck Cancer: A Multidisciplinary Approach* comes with complimentary access to supplementary videos on a PluralPlus companion website.

The companion website is located at:

http://www.pluralpublishing.com/publication/chnc

To access the videos, you must register on the companion website and log in using the access code below.

Access Code: CHNC-GA6FEE

Look for this icon throughout the text, directing you to related videos available on the companion website.

Cases in Head and Neck Cancer

A Multidisciplinary Approach

Cases in Head and Neck Cancer

A Multidisciplinary Approach

Bari Hoffman Ruddy, PhD
Henry Ho, MD
Christine Sapienza, PhD
Jeffrey J. Lehman, MD

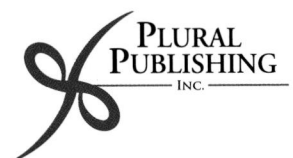

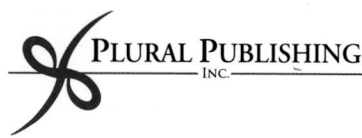
PLURAL PUBLISHING
INC.

5521 Ruffin Road
San Diego, CA 92123

e-mail: info@pluralpublishing.com
Website: http://www.pluralpublishing.com

Library of Congress Cataloging-in-Publication Data

Names: Hoffman Ruddy, Bari, editor. | Ho, Henry, editor. | Sapienza,
   Christine M., editor. | Lehman, Jeffrey J., editor.
Title: Cases in head and neck cancer : a multidisciplinary approach / [edited
   by] Bari Hoffman Ruddy, Henry Ho, Christine Sapienza, Jeffrey J. Lehman.
Description: San Diego, CA : Plural, [2016] | Includes bibliographical
   references and index.
Identifiers: LCCN 2015042630 | ISBN 9781597567152 (alk. paper) | ISBN
   1597567159 (alk. paper)
Subjects: | MESH: Head and Neck Neoplasms—therapy—Case Reports. | Head and
   Neck Neoplasms—diagnosis—Case Reports.
Classification: LCC RC280.H4 | NLM WE 707 | DDC 616.99/491—dc23
LC record available at http://lccn.loc.gov/2015042630

Contents

Preface

In general, head and neck cancer (HNC) accounts for approximately 3% of new cases of cancer in the United States with a male-to-female ratio for HNC estimated as 4:1. The incidence of patient cases with HNC resulting from the use of tobacco products is dropping due to increased societal awareness and antitobacco education. However, the overall incidence of oropharyngeal HNC is increasing as a consequence of the human papillomavirus (HPV).

Assessment and treatment of HNC requires multidisciplinary and integrative care. HNC carries a considerable burden to patients and families, including costs associated with diagnosis, treatment, hospitalization, and medications. Aside from costs that are directly attributable to HNC, there is a considerable load imposed from secondary conditions such as disordered mechanisms of airway protection (cough and swallow). These conditions are nearly ubiquitous among HNC patients at the time of diagnosis and initial treatment, and persist in over half of patients with HNC 5 or more years following diagnosis. Taken alone or together, these conditions increase the likelihood of lung infection and death. A separate financial burden in the form of physician visits, hospitalization for lung infection, medications (particularly antibiotics) to treat the lung infection, and alternative modes of nutritional support (such as tube feeds) for patients with HNC may occur. Yet, by no means is the suffering from HNC and its sequelae merely financial. Cancer, in all its forms, can exert devastating psychosocial and psycho-emotional effects on both patients and caregivers. For patients with HNC, disorders of airway protection transform eating and drinking, activities which are typically as pleasurable as they are necessary, into potential sources of embarrassment or rejection. This can lead to depression and isolation, both of which are factors that negatively impact quality of life (QoL). Health care professionals who treat patients with HNC have an obligation to continually improve the quality and effectiveness of our care. We are also obliged to explore and develop additional, effective, treatment options for our patients that can potentially lessen the financial and interpersonal burdens imposed by this disease.

There are limited resources that provide a comprehensive description of complex HNC cases. Therefore, this book was written by experts in otolaryngology, medical oncology, radiation oncology, speech pathology, nursing, radiology, and dietetics in order to provide a comprehensive presentation of the complexity of the patient with HNC. Health literacy, humanistic care approaches, and information pertaining to diagnostic and clinical concerns are presented to help successfully manage patients with HNC. The cases cover contemporary practice issues surrounding HPV, robotic or minimally invasive surgery, combined modality treatments, reflux management, and the critical role of the speech pathologist are threaded throughout the entire management process. Additionally, issues of survivorship and caregiver burden are included. Finally, unique intervention protocols are highlighted for airway protection along the continuum of prevention, pre-radiation, and post-radiation.

The multimedia component of this book is extraordinary, including complete cases with accompanying images (PET, MRI, CT), surgical video, treatment approaches, and so on. Our intended audience is for graduate education in speech pathology, medical school education, resident education, continuing education for practicing speech-language pathologists, nurse case managers, dieticians, and any person involved on a head and neck cancer team. The models of team practice demonstrate the commitment to the ideal treatment of HNC with the ultimate goal of preserving health and patient quality of life.

Acknowledgments

Florida Hospital Cancer Institute is recognized as one of America's Best Hospitals in Cancer Treatment and is accredited as a Comprehensive Cancer Care Center. The authors' affiliation with the Florida Hospital Cancer Institute, the premier nature of their care teams, and their whole person–centered approach motivated the creation of *Cases in Head and Neck Cancer: A Multidisciplinary Approach*. Ultimately, we hope our book will guide future clinicians to care for the patient with head and neck cancer in the most intelligent and respectful manner.

We are grateful to all of our authors for their wisdom and time spent creating a volume of work that documents their contemporary methods of assessment and treatment of patients with head and neck cancer. With their expert contributions, we are one step closer to helping educate the professional community on the distinct nature and needs of patients with head and neck cancer.

Contributors

Vrushali Angadi, MS, CCC-SLP
Clinical Speech-Language Pathologist
University of Kentucky Voice and Swallow Clinic
PhD Candidate, Rehabilitation Sciences
University of Kentucky
Lexington, Kentucky
Chapter 6

Carl C. Askern, MD, FACS
Director, Aesthetic Plastic Surgery Pavilion
Central California Ear, Nose & Throat
    Medical Group
Assistant Clinical Professor
Department of Surgery, Plastic Surgery Section
University of California, San Francisco
Fresno, California
Chapter 11

Annette N. Askren, MA, CCC-SLP
Speech-Language Pathologist
Department of Veterans Affairs
Washington, District of Columbia
Chapter 11

Samuel R. Atcherson, PhD
Associate Professor
Department of Audiology and Speech Pathology
University of Arkansas at Little Rock
Adjunct Clinical Associate Professor
Department of Otolaryngology-Head and Neck
    Surgery
University of Arkansas for Medical Sciences
Little Rock, Arkansas
Chapter 22

Laura J. Ball, PhD, CCC-SLP
Director of Hearing and Speech Research
Children's National Health System
Associate Professor of Pediatrics
George Washington University
Washington, District of Columbia
Chapter 19

Jeffrey E. Baylor, MD, FACS
Ear, Nose, Throat and Plastic Surgery Associates
Orlando, Florida
Chapter 17

Angela L. Campanelli, MS, CCC-SLP, BCS-S
Voice Pathologist
Dysphagia Specialist
Blaine Block Institute for Voice Analysis
    and Rehabilitation
Dayton, Ohio
Chapter 10

Keith Casper, MD
University of Michigan
Department of Otolaryngology-Head and Neck
    Surgery
Ann Arbor, Michigan
Chapter 3

Jennifer Craig, MS, CCC-SLP
Assistant in Otolaryngology
Vanderbilt Voice Center
Vanderbilt University Medical Center
Nashville, Tennessee
Chapter 15

Elizabeth Feldman, MS, DMD
Maxillofacial Prosthodontics
Dental Oncology
UF Health Cancer Center
Orlando Health
Orlando, Florida
Chapter 7

Thomas J. Gal, MD, MPH, FACS
Professor
Division of Head and Neck Surgery
University of Kentucky
Lexington, Kentucky
Chapter 6

C. Gaelyn Garrett, MD
Professor and Vice Chair
Department of Otolaryngology
Senior Executive Medical Director
Vanderbilt Voice Center
Vanderbilt University Medical Center
Nashville, Tennessee
Chapter 15

Matthew R. Garrett, MD, FACS
Southwest Ohio ENT Specialists, Inc.
Dayton, Ohio
Chapter 10

Douglas A. Girod, MD, FACS
Professor of Otolaryngology-Head and Neck Surgery
Executive Vice Chancellor
University of Kansas Medical Center
Kansas City, Kansas
Chapter 2

G. Brandon Gunn, MD
Assistant Professor
Radiation Oncology
The University of Texas
MD Anderson Cancer Center
Houston, Texas
Chapter 5

Kristie Hadden, PhD
Assistant Professor
Director, Center for Health Literacy
University of Arkansas for Medical Sciences
Little Rock, Arkansas
Chapter 22

Nancy A. Harrington, MA, CCC-SLP
Instructor
Department of Communication Sciences and
    Disorders
University of Central Florida
Florida Alliance for Assistive Services and Technology
Oviedo, Florida
Chapter 19

Henry Ho, MD, FACS
Director
Head and Neck Program
The Florida Hospital Cancer Institute

President
Ear, Nose, Throat and Plastic Surgery Associates
Associate Professor of Surgery
Florida State University College of Medicine
Associate Professor of Otolaryngology
University of Central Florida College of Medicine
Orlando, Florida
Chapters 1, 9, and 18

Bari Hoffman Ruddy, PhD, CCC-SLP
Associate Professor
Department of Communication Sciences and
    Disorders
University of Central Florida
Research Partner
Florida Hospital Cancer Institute
Director, Center for Voice Care and Swallowing
    Disorders
Ear, Nose, Throat and Plastic Surgery Associates
Orlando, Florida
Chapters 1, 9, 14, 18, and 20

Katherine A. Hutcheson, PhD
Assistant Professor
Department of Head and Neck Surgery
Associate Director of Research
Section of Speech Pathology and Audiology
The University of Texas
MD Anderson Cancer Center
Houston, Texas
Chapter 5

Kathleen Ann Kavanagh, DMH, MSN Ed RN
Director of Simulation Training Applied Research
Assistant Professor of Nursing
Brooks Rehabilitation College of Healthcare
    Sciences
School of Nursing
Jacksonville University
Jacksonville, Florida
Chapter 21

Jennifer Kent-Walsh, PhD, CCC-SLP, S-LP(C)
Professor
Communication Sciences and Disorders
Director
FAAST Atlantic Region Assistive Technology
    Demonstration Center

University of Central Florida
Orlando, Florida
Chapter 19

Bernice K. Klaben, PhD, CCC-SLP, BCS-S
Associate Professor
Department of Otolaryngology-Head and Neck
    Surgery
University of Cincinnati Medical Center
Cincinnati, Ohio
Chapter 3

Molly A. Knigge, MS, CCC-SLP, BCS-S
Manager
Adult Swallow, Voice and Swallow Clinics
University of Wisconsin, Madison
Madison, Wisconsin
Chapter 8

Mario A. Landera, SLPD, CCC-SLP, BCS-S
Instructor
Department of Otolaryngology
University of Miami
Miller School of Medicine
Miami, Florida
Chapter 4

Wendy D. LeBorgne, PhD, CCC-SLP
Voice Pathologist, Clinical Director
The Blaine Block Institute for Voice Analysis and
    Rehabilitation
The Professional Voice Center of Greater Cincinnati
Dayton, Ohio
Chapter 10

Jeffrey J. Lehman, MD, FACS
Medical Staff President
Florida Hospital
Medical Director
Center for Voice Care and Swallowing Disorders
Ear, Nose, Throat and Plastic Surgery Associates
Orlando, Florida
Chapters 1 and 14

Elizabeth Leon, MD
Physician
Malcolm Randal VA Medical Center
Assistant Professor
Department of Otolaryngology

University of Florida
Gainesville, Florida
Chapter 11

Vicki Lewis, MA, CCC-SLP
The Center for Voice Care and Swallowing
    Disorders
Ear, Nose, Throat and Plastic Surgery Associates
Orlando, Florida
Chapters 14, 17, 18 and 20

Adam T. Lloyd, MM, MA, CCC-SLP
Speech Pathologist
Ear, Nose, Throat and Plastic Surgery Associates
Voice Care Center
Orlando, Florida
Chapters 9, 13, and 14

Donna S. Lundy, PhD, CCC-SLP, BCS-S
Associate Professor
Department of Otolaryngology
University of Miami
Miller School of Medicine
Miami, Florida
Chapter 4

Kyle Mannion, MD, FACS
Assistant Professor
Department of Otolaryngology, Head and Neck
    Surgery
Vanderbilt University Medical Center
Nashville, Tennessee
Chapter 15

Annette H. May, MA, CCC-SLP, BCS-S
Speech Pathology Coordinator
Oncology
UF Health Cancer Center
Orlando Health
Orlando, Florida
Chapter 7

Timothy M. McCulloch, MD
Charles N. Ford Professor
Chairman, Division of Otolaryngology
Department of Surgery
UW School of Medicine and Public Health
Madison, Wisconsin
Chapter 8

William M. Mendenhall, MD
Professor
Department of Radiation Oncology
University of Florida
Gainesville, Florida
Chapter 11

Claudio F. Milstein, PhD, CCC-SLP
Associate Professor
Cleveland Clinic Lerner College of Medicine
Director, The Voice Center
Head and Neck Institute
Cleveland Clinic
Cleveland, Ohio
Chapter 12

Aftab H. Patni, MD
Ear, Nose, Throat and Plastic Surgery Associates
Orlando, Florida
Chapter 18

Kristen Pytynia, MD, MPH
Associate Professor
Department of Head and Neck Surgery
The University of Texas
MD Anderson Cancer Center
Houston, Texas
Chapter 5

Nikhil Rao, MD
Associate Professor of Radiation Oncology
University of Central Florida College of Medicine
Radiation Oncology Specialists
Florida Hospital
Winter Park, Florida
Chapters 1 and 18

Jennifer R. Reitz, MS, CCC-SLP
Voice Pathologist
The Blaine Black Institute for Voice Analysis and
    Rehabilitation
Dayton, Ohio
Chapter 10

Charles E. Riggs, Jr., MD, FACP
Staff Physician, Medical Division
Clinical Professor
Division of Hematology–Oncology
Department of Medicine

University of Florida College of Medicine
Gainesville, Florida
Chapter 11

Jonathon O. Russell, MD
Head and Neck Institute
Cleveland Clinic
Cleveland, Ohio
Chapter 12

Christine Sapienza, PhD, CCC-SLP
Dean
Brooks Rehabilitation College of Healthcare
    Sciences
Jacksonville University
Jacksonville, Florida
Chapters 1 and 20

Zoukaa B. Sargi, MD, MPH
Associate Professor
Department of Otolaryngology
University of Miami
Miller School of Medicine
Miami, Florida
Chapter 4

Joseph Scharpf, MD, FACS
Head and Neck Institute
Cleveland Clinic Foundation
Associate Professor of Surgery
Cleveland Clinic Lerner College of Medicine
Case Western Reserve University
Cleveland, Ohio
Chapter 12

Ilona M. Schmaulfuss, MD
Professor of Radiology
North Florida/South Georgia Veterans
    Administration
University of Florida
Gainesville, Florida
Chapter 11

Jeff Searl, PhD, CCC-SLP
Associate Professor
Hearing and Speech Department
University of Kansas Medical Center
Kansas City, Kansas
Chapter 2

Erin P. Silverman, PhD, CCC-SLP
Research Assistant Professor
Department of Physiological Sciences
University of Florida
Gainesville, Florida
Chapters 9, 13, 14, and 18

Christian E. Soto, MM, CF-SLP
The Center for Voice Care and Swallowing
    Disorders
Ear, Nose, Throat and Plastic Surgery Associates
Orlando, Florida
Chapter 17

Brian C. Spector, MD, FACS
Partner
Ear, Nose, Throat and Plastic Surgery Associates
Orlando, Florida
Chapter 13

Linda Stachowiak, MS, CCC-SLP, BCS-S
Speech Pathology Oncology Specialist
UF Health Cancer Center
Orlando Health
Adjunct Instructor
University of Central Florida
Orlando, Florida
Chapter 16

Joseph C. Stemple, PhD, CCC-SLP
Professor
Division of Communication Sciences and
    Disorders
University of Kentucky
Lexington, Kentucky
Chapter 6

Paula A. Sullivan, MS, CCC-SLP, BCS-S
Speech-Language Pathology Section, Neurology
    Service
Malcom Randall VAMC
North Florida/South Georgia Veteran's Health
    System
Gainesville, Florida
Chapter 11

Terance Ted Tsue, MD, FACS
Physician in Chief
University of Kansas Cancer Center
Douglas A. Girod MD Endowed Professor of Head
    and Neck Surgical Oncology
Vice Chairman
Department of Otolaryngology-Head and Neck
    Surgery
Interim Chairman
Department of Radiation Oncology
University of Kansas School of Medicine
Kansas City, Kansas
Chapter 2

Lee Zehenbot, MD
Florida Hospital Cancer Institute
Florida Cancer Specialists
Orlando, Florida
Chapter 18

Richard I. Zraick, PhD, CCC-SLP
Professor and Chair
Department of Communication Sciences and
    Disorders
University of Central Florida
Orlando, Florida
Chapter 22

Multimedia List

Chapter 10

Video 10–1. Video laryngo stroboscopy initial disease

Video 10–2. Video laryngostroboscopy 10 week post CRT

Video 10–3. FEES post Tx

Chapter 12

Video 12–1. Videolaryngostroboscopy at 10 months post operative visit

Video 12–2 Videolaryngostroboscopy at 45 months post operative visit

Chapter 13

Video 13–1. The initial laryngostroboscopic examination

Video 13–2. The initial postoperative laryngostroboscopic examination

Video 13–3. A repeat laryngostroboscopic examination, 5 months post treatment

Chapter 15

Video 15–1. Voice evaluation with laryngostroboscopy

Video 15–2. VLaryngostroboscopy revealing increased thickness and decreased mucosal wave of the left true vocal fold

Video 15–3. Exophytic lesion with surrounding erythema and impaired mobility of the left true vocal fold.

Chapter 16

Video 16–1. MBS pre treatment

Video 16–2. MBS post treatment

Video 16–3. Oral intake with modifications

Video 16–4. Communicating with a tracheoesophageal voice prosthesis (TEP)

Chapter 17

Video 17–1. Post treatment videofluoroscopic swallowing study video

*To patients and their families surviving with Head and Neck Cancer
and to future clinicians who will have the privilege of treating and caring for these individuals.*

PART I

Demographics and Definitions

I

Head and Neck Cancer Demographics and Team Management

Bari Hoffman Ruddy, Jeffrey J. Lehman, Nikhil Rao, Christine Sapienza, and Henry Ho

INTRODUCTION

This introductory chapter reviews cancers of the head and neck (HNC) with particular focus on the most common variety of HNC, squamous cell carcinoma (HNSCC). Specifically, this chapter reviews

- the incidence and prevalence of HNCs;
- the locations and varieties of HNCs;
- the primary causes and symptoms of HNSCC;
- the variety of HNSCC types and the disease staging process;
- treatment options for HNC, including
  - surgery,
  - radiation,
  - chemotherapy, and
  - combined modality;
- the makeup of the multidisciplinary clinical and research team involved in the assessment and treatment of patients with HNC; and
- future directions for HNC treatment.

HEAD AND NECK CANCER STATISTICS

Cancer is a class of diseases characterized as the uncontrolled growth of abnormal or malignant cells (National Cancer Institute, 2015). Cancer cells can arise anywhere in the human body, dividing beyond normal limits. Cancer cells may accumulate and form tumors, invade adjacent tissue or structures, and/or spread to other locations in the body via blood or the lymphatic system, a process referred to as *metastasis.*

In 2015, the American Cancer Society estimated that there would be 59,340 new cases of HNC and that an estimated 12,290 people will die of this disease. Overall, HNC accounts for approximately 3% of new cases of cancer in the United States. The male-to-female ratio for HNC is estimated as 4:1 (Jemal, Siegel, Xu, & Ward, 2010).

HNC SITES

HNC can affect the skin, mucous membranes, glandular structures, neurovascular elements, and supportive soft tissues and bones in the head and neck. Leukoplakia, a white patch or plaque, is often the visible presentation of a precancerous lesion or early stage carcinoma, requiring biopsy in order to determine its characteristics. HNCs frequently emerge within the

- oral cavity: lips, floor of mouth, oral tongue, buccal mucosa, gingival, retromolar trigone**, and hard palate;

- oropharynx: tonsil, soft palate, base of tongue, and lateral/posterior pharyngeal wall;
- nasopharynx;
- hypopharynx: pyriform sinus;
- larynx: glottic, supraglottic, and subglottic;
- nasal cavity and paranasal sinuses;
- salivary glands: parotid, submandibular, sublingual, and minor salivary glands;
- ear: external ear, middle ear, and temporal bone;
- neck: thyroid gland and lymph nodes; and
- regional soft tissues and supporting bones.

**The retromolar trigone is a small mucosal area behind the last molar of the lower jaw. Cancer identified in this location often rapidly spreads to adjacent oral structures.

Head and Neck Cancer Types

Squamous cell carcinoma is the most common. Other less common HNC types include the following (Mendenhall, Riggs, & Cassisi, 2005):

- Sarcoma arises from connective tissue.
- Adenocarcinoma develops in the glandular lining of an organ.
- Mucoepidermoid carcinoma develops in the salivary glands. Aggressiveness is largely dependent on histologic grade. The high grade (poorly differentiated) is associated with more aggressive behavior, and the lower grade is often associated with a more benign natural history.
- Adenoid cystic carcinoma occurs in major or minor salivary glands. It may recur many years after treatment and has a tendency to follow nerves.
- Acinic cell carcinoma occurs in the salivary glands of the head and neck.
- Lymphoma begins in cells of the immune system. There are many subtypes, and the tumor behavior varies significantly depending on the precise classification. Broadly, lymphomas are divided into Hodgkin's and non-Hodgkin's categories.

- Melanoma arises from the melanocytic system of the skin or other organs.

HEAD AND NECK SQUAMOUS CELL CANCERS

Head and neck squamous cell cancer (HNSCC) originates within the mucus membranes of the nasal cavity, sinuses, lips, oral cavity, salivary glands, tongue, soft palate, pharynx, and larynx and is the fifth deadliest cancer worldwide (Chaukar et al., 2009; Lee, Wang, Mu-Hsin, Chang, & Chu, 2013; Ma et al., 2013; Melo Filho et al., 2013) with survival rates ranging from 30% for cancers of the oral cavity and pharynx to 50% for laryngeal cancers. Five-year survival rates from 2001 to 2007 indicated a 60.8% survival rate for laryngeal cancer, oral cavity and pharynx (Chaukar et al., 2009; Lee et al., 2013; LoTempio et al., 2005; http://surveillance.cancer.gov/publications/factsheets/SEER_Cancer_Survivor_Fact_Sheet.pdf). Approximately 95% of cancers of the oral cavity and the oropharynx are squamous cell carcinomas (Hsu et al., 2008; Snow, Wackym, & Ballenger, 2009; Spitz, 1994). A portion of squamous cell cancers test positive for the human papillomavirus (HPV-16). Squamous cell histologic grading includes keratinizing versus nonkeratinizing, and well-differentiated to poorly differentiated cellular characteristics. Variants of squamous cell cancer types can include undifferentiated carcinoma, lymphoepithelioma, spindle cell carcinoma, and verrucous carcinoma.

PRIMARY CAUSES OF HNSCC

The primary risk factors linked to the development of HNSCC are inhaled cigarette or marijuana smoke, pipe and cigar smoke, as well as chewing tobacco. The greatest risk occurs when anatomical areas and their susceptible epithelium are directly exposed to these toxins. The risk level is dependent on daily consumption, type, toxicity, and manner of tobacco use (Casper & Colton, 1998; Sapienza & Ruddy, 2012).

A synergistic effect exists when tobacco use is combined with consumption of alcohol, creating a higher risk of cancer development compared to if each was consumed independently. Although tobacco use and alcohol have consistently been implicated as a causative factor for HNC, it can develop in their absence; although it is significantly less common (Spitz, 1994). Additionally, although laryngopharyngeal reflux (LPR) has been largely implicated in esophageal disease, a recently identified relationship between severe LPR and HNC disease exists (Lipan, Reidenberg, & Laitman, 2006). Recent research shows that a portion of head and neck squamous cell cancers test positive for the human papillomavirus (HPV). There are numerous types of HPV; the type most frequently associated with oropharyngeal cancer is HPV-16. HPV-18 has also been associated with this cancer (Kreimer, Clifford, Boyle, & Franceschi, 2005). Studies have also found that oral HPV infections can be acquired through sexual contact (D'Souza et al., 2007). The incidence of these HPV-positive squamous cell carcinomas has increased in recent decades, especially in younger individuals. HPV-positive tumors have been associated with better survival rates than HPV-negative tumors (Ang et al., 2010). Please see Chapter 5 for contemporary and detailed information regarding HPV-positive tumors in the oropharynx.

GENERAL CANCER STAGING

American Joint Committee on Cancer Staging (AJCC) Guidelines

The TNM staging system developed by the American Joint Committee on Cancer (AJCC) Staging (http://www.cancerstaging.org) correlates with survival outcomes and is organized as follows:

T: Tumor (extent of primary tumor)

N: Nodal disease (lymphatic spread; regional metastasis)

M: Metastasis (distant; spread outside head and neck region)

- Primary tumor (T)
  - TX: Primary tumor cannot be assessed
  - T0: No evidence of primary tumor
  - Tis: Carcinoma in situ
- Stage 0
  - Tis, N0, M0
- Stage I
  - T1, N0, M0
- Stage II
  - T2, N0, M0
- Stage III
  - T3, N0, M0
  - T1, N1, M0
  - T2, N1, M0
  - T3, N1, M0
- Stage IVA
  - T4a, N0, M0
  - T4a, N1, M0
  - T1, N2, M0
  - T2, N2, M0
  - T3, N2, M0
  - T4a, N2, M0
- Stage IVB
  - T4b, any N, M0
  - Any T, N3, M0
- Stage IVC
  - Any T, any N, M1

Tumor staging takes into account the size of a tumor, how deep it has penetrated, whether it has invaded adjacent organs, if it has metastasized to lymph nodes, and whether it has spread to distant organs. Management is typically prescribed and/or changed based on the stage at initial diagnosis or recurrence, and remains a powerful predictor of survival. The staging system is clinical, based on the best possible estimate of disease extent recorded before treatment. The assessment of the primary tumor is based on inspection and palpation, when possible, and by visual endoscopic/stroboscopic examination. In order to accurately stage the cancer, the tumor must be confirmed histologically by biopsy. Radiographic studies such as CT, MRI, or PET scans help delineate the degree of local extent, as well as potential regional lymphatic and distant metastatic spread (Mendenhall, Riggs, & Cassisi, 2005).

PRIMARY TUMOR STAGING

Staging Supraglottic (Above the Vocal Folds) Cancer

- T1: Tumor limited to one subsite of supraglottis with normal vocal fold mobility
- T2: Tumor invades mucosa of more than one adjacent subsite[1] of supraglottis or glottis or region outside the supraglottis (e.g., mucosa of base of tongue, vallecula, or medial wall of piriform sinus) without fixation of the larynx
- T3: Tumor limited to larynx with vocal fold fixation and/or invades any of the following: postcricoid area, pre-epiglottic tissues, paraglottic space, and/or minor thyroid cartilage erosion (e.g., inner cortex)
- T4a: Tumor invades through the thyroid cartilage, and/or invades tissues beyond the larynx (e.g., trachea, soft tissues of the neck including deep extrinsic muscle of the tongue, strap muscles, thyroid, or esophagus)
- T4b: Tumor invades prevertebral space, encases carotid artery, or invades mediastinal structures

[1]Determination varies for different parts of the head and neck.

Subsites Include the Following

- False vocal folds
- Arytenoids
- Suprahyoid epiglottis
- Infrahyoid epiglottis
- Aryepiglottic folds (laryngeal aspect)

Note: Supraglottis involves many individual subsites. Patients with supraglottic cancers typically present with symptoms of sore throat, painful and effortful swallowing, referred ear pain, change in voice quality, or neck mass. Early vocal fold cancers are associated with chronic and progressive hoarseness. Cancers arising in the subglottic area commonly involve the vocal fold(s) once they become symptomatic, and thus, symptoms usually relate to a contiguous spread (Castellanos, Spector, & Kaiser, 1996).

Staging Glottic (at the Level of the Vocal Folds) Cancer

Glottic presentation may vary by volume of tumor, anatomic region involved, and the presence or absence of normal vocal fold mobility:

- T0: No evidence of primary tumor
- Tis: Carcinoma in situ: confined to tissues lining the larynx
- T1: Tumor limited to the vocal fold(s), which may involve anterior or posterior commissure, with normal mobility
- T1a: Tumor limited to one vocal fold
- T1b: Tumor involves both vocal folds
- T2: Tumor extends to supraglottis and/or subglottis and/or with impaired vocal fold mobility
- T3: Tumor limited to the larynx with vocal fold fixation and/or invades paraglottic space, and/or minor thyroid cartilage erosion (e.g., inner cortex)
- T4a: Tumor invades through the thyroid cartilage and/or invades tissues beyond the larynx (e.g., trachea, soft tissues of neck, including deep extrinsic muscle of the tongue, strap muscles, thyroid, or esophagus)
- T4b: Tumor invades prevertebral space, encases carotid artery, or invades mediastinal structures

Staging of Subglottic (Below the Vocal Folds) Cancer

- T1: Tumor limited to the subglottis
- T2: Tumor extends to vocal fold(s) with normal or impaired mobility
- T3: Tumor limited to larynx with vocal fold fixation
- T4a: Tumor invades cricoid or thyroid cartilage and/or invades tissues beyond

the larynx (e.g., trachea, soft tissues of neck, including deep extrinsic muscles of the tongue, strap muscles, thyroid, or esophagus)
- T4b: Tumor invades prevertebral space, encases carotid artery, or invades mediastinal structures

Staging of Oropharyngeal Cancer

- T1: Tumor is 2 cm (about three-quarter inch) across or smaller
- T2: Tumor is larger than 2 cm across but smaller than 4 cm (about 1 ½ inch)
- T3: Tumor is larger than 4 cm across. For cancers of the oropharynx, T3 also includes tumors that are growing into the epiglottis.
- T4a: Tumor is growing into nearby structures. This is known as *moderately advanced local disease*.
  - For oral cavity cancers: the tumor is growing into nearby structures, such as the bones of the jaw or face, deep muscle of the tongue, skin of the face, or the maxillary sinus.
  - For lip cancers: the tumor is growing into nearby bone, the inferior alveolar nerve (the nerve to the jawbone), the floor of the mouth, or the skin of the chin or nose.
  - For oropharyngeal cancers: the tumor is growing into the larynx (voice box), the tongue muscle, or bones such as the medial pterygoid, the hard palate, or the jaw.
- T4b: The tumor has grown through nearby structures and into deeper areas or tissues. This is known as *very advanced local disease*. Any of the following may be true:
  - The tumor is growing into other bones, such as the pterygoid plates and/or the skull base (for any oral cavity or oropharyngeal cancer).
  - The tumor surrounds the internal carotid artery (for any oral cavity or oropharyngeal cancer).

- For lip and oral cavity cancers: the tumor is growing into an area called the *masticator space*.
- For oropharyngeal cancers: the tumor is growing into a muscle called the *lateral pterygoid muscle*.
- For oropharyngeal cancers: the tumor is growing into the nasopharynx (the area of the throat that is behind the nose).

Staging of Nasopharyngeal Cancer

- T1: Tumor confined to the nasopharynx, or tumor extends to oropharynx and/or nasal cavity without parapharyngeal extension (e.g., without posterolateral infiltration of tumor)
- T2: Tumor with parapharyngeal extension (posterolateral infiltration of tumor)
- T3: Tumor involves bony structures of skull base and/or paranasal sinuses
- T4: Tumor with intracranial extension and/or involvement of cranial nerves, hypopharynx, or orbit, or with extension to the infratemporal fossa/masticator space

CANCER SPREAD

Cancer spread or *metastasis* refers to the migration of cancer cells from the site of initial presentation, to other areas of the body not previously involved. Cancer spread can be characterized as local, lymphatic, or hematogenous. Initial spread is usually regional, involving tissues adjacent to the tumor cells. Most primary tumors arise as surface lesions and spread by local invasion laterally as well as deeply, following a pathway of least resistance between fascial planes. Muscle tissue frequently becomes invaded by laryngeal and tongue cancers. Bone and cartilage can become invaded in serious, advanced cases.

Lymphatic and hematogenous spread refers to the processes of transport of cancer cells from the primary tumor, to remote locations throughout the body through lymph or blood. Lymphatic spread is the most common means of metastasis and occurs through lymph channels, with frequent involvement of regional lymph nodes. The lymphatic system is closely related to the circulatory system and constitutes an intricate network of lymphatic vessels, which transport a clear fluid (lymph) containing lymphocytes, white blood cells, and waste products from body tissues and toward the heart, where these products are transferred into the subclavian veins. Lymph nodes filter this fluid, and contain white blood cells that can generate immune responses to organisms or cancer cells contained in the lymph. Cancer spreads readily through the lymphatic system due to the density in lymphatic tissue and richness in lymphatic drainage (Spaulding, Hahn, & Constable, 1987). Because the lymphatic system eventually empties into the venous system, tumor cells transported via lymphatic spread can eventually spread via hematogenous mechanisms. Hematogenous spread refers to transport of cancer cells through the blood. Cancer cells enter the bloodstream through the walls of veins or (less commonly) arteries as well as through associations with the lymphatic system.

Definition of Regional Lymph Nodes (N)

- NX: Regional lymph nodes cannot be assessed
- N0: No regional lymph node metastasis
- N1: Metastasis in a single ipsilateral lymph node 3 cm or smaller in greatest dimension
- N2: Metastasis in a single ipsilateral lymph node, larger than 3 cm but 6 cm or smaller in greatest dimension, or in multiple ipsilateral lymph nodes 6 cm or smaller in greatest dimension, or in bilateral or contralateral lymph nodes 6 cm or smaller in greatest dimension:
  - N2a: Metastasis in a single ipsilateral lymph node larger than 3 cm but 6 cm or smaller in greatest dimension
  - N2b: Metastasis in multiple ipsilateral lymph nodes 6 cm or smaller in greatest dimension
  - N2c: Metastasis in bilateral or contralateral lymph nodes 6 cm or smaller in greatest dimension

- N3: Metastasis in a lymph node larger than 6 cm in greatest dimension

In the clinical evaluation, the actual size of the nodal mass is measured to complete staging, and allowance should be made for intervening soft tissues.

Defining Distant Metastasis (M)

- MX: Distant metastasis cannot be assessed
- M0: No distant metastasis
- M1: Distant metastasis

Specific Mechanisms and Sites of Laryngeal Cancer Spread

The true vocal folds are devoid of lymphatics. As a result, early stage laryngeal cancer confined to the vocal folds rarely presents with involved lymph nodes. Cancer that extends above or below the vocal folds may lead to lymph node involvement (Spaulding et al., 1987). Primary subglottic cancers (which are rare) drain through the cricothyroid and cricotracheal membranes to the pretracheal, paratracheal, and inferior jugular nodes, and occasionally to the mediastinal nodes (Spaulding et al., 1987).

SURGICAL TREATMENT OPTIONS FOR TREATING HEAD AND NECK CANCER

Although some patients are not offered surgery due to anatomic unresectability or prohibitive comorbidities such as end-stage lung or cardiac disease, a variety of curative surgical procedures are used to treat head and neck cancers, some of which allow for preservation of function (Carew & Shah, 1998; Maddox & Davies, 2012). The selection of surgical procedure is individualized for each patient, taking into consideration the anatomic region affected by the cancer, the stage of cancer, voice and swallowing status, cognitive status, motor function and coordination, quality of life factors, training and clinical expertise of the treatment team, as well as patient preference. Please refer to Chapters 2 through 18 for in-depth presentation of HNC case studies that highlight the specific surgical approaches and are selected for each case.

Small superficial cancers throughout the head and neck region without deeper tissue invasion or lymph node involvement are often successfully treated by surgery alone. By eliminating or reducing radiation therapy dose following surgery, the late toxicity of tissue scarring and resultant diminished swallowing function, may be reduced as well. Less invasive techniques can be used to remove early stage tumors restricted to superficial tissues. Examples of these are vocal fold stripping (removal of outermost layers of the vocal folds) or laser surgery where cancer cells are ablated via a high-intensity laser that is coupled with an endoscope or operating microscope and directed down to the laryngeal vestibule. Recovery from these types of procedures is typically rapid, and in many cases, normal or near-normal voicing is resumed relatively quickly. In some cases where the tumor has invaded deeper layers of the vocal fold, a partial or complete removal of the fold itself, referred to as *cordectomy,* is indicated. Recovery time and postsurgical voice and/or swallow status will vary relative to the extent of the procedure. Surgical procedures such as *partial* or *total laryngectomy* involve removal of part or all of the larynx and, once again, will vary relative to the stage of the tumor. Every effort is made to retain uninvolved structures meaning that laryngectomy procedures are highly individualized with the goal of disease resolution while minimizing postsurgical recovery and side effects. Ongoing evolution of surgical procedures has seen the rise in approaches involving laser technology. These techniques are typically referred to as transoral laser microsurgery (TOLM) (Zeitels & Burns, 2006) and microflap reconstruction (Anthony, Singer, & Mathes, 1994; Aryan, 1979).

A relatively new surgical technique, transoral robotic surgery (TORS), was approved by the FDA for use in the HNC population in 2009. With the use of this system, a specially trained surgeon sits at a robotic console and controls robotic arms that hold miniaturized surgical tools. This less-invasive surgical technique can be utilized to remove lesions of the oropharynx, hypopharynx, tongue base, and supraglottic larynx without the need to create large incisions for access and exposure. Studies have shown that effective resection of HNCs can be completed with TORS while preserving function. En bloc (together or "at the same time") surgical resection completed by this system may eliminate the need for radiation therapy following surgery. If radiation therapy is required, lower doses may be able to be used. Eliminating or reducing radiation exposure following surgery helps maximize organ function and preserve head and neck structures (Leonhardt et al., 2012). TORS is used to resect lesions of the oral, oropharyngeal, and supraglottic cavities. At present, resection of lesions in the glottic or subglottic regions cannot be completed with TORS. TORS offers increased accessibility to anatomic locations that were previously managed by highly invasive, open surgical techniques and holds great promise for the future of HNC treatment (Van Abel & Moore, 2012).

Role of the Speech-Language Pathologist (SLP) in Surgical Protocols

Although speech-language pathologists (SLPs) do not make surgical decisions, their involvement in the surgical process is critical to patients' overall rehabilitation. The SLP must have an understanding of the exact nature and extent of the resection and reconstruction that will occur during surgery so that accurate and informative counseling is administered and effective communication with the patient occurs prior to and following surgery.

ORGAN PRESERVATION THROUGH RADIATION AND/OR CHEMOTHERAPY

Radiation Therapy

Radiation is energy in the form of waves or moving subatomic particles emitted by an atom or other body as it changes from a higher energy state to a lower energy state. These particles are harnessed and used to kill cancer cells during a process known as radiation therapy. Radiation therapy, either alone or in combination with chemotherapy (chemoradiation; chemotherapy plus radiation) protocols allow for preservation of structures and function within affected regions of the head and neck. Curative radiation therapy administered alone (e.g., without surgery or chemotherapy) to treat HNC is referred to as a *definitive therapy*. Additionally, radiation therapy is commonly used as a *concomitant* (used alongside another approach such as surgery or chemotherapy) or *adjuvant* (used after another approach) therapy in order to enhance treatment response.

Historically, treatment with radiation therapy commonly resulted in unwanted and long-term side effects including tissue hardening or *fibrosis* (Forastiere et al., 2003; Stupp, Weichselbaum, & Vokes, 1994; Taylor, 1987). When laryngeal and pharyngeal regions fall within the radiation treatment field, fibrosis can result in reduced movement within jaw, tongue, and laryngeal tissues during speech and swallow. Additionally, fibrotic changes to muscles lining the pharynx reduce contractile capabilities in these muscles, potentially impairing bolus transfer during swallow (Fung et al., 2005). In severe cases where the larynx is rendered nonfunctional as a result of radiation treatment and dysphagia is severe and vocal quality poor, a patient may undergo a total salvage laryngectomy. In these cases, total laryngectomy serves to assist swallowing and development of alaryngeal communication above and beyond that which might be achievable with an altered, but preserved, larynx after treatment.

Modern radiation therapy for HNC uses intensity-modulated radiation therapy (IMRT; Nutting et al., 2011). This technique has resulted in a much lower rate of late complications and xerostomia after radiation. IMRT requires great care in delineating the target volumes and avoidance structures and when used appropriately allows for significant improvements in control with diminished late toxicity (May et al., 2013).

Methods of Delivering Radiation

- Conventional dosages: This involves a daily dose of radiation to tumor or areas at risk for recurrence as described above. This method is used for most cases including those receiving combined modality chemotherapy. Selected cases may benefit from other fractionation schedules as described below.

- Hypofractionation: This involves fewer fractions, higher doses, and shorter treatment duration.
  - This approach divides the daily dose into one per day or every few days resulting in a higher overall daily dose and lower total dose.
- Accelerated fractionation: An example of this is the "concomitant boost" technique used after conventional fractionation. The intent is to decrease the total duration of the radiotherapy course to account for theoretical cancer repopulation.
- Hyperfractionation: With this, more than one dose of radiation is administered within the same day but in smaller dosage amounts, allowing for a higher total dose of radiation.

Typical Schedules of Radiation Therapy

Radiation dosage is measured in gray (Gy) which is a measurement of joules per kilogram—100 cGy is equal to the previously used 100 rads terminology. A rad defines the rate of absorption of radiation energy. Fractionation refers to dosing radiation in small increments over a specific time period with intervals between the small-dose fractions (Bastholt & Berthelsen, 1997; Clifford Chao, Ozyigit, Low, Wippold, & Thorstad, 2002).

- Conventional dosages
  - Dose per fraction (treatment) 1.8 to 2 Gy
  - Doses to gross disease 66 to 70 Gy
  - Subclinical doses 50 to 54 Gy
  - Postoperative doses 50 to 66 Gy

Postradiation Symptoms

- Dental loss and tooth decay (caries)
- Dysgeusia: Bad taste in the mouth
- Dysphagia: Difficulty swallowing
- Dysphonia: Difficulty producing voice, including hoarseness and change in pitch, loudness, or quality
- Edema: Swelling caused by excess fluid in body tissues

- Erythema: Redness of the tissue
- Fatigue: Condition marked by extreme tiredness and inability to function due to lack of energy; fatigue is usually acute
- Fibrosis: Thickening of fibrous tissue
- Fistulas: An abnormal passage, opening, or connection between two internal organs or from an internal organ to the surface of the body
- Hypersensitive gag/oral aversion: Increased/exaggerated response to oral stimuli due to increased sensitivity
- Inflammatory reactions: Local response to cellular injury that is marked by capillary dilatation, redness, heat, pain, swelling, and often loss of function
- Loss of appetite
- Mucositis: Complication of some cancer therapies in which the lining of the digestive system becomes inflamed, resulting in sores in the mouth
- Nausea: Feeling of sickness or discomfort in the stomach that may come with an urge to vomit
- Necrosis: Death of living tissues
- Odynophagia: Pain produced by swallowing
- Stricture/stenosis: Narrowing (stricture) of a duct or canal
- Thick secretions: Heavy substance of mucus
- Thrush: Type of yeast (*Candida*), that may proliferate in moist skin areas and mucosa of the body
- Trismus: Spasm of the muscles of mastication resulting from any of various abnormal conditions or diseases; can be caused by postradiation fibrosis, which results in decreased jaw opening
- Xerostomia: Dry mouth

Chemotherapy

Chemotherapy is not considered a *definitive* treatment for the management of HNC. That is, chemotherapy is not used as an isolated treatment approach. Chemotherapy is frequently used as a concomitant or adjuvant therapy to surgery or radiation. Chemotherapy used in combination with radiation therapy ("chemoradiation") improves survival rates in patients with HNSCC, particularly when administered concurrently (Vokes, 2010).

Induction chemotherapy uses high doses of anticancer compounds early in treatment, particularly of larger or more invasive tumors, in order to "weaken" the tumor and allow for greater impact from treatments that follow (typically surgery or radiation therapy). Emerging techniques for cancer treatment are exploring the use of induction chemotherapy, in combination with concomitant chemoradiation, to enhance treatment outcomes relative to those attained through use of chemoradiation alone.

Side Effects of Organ Preservation Techniques

Although radiation therapy and chemotherapy are considered organ preservation approaches, preservation of the anatomic structure does not always equal preservation or improvement of function, and in most cases, organ preservation results in significant sequelae and a decrease in quality of life (Logemann et al., 2008). Sequelae are morbid conditions following the consequences of disease and could include pain, bleeding, ulcerations to mucosa, bone damage, permanent damage to salivary glands, chewing difficulty, and/or dysphagia.

Role of the SLP in Organ Preservation Protocols

The SLP is involved, on an as-needed basis, in the care of HNC patients prior to, during, and after treatment. Prior to chemoradiation, the speech pathologist performs a clinical evaluation of speech, voice, and swallowing, including an instrumental assessment with endoscopy, laryngostroboscopy, fiberoptic endoscopic evaluation of swallowing (FEES), and/or modified barium swallow (MBS), as indicated.

Patient counseling includes explaining the normal anatomy and physiology of the head and neck to the patient while providing information about the potential changes that may occur from radiation or combined modality chemoradiation. Additionally, possible changes that may be evident upon examination due to the presence of the tumor itself are often discussed with the patient. The SLP often provides details that help the patient understand the timelines associated with realistic expectations for recovery and return to work, reducing fears or misconceptions about the process and outcomes associated with radiation. Prior to radiation the patient should be provided with a swallow rehabilitation plan and vocal and oral hygiene protocol to help with the management of any side effects. It is critical that the patient understands his or her responsibility in complying with the rehabilitation program. During treatment, and in the post treatment phase of chemoradiation, the SLP may recommend saliva substitutes as needed, or provide suggestions to alleviate symptoms of xerostomia, introduce swallow strategies or diet modification as needed, establish a swallowing schedule, reinforce swallow exercises, promote vocal hygiene, and assist with oral care. Please refer to Chapters 2 through 18 for in-depth presentation of HNC case studies that highlight the specific contributions of the SLP to the treatment of individuals with HNC, from diagnosis through follow-up and ongoing management.

COMBINED MANAGEMENT APPROACHES

Advanced laryngeal cancers are often treated by combining radiation, chemotherapy, and/or surgery (Fowler & Lindstrom, 1992; Mendenhall et al., 2005; Silver & Ferlito, 1996; Thawley, Panje, Batsakis, & Lindberg, 1999; Wang, 1997). There are at least three types of combined management approaches for treating HNC. The selection of treatment modality is usually dependent on the site and extent of tumor, likely functional outcomes, and preference of the patient being treated:

- surgery followed by radiation or chemoradiation;
- chemotherapy followed by surgery, radiation, or chemoradiation; or
- chemoradiation followed by surgery.

MULTIDISCIPLINARY CLINICAL AND RESEARCH TEAM

A multidisciplinary team of medical and allied health care professionals is critical for the successful and coordinated rehabilitation plan for the patient diagnosed with HNC.

Medical Team Members

Head and Neck (HNC) Surgeon

The HNC surgeon is usually involved in the initial assessment of the patient with HNC, frequently acting as case manager. At times patients bypass the HNC surgeon and are referred directly to radiation or medical oncology by the primary care physician. In these cases, initial diagnosis and biopsy may have been made by an oral surgeon, a dentist, or through interventional radiology during a fine-needle biopsy. The responsibilities of the HNC surgeon include diagnosis of the disease and organization of the treatment plan. Following removal of the tumor or tumors, the HNC surgeon will lead reconstruction efforts. In complex cases (such as patients who require free flap reconstructions), a separate reconstruction team may be involved. This can include coordinating consultations with other health care professionals and facilitating interdisciplinary communication pertaining to determining all available treatment options for the patient.

Plastic Surgeon

When not completed by the HNC surgeon, a plastic surgeon may perform reconstructive surgery following tumor removal. Extensive surgical resections are often performed with a two-team (HNC surgical plus plastic surgery) approach, utilizing a reconstructive plastic surgery specialist to perform microvascular free-flap transfer or other reconstructive techniques after tumor resection by the head and neck surgical team.

Radiation Oncologist

The radiation oncologist works with the HNC surgeon to stage the tumor or tumors and determine the potential for involvement of structures adjacent to the primary tumor, as well as regional and distant spread of disease. The radiation oncologist decides if radiation therapy is a viable treatment option for the patient, and communicates with other members of the team to formulate options to present to the patient. If radiation is elected by the patient, the radiation oncologist decides the optimal treatment, dosage levels, and type.

Medical Oncologist

As a nonsurgical cancer specialist, the medical oncologist is responsible for the administration of chemotherapeutic agents, often used in conjunction with radiation therapy in more advanced tumors. He is also involved in general aspects of patient care when disease is advanced, including staging of the cancer, supportive care, psychological aspects, and palliative or pain care.

Radiologist/Nuclear Medicine Specialist

The radiologist interprets the results of imaging studies including magnetic resonance imaging (MRI), computed tomography (CT), positive emission tomography (PET) scans, and ultrasound studies completed during diagnostic or post treatment assessments. Radiologists may help with initial diagnosis by obtaining image-guided fine-needle aspiration (FNA) specimens, where appropriate.

Pathologist

The pathologist examines any tissue removed during treatment for anatomical abnormalities. A report is sent to the treating physician as to the type of cancer tissue, histologic grade, and completeness of surgical excision. Each of these elements, along with other factors such as P16 status and microscopic invasion of structures, affects the choices that are made by the treatment team.

Internal Medicine Physician

The internal medicine physician contributes to pre- and postoperative management of medical comorbidities, such as heart disease, diabetes, and high blood pressure, along with the primary care practice physician or nurse practitioner. Preoperatively, the Internal Medicine physician works with patients to identify those who are at risk for postsurgical complication(s) and assist with treatment complications following radiation or surgery including hypothyroidism, metabolic imbalance due to nutritional inadequacy, and cardiovascular events such as myocardial infarction or stroke. Internal medicine subspecialties are involved on an as-needed basis to address specific issues. An example of this could be an infectious disease specialist consulted to assist in the treatment of postoperative infections such as methicillin-resistant *Staphylococcus aureus* (MRSA).

Dental-Maxillofacial Prosthodontist

This team member is a dentist specializing in the creation and placement of prosthetic teeth or other oral cavity structures to restore comfort, health, and physical appearance to patients post treatment. In some cases, use of prosthetics can provide functional and cosmetic restoration superior to results obtainable by surgical reconstruction.

Allied Health Care Members

Speech-Language Pathologist

The role of the speech-language pathologist within the multidisciplinary team was discussed in detail during earlier sections presenting specific treatment approaches (e.g., surgical, radiation therapy, or combined modality). In general, the speech-language pathologist's role is to evaluate and provide treatment for head and neck cancer patients with short- and long-term communication needs. The speech-language pathologist is also responsible for evaluating and treating dysphagia symptoms that occur as a result of surgery and/or radiation treatments. For the patient who has had a total laryngectomy, the speech pathologist will entrain alaryngeal speech or show the patient how to use assistive devices to restore speech communication following removal of the vocal folds during laryngectomy.

Nurse

Nurses care for the patient throughout all phases of HNC diagnosis and treatment and are frequently often involved in case management within outpatient settings. Nurses collaborate with other team members to implement an individualized care plan. They assist and support the patients during treatment procedures, therapies, surgery, and hospital stays. In addition to the speech-language pathologist, the nurse may function to provide patient education prior to release from the hospital, particularly pertaining to postsurgical stoma care.

Registered Dietitian

A registered dietician is responsible for evaluating the patient's nutritional health prior to and following surgery, radiation, or combined modality treatments. Dietitians make recommendations regarding caloric intake necessary to gain or maintain a patient's weight, and counsel the patient and caregivers regarding nutritional health and well-being.

Mental Health Counselor/ Social Worker/Case Manager

These team members are responsible for providing counseling to the patient or family or to assist with coping strategies for a range of issues, including potential death, serious illness, end-of-life care, postoperative depression, role of family or caregivers, self-image, anger, and anxiety. Counselors are adept at helping people "work through" complex emotional states, develop strategies to cope with the myriad changes that occur during cancer treatment, and adapt to these changes moving forward. Social workers assist with adapting the patient's environment to his or her unique set of needs post treatment.

Physical and Occupational Therapists

Physical and occupational therapists work with patients to restore movement or functional skills impaired as a result of cancer, and/or cancer treatment. Patients who have undergone extensive surgery to the head or neck frequently experience limited postsurgical mobility of the shoulder, neck, arm, or hand ipsilateral to the surgical site. Physical therapists work with the patients to rehabilitate gross motor movement, whereas occupational therapists concentrate on the vital activities of daily living (ADLs) necessary for functional engagement in home, social, or professional settings.

Lymphedema Therapist

Lymphedema therapists are specialists who hail from varied backgrounds including physical therapy, occupational therapy, massage therapy, and nursing. Specialty training is required for certification in this specialty. Patients who have undergone removal of lymphatic structures, such as dissection of lymph nodes in the neck, or who have sustained damage to the head or neck as a result of the tumor, or radiation treatment, frequently experience reduced drainage of lymphatic fluid. Accumulation of lymphatic fluid can result in swelling and discomfort of the head and neck area. Lymphedema therapy promotes drainage of lymphatic fluid into the bloodstream and results in decreased swelling in the head and neck region.

Respiratory Therapist

The respiratory therapist evaluates, treats, and cares for breathing or respiratory disorders. These disorders can include ventilator management, tracheostomy care, and delivery of nebulized medications to treat asthma or other pulmonary diseases.

Other Members: The Laryngectomized Visitor

Finally, an important nonprofessional team member is the person who has experienced the patient's situation (or similar). In the case of total laryngectomy, this individual is referred to as a *laryngectomized* or *laryngectomee visitor*. The laryngectomee visitor serves to help boost the patient's morale by showing ease of communication through mastered alaryngeal speech. In many cases, the visit provides motivation to become engaged in the rehabilitation process. Often, the visitor's spouse or caregiver will visit with the patient's spouse/caregiver providing support. These interactions are valuable as patient-to-patient support (Stemple, Glaze, & Klaben, 2000).

DEVELOPING A SYSTEM TO TRACK OUTCOMES WITH THE HEAD AND NECK CANCER POPULATION

Evaluation of treatment outcomes for HNC patients can be achieved in a variety of ways: locoregional control, disease-free survival, overall survival at 2 to 5 years, functional outcomes related to ADLs, and quality of life. Outcomes should be reported after treatment (typically surgery, radiation, or combined modality) and at specified post treatment time points. Databases used to track HNC treatment outcomes typically include patient demographic data including age, gender, and racial or ethnic identity as well as information on the cancers being tracked, including grade or stage. Finally, information pertaining to treatment approaches, survival rates, and other noteworthy features of each case are recorded. Individual facilities frequently will develop and maintain their own databases composed of local and regional data, including

- functional outcomes following surgery, such as
  - types of surgical approaches and
  - medical management;
- functional outcomes following radiotherapy, including
  - audit of complications of radiation therapy via clinical and instrumental exam;
- proportion of patients undergoing laryngectomy who receive surgical voice restoration or use other methods of alaryngeal speech;
- patient satisfaction with medical and behavioral support services during treatment;
- audit of patient performance status (based on specified time intervals);
- audit of therapy protocol/therapy compliance; and
- quality of Life (QOL) outcomes, including
  - QOL related to swallowing function and
  - QOL related to vocal function.

FUTURE DIRECTIONS

New technologies including molecular imaging are transforming oncological patient care and expanding our understanding of tumor biology as well as the manner in which tumors interact with their host tissues. Molecular imaging and biological characterization of tumor cells allow for exceptionally detailed characterization of the tumor, opening the door to increasing personalization of treatment planning. In addition, these technologies serve as a therapeutic tool for guiding targeted therapies in real time and assisting in the selection of pharmacological agents with maximum potential impact on preventing tumor growth. Moving forward, these technologies will likely contribute to the development and optimization of new and less invasive therapies for cancer and will serve as objective measures of treatment efficacy.

CONCLUSIONS

The successful treatment of HNC with restoration of maximal function requires a team effort. This includes a knowledgeable and skilled SLP who is involved in the rehabilitation of speech and swallowing. Because both quantity and quality of life are highly influenced by the functional status of speech and swallowing, clinicians must continue to objectively evaluate treatment results to improve functional outcomes and allow evidence-based comparisons of different forms or combinations of cancer management protocols.

USEFUL WEBSITES

A wealth of peer-reviewed information and updated quarterly reports can be found under the HNC section on the National Cancer Institute website (http://www.cancer.gov). Specific information is provided on the site for the clinician working with patients with cancer as well as a separate section for patient information.

The Surveillance Epidemiology and End Results (SEER) section of the National Cancer Institute website provides the SEER Cancer Statistics Review that reports incidence, mortality, survival, prevalence, and lifetime risk statistics (http://seer.cancer.gov/csr/1975_2008/index.html).

Websites Helpful for Head and Neck Cancer Information and Support

Support for People With Head and Neck Cancer: http://www.spohnc.org/; http://www.oralcancersupport.org

Scott Hamilton CARES initiative: http://www.chemocare.com

The Head and Neck Cancer Alliance: http://www.headandneck.org

Oral Cancer Foundation: http://www.oralcancerfoundation.org

National Cancer Institute: http://www.cancer.gov

American Cancer Society: http://www.cancer.org

The International Association of Laryngectomees: http://www.theial.com

CancerCare: http://www.cancercare.org

WebWhispers: http://www.webwhispers.org

REFERENCES

Ang, K. K., Harris, J., Wheeler, R., Weber, R., Rosenthal, D. I., Nguyen-Tân, P. F., . . . Gillison, M. L. (2010). Human papillomavirus and survival of patients with oropharyngeal cancer. *New England Journal of Medicine, 363*(1), 24–35.

Anthony, J. P., Singer, M. I., & Mathes, S. J. (1994). Pharyngoesophageal reconstruction using the tubed free radial forearm flap. *Clinics in Plastic Surgery, 21*(1), 137–147.

Aryan, S. (1979). The pectoralis major myocutaneous flap. A versatile flap for reconstruction of cervical esophagus by revascularized isolated jejunal segment. *Annals of Surgery, 149*, 162.

Bastholt, L., & Berthelsen, A. (1997). Importance of overall treatment time for the outcome of radiotherapy of advanced head and neck carcinoma: Dependency on tumor differentiation. *Radiotherapy and Oncology, 43*(1), 47–51.

Carew, J. F., & Shah, J. P. (1998). Advances in multimodality therapy for laryngeal cancer. *Cancer Journal for Clinicians, 48*(4), 211–228.

Casper, J., & Colton, R. (1998). *Clinical manual for laryngectomy and head/neck cancer rehabilitation* (2nd ed.). San Diego, CA: Singular.

Castellanos, P., Spector, G., & Kaiser, T. (1996). *Tumors of the larynx and laryngopharynx: Otorhinolaryngology-head and neck surgery* (15th ed., pp. 585–652). Baltimore, MD: Williams & Wilkins.

Chaukar, D. A., Walvekar, R. R., Das, A. K., Deshpande, M. S., Pai, P.,S., Chaturvedi, P., . . . D'Cruz, A. K. (2009). Quality of life in head and neck cancer survivors: A cross-sectional survey. *American Journal of Otolaryngology, 30*(3), 176–180.

Clifford Chao, K. S., Ozyigit, G., Low, D. A.,Wippold, F. J., & Thorstad,W. L. (2002). *Intensity modulated radiation therapy for head and neck cancers.* St. Louis, MO: Lippincott Williams & Wilkins.

D'Souza, G., Kreimer, A. R., Viscidi, R., Pawlita, M., Fakhry, C., Koch, W. M., . . . Gillison, M. L. (2007). Case-control study of human papillomavirus and oropharyngeal cancer. *New England Journal of Medicine, 356*(19), 1944–1956.

Forastiere, A. A., Goepfert, H., Maor, M., Pajak, T. F., Weber, R., Morrison, W., . . . Cooper, J. (2003). Concurrent chemotherapy and radiotherapy for organ preservation in advanced laryngeal cancer. *New England Journal of Medicine, 349*(22), 2091–2098.

Fowler, J. F., & Lindstrom, M. J. (1992). Loss of local control with prolongation in radiotherapy. *International Journal of Radiation Oncology, Biology, and Physics, 23*(2), 457–467.

Fung, K., Lyden, T., Lee, J., Urba, S., Worden, F., Eisbruch, A., . . . Wolf, G. T. (2005). Voice and swallowing outcomes of an organ preservation trial for advanced laryngeal cancer. *International Journal of Radiation Oncology, Biology, and Physiology, 63*(5), 1395–1399.

Hsu, Y. B., Chang, S. Y., Lan, M. C., Huang, J. L., Tai, S. K., & Chu, P. Y. (2008). Second primary malignancies in squamous cell carcinomas of the tongue and larynx: An analysis of incidence, pattern, and outcome. *Journal of the Chinese Medical Association, 71*(2), 86–91.

Jemal, A., Siegel, R., Xu, J., & Ward, E. Cancer statistics, 2010. *CA: A Cancer Journal for Clinicians 2010, 60*(5), 277–300.

Kreimer, A. R., Clifford, G. M., Boyle, P., & Franceschi, S. (2005). Human papillomavirus types in head and neck squamous cell carcinomas worldwide: A systematic review. *Cancer Epidemiology, Biomarkers, and Prevention, 14*(2), 467–475.

Lee, T. L., Wang, L. W., Mu-Hsin Chang, P., & Chu, P. Y. (2013). Quality of life for patients with hypopharyngeal cancer after different therapeutic modalities. *Head & Neck, 35*(2), 280–285.

Leonhardt, F. D., Quon, H., Abrahão, M., O'Malley, B. W. Jr., & Weinstein, G. S. (2010). Transoral robotic surgery for oropharyngeal carcinoma and its impact on patient-reported quality of life and function. *Head & Neck, 34*(2), 146–154.

Lipan, M. J., Reidenberg, J. S., & Laitman, J. T. (2006). Anatomy of reflux: A growing health problem affecting structures of the head and neck. *Anatomical Record Part B: The New Anatomist, 289*(6), 261–270.

Logemann, J. A., Pauloski, B. R., Rademaker, A.W., Lazarus, C. L., Gaziano, J., Stachowiak, L., . . . Mittal, B. (2008). Swallowing disorders in the first year after radiation and chemoradiation. *Head & Neck, 30*(2), 148–158.

LoTempio, M. M., Wang, K. H., Sadeghi, A., Delacure, M. D., Juillard, G. F., & Wang, M. B. (2005). Comparison of quality of life outcomes in laryngeal cancer patients following chemoradiation vs. total laryngectomy. *Otolaryngology-Head and Neck Surgery, 132*(6), 948–953.

Ma, Y., Liu, L., Huang, D., Wang, J., Wu, W., Liu, M., & Zhao, J. (2013). [Research of postoperative quality of life of laryngeal carcinoma patients]. *Lin Chung Er Bi Yan Hou Tou Jing Wai Ke Za Zhi, 27*(4), 169–174.

Maddox, P. T., & Davies, L. (2012). Trends in total laryngectomy in the era of organ preservation: A population based study. *Otolaryngology-Head and Neck Surgery, 147*(1), 85–90.

May, J. T., Rao, N., Sabater, R., Boutrid, H., Caudell, J., Merchant, F., . . . Trotti, A. (2013). Intensity-modulated radiation therapy as primary treatment for oropharyngeal squamous cell carcinoma. *Head & Neck, 35*(12), 1796–1800.

Melo Filho, M. R., Rocha, B. A., Pires, M. B., Fonseca, E. S., Freitas, E. M., Martelli Junior, H., & Santos, F. B. (2013). Quality of life of patients with head and neck cancer. *Brazilian Journal of Otorhinolaryngology, 79*(1), 82–88.

Mendenhall, W. M., Riggs, C. E., Jr., & Cassisi, N. J. (2005). Treatment of head and neck cancers. In V. T. DeVita Jr., S. Hellman, & S. A. Rosenberg (Eds.), *Cancer: Principles and practice of oncology* (7th ed., pp. 662–732). Philadelphia, PA: Lippincott Williams & Wilkins.

National Cancer Institute. (2015). *What is cancer.* Retrieved from http://www.cancer.gov/about-cancer/what-is-cancer

Nutting, C., Morden, J., Harrington, K., Urbano, T., Bhide Clark, C., Miles, E., . . . Hall, E., PARSPORT trial management group. (2011). Parotid-sparing intensity modulated versus conventional radiotherapy in head and neck cancer (PARSPORT): A phase 3 multicenter randomized controlled trial. *Lancet Oncology, 12*(2), 127–136. doi:10.1016/S1470-2045(10)70290-4

Sapienza, C., & Hoffman Ruddy, B. (2012). *Voice disorders.* San Diego, CA: Plural.

Silver, C. E., & Ferlito, A. (1996). *Surgery for cancer of the larynx and related structures* (2nd ed.). Philadelphia, PA: Saunders.

Snow, J. B., Wackym, P. A., & Ballenger, J. J. (2009). *Ballenger's otorhinolaryngology: Head and neck surgery.* Shelton, CT: People's Medical/B.C. Decker.

Spaulding, C. A., Hahn, S. S., & Constable, W. C. (1987). The effectiveness of treatment of lymph nodes in cancers of the pyriform sinus and supraglottis. *International Journal of Radiation Oncology, Biology, and Physics, 13*(7), 963–968.

Spitz, M. R. (1994). Epidemiology and risk factors for head and neck cancer. *Seminars in Oncology, 21*(3), 281–288.

Stemple, J. C., Glaze, L. E., & Klaben, B. G. (2000). *Clinical voice pathology: Theory and management* (3rd ed.). San Diego, CA: Singular.

Stupp, R., Weichselbaum, R. R., & Vokes, E. E. (1994). Combined modality therapy of head and neck cancer. *Seminars in Oncology, 21*(3), 349–358.

Taylor, S. G., IV. (1987). Integration of chemotherapy into the combined modality therapy of head and neck squamous cancer. *International Journal of Radiation Oncology, Biology, and Physics, 13*(5), 779–783.

Thawley, S. E., Panje, W. R., Batsakis, J. G., & Lindberg, R. D. (Eds.). (1999). *Comprehensive management of head and neck tumors* (2nd ed.). Philadelphia, PA: W. B. Saunders.

Van Abel, K. M., & Moore, E. J. (2012). The rise of transoral robotic surgery in the head and neck: Emerging applications. *Expert Review of Anticancer Therapy, 12*(3), 373–380.

Vokes, E. E. (2010). Induction chemotherapy for head and neck cancer: Recent data. *Oncologist, 15*(3), 3–7.

Wang, C. C. (Ed.). (1997). *Radiation therapy for head and neck neoplasms* (3rd ed.). New York, NY: Wiley-Liss.

Zeitels, S., & Burns, J. A. (2006). Laser applications in laryngology: Past, present, and future. *Otolaryngologic Clinics of North America, 39*(1), 159–172.

PART II

Oral Cavity Cases

2

Lip, Anterior Floor of Mouth, and Mandibular Cancer

Jeff Searl, Terance Ted Tsue, and Douglas A. Girod

INTRODUCTION AND MEDICAL HISTORY

Patient M was 38 years old when he first presented to our otolaryngology practice with complaints of a persistent cold sore on his right lower lip. His medical history was unremarkable and he denied any prior cancers or medical diagnoses. He took an over-the-counter anti-inflammatory for self-diagnosed chronic lower back pain. There was no family history of cancer.

Social History

Patient M was an unmarried Caucasian who lived alone yet maintained an active social life. His parents and two siblings were alive and supportive of Patient M as he dealt with the cancer diagnosis and treatment. He graduated from high school and worked in various capacities as a heavy machine operator on farms for 20 years.

Risk Factors

Interview of Patient M on intake revealed several risk factors associated with oral cancer. These included 20 years of daily snuff use. He placed the snuff in his lower right lip, typically spitting rather than swallowing saliva. Second, he had one to two alcoholic drinks per day, usually beer (moderate alcohol consumption per U.S. Department of Health and Human Services). A third risk factor was sun and wind exposure on nearly a daily basis from his job. He denied using sunscreen or UV protection on his lips. He said his lips were "always dry and cracked." He pursued medical help because his lip sores would get better but never really heal for several weeks. He was queried about human papillomavirus (HPV) exposure and risk factors including oral sex practice, but he evaded answering such questions (later testing indicated the cancer was not HPV-positive).

Timeline

Patient M's cancer diagnosis was made at another facility. Following a presumptive diagnosis of lip cancer in the clinical setting, he was seen by an otolaryngologist who recommended biopsy and head, neck, and chest magnetic resonance imaging (MRI). He ultimately was diagnosed with squamous cell carcinoma of the lip staged as T2 N0 M0. External beam radiation and chemotherapy were recommended, and prior to that a percutaneous endoscopic gastrostomy (PEG) tube was placed. A total of 38 radiation and 17 chemotherapy treatments were completed at that facility (72 Gy [Gray] to the primary site).

Unfortunately, the tumor continued to grow aggressively, and by the end of the radiation the tumor had ulcerated through the full thickness of the lower lip off midline to the right. At this point (8 weeks after diagnosis) he failed to keep a follow-up appointment with his otolaryngologist. After 10 days the patient presented to the otolaryngology clinic and was referred to our facility. Because of the aggressive nature of the tumor, the diagnostic workup (described below) was completed quickly and a surgical treatment approach was finalized within a week.

DIAGNOSTIC WORKUP

Records from the outside facility were reviewed. Biopsy was not repeated given the definitive diagnosis made previously. The tumor had, by all accounts from the patient and referring physician, grown substantially both during and after the radiation therapy. During an oral exam completed at the first clinic visit with the head and neck surgeon at our facility, the tumor was noted to extend through the lower lip, with anterior facial skin and submentum involvement. A mass on the anterior floor of the mouth also was noted.

Assessment of the head, neck, and chest confirmed a very large tumor of the lower lip with extension into the floor of mouth, mandible and lower right buccal mucosa; regional lymph nodes also were involved. The tumor was staged as T4a N2 M0. Heart, lung, gut, and neurological function were normal per clinical exam. He was 5'8" and weighed 120 lbs which represented a weight loss of 54 lb from the time he started radiation therapy. His body mass index (BMI) of 18 and blood lab results (e.g., low serum albumin and prealbumin, etc.) suggested early malnutrition. No other comorbidities were identified.

Tumor Board Discussion

Tumor board discussion ultimately concluded with a plan for aggressive surgical resection and reconstruc-

tion. Specifically, direct laryngoscopy to determine the extent of the ulcerating lesion, bronchoscopy to inspect the lower airway, esophagoscopy to evaluate the integrity of the mucosa of the esophagus, segmental composite resection of the lower lip, anterior floor of mouth, anterior mandible and right buccal region, and modified radical neck dissection for cervical lymph node involvement. The planned reconstruction was microvascular free radial forearm flap, microvascular osteocutaneous fibular free flap, bilateral reconstruction of the mandible, Alloderm graft to the carotids bilaterally, and lower lip reconstruction with palmaris tendon suspension bilaterally.

Presurgical workup (besides ENT and anesthesiology) included evaluation by dietetics given the early signs of malnutrition. PEG feedings were adjusted in preparation for the surgery. The team psychologist assessed the patient to prepare him for the extensive surgery that would result in obvious changes to his face. Mild depression, general fatigue, and malaise were noted. Supportive counseling while an inpatient and as needed postdischarge was recommended. The speech language pathologists (SLP) was part of the tumor board discussion and met with the patient to do a baseline assessment of speech and swallowing abilities (described below).

SURGICAL INTERVENTION

Resection

After sedation and intubation, esophagoscopy was attempted, but the scope could only be passed to the midcervical esophagus due to restricted neck movement believed to be related to the prior radiation. The scope was removed and the oral lesion was noted to involve the through-and-through thickness of the lower lip with extension to buccal mucosa, anterior floor of mouth, and mandible. The pharynx, larynx, subglottis, and trachea were free of visible abnormality.

Bilateral neck dissection (levels 2 through 5) was completed with preservation of cranial nerves X, XI, and XII. The full lower lip, from commissure to commissure, was removed down to the mandible with preservation of the lingual and hypoglossal nerves in the region. The right lower buccal mucosa with tumor involvement was resected. With the mandible exposed, osteotomies were made to remove the mandible back to the angle on the right around to the body of the mandible on the left. With the mandible freed, the soft tissue of the anterior floor of the mouth (including submandibular glands) was removed in total with the mandible resection. A total of 12 cm of mandible was removed.

RECONSTRUCTION

Reconstruction continued immediately from the resection. The process was extensive and proceeded as follows:

1. harvesting of the radial forearm (fasciocutaneous) free flap from the right forearm (9 × 14 cm paddle; healed forearm shown in Figure 2–1A);
2. harvesting of osteocutaneous fibular free flap from the right leg (15 cm of bone and 6 × 14 cm tissue paddle; healed leg shown in Figure 2–1B);
3. placement of the fibular flap using the bone to reconstruct the mandibular defect; after the bony graft was set, the musculocutaneous paddle was utilized to reconstruct the floor of mouth, alveolus, and buccal defect using microvascular techniques (healed flaps shown in Figure 2–2);
4. placement of the fadial forearm flap to reconstruct the lower lip and chin—the palmaris longus tendon was harvested from the right forearm and secured to the malar prominences on each side, and then the forearm flap was draped over the tendon and sutured into place to reconstruct the inner lip, outer lip, lower right cheek, and chin (healed flap shown in Figure 2–3);
5. Alloderm sheets were used to cover the carotids bilaterally (these were exposed by removal of the sternocleidomastoid muscles during the radical neck dissection), and the neck incisions were closed in multiple layers including approximation and attachment of the radial forearm flap in the chin to the surrounding neck tissue; and
6. split thickness skin grafts were harvested (left thigh) and used to cover flap donor sites in the right forearm and the right lower leg.

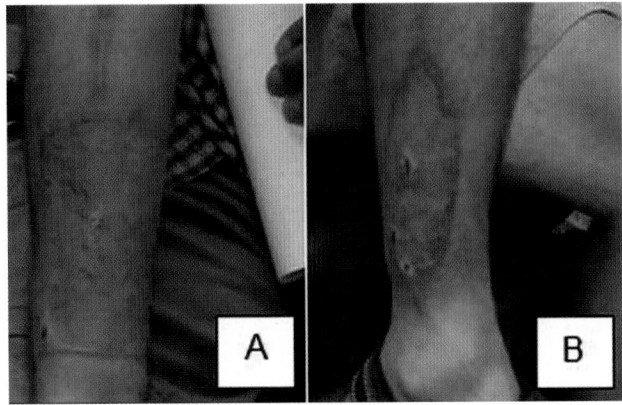

Figure 2–1. A. Healed forearm flap donor site. **B.** Healed fibula flap donor site.

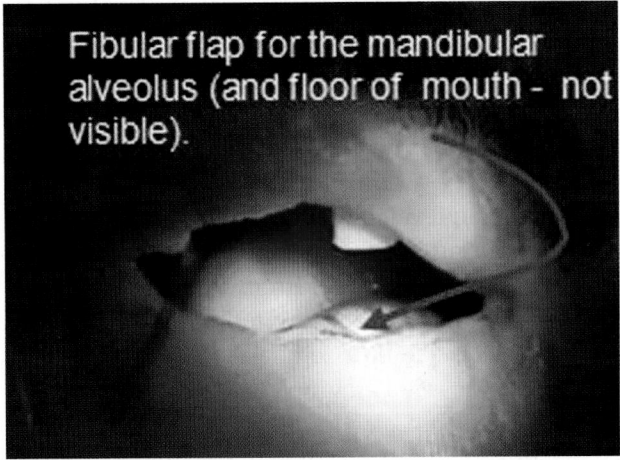

Figure 2–2. Maximal mouth opening showing a portion of the fibular osteocutaneous flap inside the oral cavity. Note the hair on the reconstructed mandibular arch.

POSTOPERATIVE MEDICAL COURSE AND COMPLICATIONS

Patient M's 7-day hospital course was uneventful. He was discharged with the PEG in place to meet 100% of nutritional needs. The tracheostomy tube also was in place. Daily physical therapy was occurring, and the SLP was following the patient primarily for immediate communication issues. Patient M was readmitted to the hospital 13 days later due to a foul smell from the right neck and fistula development

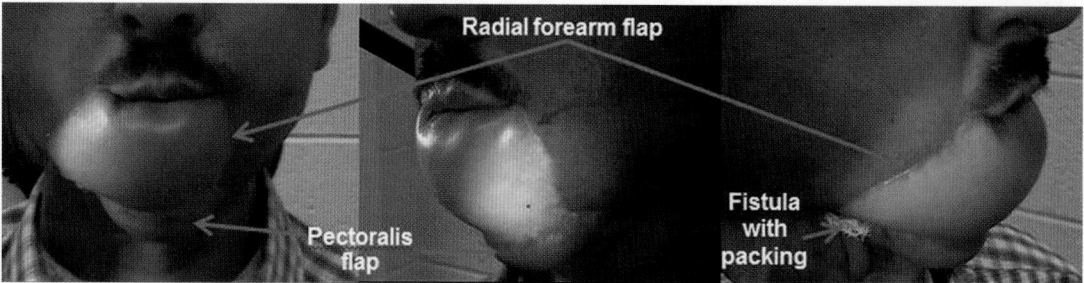

Figure 2–3. Radial forearm flap reconstructing lower lip, chin, and lower right cheek. Pectoralis flap also shown which occurred after the original reconstruction to address wound breakdown and fistula. Remnant of the fistula (does not communicate with oral cavity) with packing is shown on the right image.

that ran from the anterior floor of the mouth to the anterior neck. In the operating room the prior neck incision was opened and the wound was débrided and irrigated with antibiotics. In order to close the fistula, a small pectoralis major myofascial flap was elevated and run through a skin tunnel up the neck and into the region (flap is visible in Figure 2–3).

Unfortunately, he had further wound breakdown resulting in a pharyngocutaneous fistula requiring another surgical procedure 20 days after the pectoralis flap. A second rotation flap using pectoralis myofascial flap remnants was completed. During this hospital stay he began hyperbaric oxygen treatments that were done twice daily while in the hospital and continued for 20 treatments postdischarge.

SPEECH-LANGUAGE THERAPY ASSESSMENT AND TREATMENT

Presurgery

Prior to and during the radiation and chemotherapy done at the outside facility, Patient M did not receive SLP evaluation or treatment. This is unfortunate given the growing evidence that completing oral and swallowing movements prior to and during radiation is likely to optimize swallowing outcomes (Carnaby-Mann et al., 2012; Carroll et al., 2008; Hutcheson et al., 2013; Kotz et al., 2012; Kul-

bersh et al., 2006). Once his care was transitioned to our facility, the SLP established ongoing contact with Patient M

Because of the severity of his situation requiring immediate surgery, the SLP's presurgical meeting was brief. This meeting included the following:

1. The oral mechanism exam revealed weakness of the lips during maximum compression possibly as protective to the tumors presence, limited range of motion of upper and lower lips on protrusion, normal retraction of the lips during smiling, normal tongue range of motion and strength. Maximal jaw opening was reduced (TheraBite Range of Motion scale was 30 mm [less than 35 mm from incisor-to-incisor was considered trismus; Steiner et al., 2015]), presumably from the prior radiation therapy. All of his teeth on the mandibular arch had been extracted prior to radiation as were the maxillary central and lateral incisors.

2. Speech intelligibility was 99% on the sentence portion of the Sentence Intelligibility Test (SIT) and 95% on the word portion.

3. Swallowing status was initially addressed through an interview of his recent history. He was nearly 100% tube fed at this time, describing occasionally taking small sips of water or coffee without coughing or choking. He denied having been given, or having done on his own, any jaw, lip, tongue or swallowing exercises before, during, or after his radiation therapy. He was observed

swallowing 5 cc and 10 cc drinks of water without obvious indications of difficulty. No drooling, oral residue, voice change, or coughing/choking occurred on multiple swallow attempts. The clinician could feel laryngeal elevation during these attempts. Patient M denied any sensation of material "hanging up" in the throat. Because of time constraints it was not possible to obtain a flexible endoscopic evaluation or a modified barium swallow (MBS) study.

OUTCOMES DURING HOSPITALIZATIONS

Patient M was in the hospital for 7 days after his resection and reconstruction. The extent of his reconstruction, postoperative edema, and concern about healing due to prior radiation therapy, led to a restriction from his doctors in terms of jaw, lip, or tongue movements with the SLP. Throughout that stay the SLPs primary role was establishing a functional way to communicate with the health care team and family members. He verbalized in response to questions and could be understood approximately 60% of the time when constrained to short responses. He used gestures and facial expressions for much of his communicating, along with a simple dry erase board for more extended or specific responses. He continued on 100% tube feeding during this hospital stay.

A week after his discharge he returned to the outpatient Ear Nose and Throat Clinic. Although doing well, he still had a fair amount of oral swelling and pain. The restriction on starting oral movements in therapy was maintained. Unfortunately, he was readmitted to the hospital before his next outpatient visit with the SLP due to the foul smell from his neck that required débridement and pectoralis flap to manage the fistula. This began a treacherous time period for Patient M in terms of his healing and recurrent fistula. While the SLP maintained contact with Patient M, the primary focus was on promoting good healing in the mouth and neck. Toward that goal, there was concern about placing undue pressure on suture lines prompting continued tube feeding and deferred speech therapy.

Postdischarge From Last Hospitalization

Reevaluation

The first time that a complete postdischarge SLP evaluation could be completed was nearly 7 weeks from the original resection and reconstruction due to the complicated healing process. Patient M was still 100% PEG dependent. Observations and evaluation data at this postdischarge visit were as follows:

1. Oral mechanism (Figure 2–4): Patient M presented with severely restricted mouth opening measured at 20 mm (estimation of upper central incisor to reconstructed mandibular alveolus); immobility of the lower lip flap on all tasks, but the upper lip could make complete closure with the lower lip flap; retracting the lips in a smile resulted in raising of the upper lip but no corner of the mouth movement; restricted tongue protrusion with inability to extend tip to the lips; very limited ability to lateralize the tongue. The presence of the fibula flap inside the oral cavity created difficulty with most tongue movements but Patient M was able to reach the maxillary alveolar ridge and hard palate with the tongue during nonspeech and speech movements. The lower lip flap and the anterior floor of the mouth were de-sensate (see Video 2–1).

2. Sentence Intelligibility Test (SIT; Yorkston, Beukelman, & Hakel, 1996): Sentence intelligibility was 74% and word intelligibility was 86%.

3. Other observations of communication: Patient M's speaking rate was perceived to be fast in conversational exchange. Visually he appeared to be using significant upper lip movement upward that tended to be visually distracting. Additionally, he avoided eye contact and routinely furrowed his brow or maintained a raised eyebrow when speaking. When asked, he indicated he felt he was "working hard" to talk clearly (see Video 2–2).

4. Swallowing: Observations of swallowing small sips of water were as follows: difficulty sipping from a cup, which the patient attributed to numb lips and floor of mouth; incomplete seal

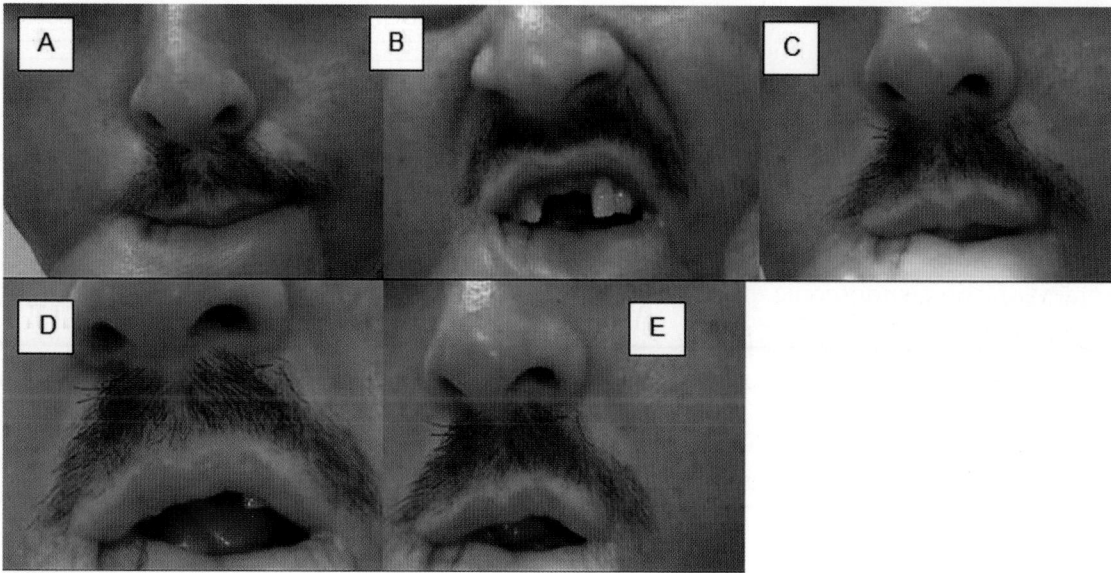

Figure 2–4. A. Lip press. **B.** Attempt at lip retraction. **C.** Maximal tongue protrusion. **D.** Attempt to lateralize tongue to the left. **E.** Attempt to lateralize tongue to the right.

around a drinking straw; minimal oral escape of water out the lips (various locations from corner to corner); difficulty initiating movement of the water from the oral cavity to the pharynx as evidenced by whole head movements forward and back and self-reported by Patient M throughout the trials; perceptible elevation of the larynx visually and with light finger placement on his neck; no change in vocal quality after any trial; no coughing or choking; patient report of having to swallow hard to get water to go down the throat.

A modified barium swallow study was completed that same day and scored using the Modified Barium Swallow Impairment Profile (MBSImP, see Martin-Harris et al., 2008). Only small sips (5 mL × 6 trials) could be completed due to the severity of the deficits observed. Primary findings in the oral ratings were incomplete lip closure with escape (component 1 rating of 2), poor bolus holding (component 2 rating = 1); poor bolus transport (component 4 rating = 3), oral residue (component 5 rating = 1). During pharyngeal transit the findings were minimally reduced laryngeal elevation (component 8 rating = 1); no discernable anterior hyoid movement (component 9 rating = 0); partial epiglottic inversion (component 10 rating = 1); reduced pharyngoesophageal (PE) segment opening (component 14 rating = 2); and pharyngeal residue in the pyriforms and pharyngeal wall (component 16 rating = 2c, e). An anterior–posterior view revealed that the oral residue was primarily on the floor of the mouth on the right side; pharyngeal residues were symmetrical. Effortful and repeated swallows eventually cleared the pharyngeal residue but not the oral, which at times trickled into the pharynx. Trials with the Mendelsohn maneuver (goal of extending laryngeal elevation and therefore PE segment opening) were attempted, but he was not able to consistently execute the maneuver.

On the Penetration-Aspiration Scale (PAS; Rosenbek, Robbins, Roecker Coyle, & Wood, 1996), he was scored a 3 (enters airway above the folds/not ejected). His Functional Oral Intake Scale (FOIS; Crary, Carnaby Mann, & Groher, 2005) was Level 1, "nothing by mouth." Finally, Patient M completed the M.D. Anderson Dysphagia Inventory (MDADI; Chen et al., 2001) with an overall score of 45 (severe swallow related impact on his quality of life).

RECOMMENDED SWALLOWING TREATMENT

Based on these findings, individual therapy was recommended with the following two goals within the next 6 to 8 weeks:

1. Patient M will be able to safely take liquids and soft solids by mouth for pleasure on a daily basis (i.e., increase FOIS score from 0 to 3).
2. Patient M will increase his speech intelligibility at the sentence level to greater than 85% as measured by the sentence portion of the SIT.

He was seen twice a week for individual therapy for an initial block of 15 sessions (missed once due to transportation issues). He was trained to complete a series of jaw, lip, and tongue range of motion movements. The decision to utilize nonspeech and nonswallow specific movements for a portion of his exercise program was based principally on the literature on such exercises for individuals with head and neck cancer who have had radiation therapy (e.g., Carnaby Mann et al., 2012; Hutcheson et al., 2013; Kotz et al., 2012). It was unfortunate that he had not been doing these exercises prior to and during his radiation therapy, but given the aggressiveness of his tumor and the complicated surgical history after radiation, it is unlikely that he could have, or would have been allowed to complete such exercises over time. The intention now was to maximize range of movements of all structures and potentially to limit further fibrosis.

For the jaw, the TheraBite device was utilized after training in its use in the clinic. The lip exercises included protrusion, retraction, and maximal lip press; the tongue exercise included maximal protrusion, tip lateralization, tip movement as far around the mandibular buccogingival sulcus as possible, and tip and dorsum pressing against the hard palate. He was instructed to complete short exercise periods (~10–15 min) five times daily; within each period he cycled through 5 to 10 repetitions of each exercise.

Specific to swallowing, three items were trained:

1. Mendelsohn maneuver (Lazarus, Logemann, & Gibbons, 1993; McCullough et al., 2012; Men-delsohn & McConnell, 1987). These maneuvers were initially completed with just saliva swallows with moistening of the tongue as needed.
2. Anticipating taking small sips from a cup or straw, he worked at obtaining complete seal around a straw. This was done in front of a mirror. With visual feedback he could assess the seal and adjust as needed. The adjustments were either increased jaw elevation to push the lower lip flap more completely into the upper lip conforming around the straw, or slightly effortful pursing of the upper lip. Over time the visual cue was faded and he could better sense the effort required for complete closure. Similar work occurred with completing a seal around the edge of a cup. He expressed preference for the straw once he progressed to taking small amounts of liquid in the clinic because he felt he did not have to work so hard to move the liquid to the throat. A flexible scope was passed nasally when first shifting to the small water bolus attempts and no instances of undue spillage or penetration/aspiration on either straw or cup sips was noted.
3. Effortful swallow (Hind, Nicosia, Roecker, Carnes, & Robbins, 2001; Lazarus et al., 1993) was also trained in the first week of therapy, and he continued to execute sets of 5 to 10 such swallows scattered throughout his day (minimum of five times but was instructed to do it as often as possible).

Specific to his speech in addition to the oral movements, therapy focused on the following:

1. Consistent use of general intelligibility strategies including slower speaking rate, heightened awareness of intelligibility breakdown by observing the listener and asking for confirmation of understanding, and improved eye contact from Patient M
2. Reduction of the visually distracting forehead, eyebrow, and excessive upper lip movement was targeted. This began toward the end of the 15 sessions because Patient M indicated that his family always thought he was angry when talking with them because of his facial expression. First, he was made aware of these movements in

front of a mirror and subsequently with clinician cuing when he was not in front of the mirror. He ultimately verbalized that he could feel when he was tensing his face and then he consciously could halt the distracting movements.

REASSESSMENT FOLLOWING TWO MONTHS OF SWALLOWING TREATMENT

Patient M was diligent in completing his at-home exercises. At the end of 2 months he was taking sips of liquids (water primarily, but also coffee, juices) for pleasure while meeting his nutrition needs via the PEG. His FOIS rating had increased to a 3 based on his report, and a new goal was set to achieve a rating of 5. MDADI score had increased from 45 to 60 (34% increase from baseline) mostly based on an improvement in the "emotional" component on the MDADI. A repeat MBS indicated no loss of material out the lips; minimal oral residue on the floor of the mouth persisted; during Mendelsohn attempts he was able to increase the duration of the maximal laryngeal elevation by approximately 0.5 s in most instances resulting in prolonged PE opening. When prolonging laryngeal elevation, minimal pyriform sinus residue was noted on thin, nectar, and thick liquids, but serve residue on paste (solids not attempted) with consistent penetration and aspiration on the paste attempts. Based on these findings, his diet was advanced slowly to include not just water but other liquids (up to milkshake thick) while at home for partial nutrition and pleasure. The dietician met with him to plan adjustments to the PEG feedings depending on his oral liquid intake. Over the next 2 months he continued to be seen in the clinic approximately once a week to slowly advance his diet safely.

Patient M's SIT score increased to 92% exceeding the goal that was set. His intelligibility in less structured testing in a quiet clinic room was judged to be lower than this by the clinician (~85% depending on context and visual cues). Continued use of a fast speaking rate was the most likely cause of the further intelligibility reduction (see Video 2–3). He was not working at this point but expressed that he

was now talking on the telephone and engaging in some social activities outside of the house, although still self-conscious of his appearance.

Patient M continued to be followed for the next 3 months with SLP visits spaced out to once every 2 weeks. He eventually transferred his care back to his home community which was approximately 60 minutes from our facility because transportation was increasingly an issue. He ultimately moved several states away, and his care (ENT and SLP) was transferred to another teaching hospital.

Despite not having final outcome data beyond the several months that he was followed by the authors, there was much that the team learned in working with Patient M In spite of the complicated nature of his radiation, surgery, and healing, meaningful improvement in both swallowing and communication was accomplished. Close communication between the surgeons and the SLPs was required to safely begin a SLP therapy regimen given his issues with wound breakdown and fistula. Multidisciplinary approach extending beyond ENT and SLP also was critical in his case. Dietetics and psychology played important roles in his total rehabilitation. For the SLP treatment planning, Patient M presented in a manner that did not closely match what is presented in the peer-reviewed literature. This is not uncommon when dealing with advanced oral cancer patients where very individualized surgeries are necessary. However, solid understanding of normal speech and swallowing along with detailed understanding of the radiation and surgical treatments that he underwent served as the basis for understanding and then targeting his deficits. There was available literature to be applied to his case in terms of addressing swallowing problems in individuals who have had radiation to the head and neck, and more generally about the possible benefits of the Mendelsohn maneuver. The literature to guide the work on Patient M's speech is more limited. Given the significant restrictions to his tongue movements, however, information on rehabilitation after partial and near-total glossectomy was reviewed and utilized in treatment planning. This included work by Furia et al. (2010) that focused on maximizing residual mobility of the articulators as well as eliminating maladaptive behaviors (fast rate and visual distractors in Patient M's case). Older literature with partial glossectomees by Skelly et al. (Skelly, Spector, Donaldson, Brodeur, & Paletta, 1971; Skelly, Donaldson, Fust, & Townsend, 1972) also was reviewed and incorporated into the treatment approach.

REFLECTION AND ANALYSIS FOR FURTHER STUDY

1. What is the role of biofeedback approaches in the treatment of speech and swallow impairments in this population?

2. In the presented case, mirror work was used for biofeedback during speech tasks. What other approaches are possible? Be sure and think about all sensory modalities as well as various technologies for the provision of biofeedback. How might these be implemented in both the home and clinical setting?

3. As with this case, wound healing frequently interferes with or even delays rehabilitation efforts. When this is the case, how can the SLP maintain therapeutic contact with the patient, and what factors are crucial for determining when and how therapy can resume?

REFERENCES

Carnaby-Mann, G., Crary, M. A., Schmalfuss, I., & Amdur, R. (2012). "Pharyngocise": Randomized controlled trial of preventative exercises to maintain muscle structure and swallowing function during head-and-neck chemoradiotherapy. *International Journal of Radiation Oncology, Biology, Physics, 83*(1), 210–219.

Carroll, W. R., Locher, J. L., Canon, C. L., Bohannon, I. A., McColloch, N. L., & Magnuson, J. S. (2008). Pretreatment swallowing exercises improve swallow function after chemoradiation. *Laryngoscope, 118,* 39–43.

Chen, A. Y., Frankowski, R., Bishop-Leone, J., Hebert, T., Leyk, S., Lewin, J., & Helmuth, G. (2001). The development and validation of a dysphagia-specific quality-of-life questionnaire for patients with head and neck cancer. *Archives of Otolaryngology-Head and Neck Surgery, 127,* 870–876.

Crary, M., Carnaby-Mann, G., & Groher, M. (2005). Initial psychometric assessment of a functional oral intake scale for dysphagia in stroke patients. *Archives of Physical Medication and Rehabilitation, 86,* 1516–1520.

Furia, C. L., Kowalski, L. P., Latorre, M. R., Angelis, E. C., Martins, N. M., Barros, A. P., & Ribeiro, K. C. (2010). Speech intelligibility after glossectomy and speech rehabilitation. *Archives of Otolaryngology-Head and Neck Surgery, 127,* 877–883.

Hind, J. S., Nicosia, M. A., Roecker, E. B., Carnes, M. L., & Robbins, J. (2001). Comparison of effortful and noneffortful swallows in healthy middle-aged and older adults. *Archives of Physical Medicine and Rehabilitation, 82,* 1661–1665.

Hutcheson, K. A., Bhayani, M., Beadle, B. M., Gold, K. A., Shinn, E. H., Lai, S. Y., & Lewin, J. S. (2013). Eat and exercise during radiotherapy or chemoradiotherapy for pharyngeal cancer: Use it or lose it. *JAMA Otolaryngology-Head and Neck Surgery, 139*(11), 1127–1134. doi:10.1001/jamaoto.2013.4715

Kotz, T., Federman, A. D., Kao, J., Milman, L., Packer, S., Lopez-Prieto, C., Forsythe, K., & Genden, E. M. (2012). Prophylactic swallowing exercises in patients with head and neck cancer undergoing chemoradiation: A randomized trial. *Archives of Otolaryngology-Head and Neck Surgery, 138*(4), 376–382.

Kulbersh, B. D., Rosenthal, E. L., McGrew, B. M., Duncan, R. D., McColloch, N. L., Carroll, W. R., & Magnuson, J. S. (2006). Pretreatment, preoperative swallowing exercises may improve dysphagia quality of life. *Laryngoscope, 116,* 883–886.

Lazarus, C., Logemann, J. A., & Gibbons, P. (1993). Effects of maneuvers on swallow function in a dysphagic oral cancer patient. *Head & Neck, 15,* 419–424.

Martin-Harris, B., Brodsky, M. B., Castell, D. O., Schleicher, M., Sandidge, J., Maxwell, R., & Blair, J. (2008). MBS measurement tool for swallow impairment—MBSImp: Establishing a standard. *Dysphagia, 23*(4), 392–405.

McCullough, G. H., Kamarunas, E., Mann, G. C., Schmidley, J. W., Robbins, J. A., & Crary, M. (2012). Effects of Mendelsohn maneuver on measures of swallowing duration post-stroke. *Topics in Stroke Rehabilitation, 19,* 234–243.

Mendelsohn, M. S., & McConnell, F. M. (1987). Function in the pharyngoesophageal segment. *Laryngoscope, 97,* 483–489.

Rosenbek, J. C., Robbins, J. A., Roecker, E. B., Coyle, J. L., & Wood, J. L. (1996). A penetration-aspiration scale. *Dysphagia, 11*(2), 93–98.

Skelly, M., Donaldson, R. C., Fust, R. S., & Townsend, D. L. (1972). Changes in phonatory aspects of glossectomee intelligibility through vocal parameter manipulation. *Journal of Speech and Hearing Disorders, 37*(3), 379–389.

Skelly, M., Spector, D. J., Donaldson, R. C., Brodeur, A., & Paletta, F. X. (1971). Compensatory physiologic phonetics for the glossectomee. *Journal of Speech and Hearing Disorders, 36*(1), 101–114.

Steiner, F., Evans, R., Marsh, R., Rigby, P., James, S., Sutherland, K., . . . Tan, S. T. (2015). Mouth opening and trismus in patients undergoing curative treatment for head and neck cancer. *International Journal of Oral Maxillo-Facial Surgery, 44,* 292–296.

Yorkston, K., Beukelman, D., & Hakel, M. (1996). *Sentence Intelligibility Test©.* Lincoln, NE: Communication Disorders Software.

3

Speech and Swallowing After Hemiglossectomy With Radial Forearm Free Flap Reconstruction

Bernice K. Klaben and Keith Casper

INTRODUCTION AND MEDICAL HISTORY

Patient C is a 55-year-old female who presented to our otolaryngology practice with a prior history of non-Hodgkin's lymphoma, approximately 10 years ago, and bone marrow transplant with graft versus host disease. Medical history was otherwise positive for stage I colon cancer (2005), type II steroid-induced diabetes (diagnosed in 2007), esophageal reflux (2009), stage III chronic kidney disease secondary to the lymphoma treatment, and dermatomyositis lichen planus. She never smoked or used smokeless tobacco, alcohol, or illicit drugs. Additional past medical history is presented in Table 3–1.

DIAGNOSTIC WORKUP

Biopsies of the left oral tongue lesions were positive for squamous cell carcinoma. In the past, she had a history of multiple lesions on the left lateral tongue which would go away with topical creams. Beginning in December 2013, one of these lesions did not

resolve. She did not present with any bleeding from the lesions, weight loss, dysphagia, odynophagia, dyspnea, or neck masses.

Table 3–1. Summary of the Complex Surgical History of This Patient

Cesarean section	1992
Cataract extraction, bilateral	2004
Small intestine surgery, ileocecal resection for Stage I (T1, N0, M0) adenocarcinoma of the colon	12/2004
Right colectomy	2005
Left hip arthroplasty	2005
Anterior cervical discectomy with fusion	03/2010
Cholecystectomy	08/2011
Shoulder arthroscopy, right	11/2013
L hemiglossectomy (T2N0Mx squamous cell carcinoma), R RFFF, L selective neck dissection (Levels I–IV)	03/2014
Colonoscopy	11/2014
Transoral CO$_2$ laser ablation of granulation tissue	01/2015

Speech-Language Pathology (SLP) Preoperative Counseling

Patient C was seen prior to surgery for a hemiglossectomy. She was eating a normal diet. During the consultation the speech-language pathologist (SLP) gathered information pertaining to the patient's understanding of the surgery, risks and benefits, and expected outcomes. Information regarding potential postsurgical effects of voice, speech, and swallowing were discussed with Patient C. An explanation of the SLP's role, as well as Patient C's role, in rehabilitation following surgery was provided. Patient C was given information on planned nasal gastric feeding to provide nutritional intake following surgery. She was counseled on management of oral secretions and postsurgical swallowing of secretions in addition to the importance of maintaining good oral care. Tables 3–2 and 3–3 present the results of the presurgical evaluations. Oral motor examination results are presented in Table 3–4.

Table 3–2. Evaluation Scores: Initial Visit and 1 Year Postsurgery

MD Anderson Dysphagia Index (MDADI)	4/2014	5/2015
Physical scale	70	54
Functional scale	68	59
Emotional scale	87	48
Global	60	40

Note. 0 = extremely low functioning, 100 = high functioning

Table 3–3. Questionnaire: Initial Visit and 1 Year Postsurgery

	4/2014	5/2015
Reflux Symptom Index Score (<13 WNL)	12	8
Glottal Function Index (score >4 reflects problems in vocal function)	0	7
Sydney Swallow Questionnaire (Total: 1700)	1408	257

SURGICAL REPORT FOR LEFT HEMIGLOSSECTOMY

Patient C underwent a left hemiglossectomy in March 2014. A right radial forearm free flap (skin paddle dimension 9 × 5 cm) was used for reconstruction of the surgical site. Microvascular anastomosis was achieved with the left facial artery anastomosed to the radial artery, venae comitantes anastomosed to branch of the internal jugular vein with a 2.0 coupling device, and cephalic vein anastomosed to a branch of the internal jugular vein with a 3.0 coupling device. A split-thickness skin graft (dimensions 9 × 5 cm) was taken from the right thigh and was sutured to the donor site.

POSTOPERATIVE EVALUATION

Patient C was referred by her otolaryngologist 3 weeks after her surgery for a repeat speech evaluation and initial dysphagia assessment with recommendations. A nasogastric tube (NGT) was placed at the time of surgery for all nutritional needs. The patient experienced excessive secretions in the oral cavity after surgery and used suction throughout the day.

A fiberoptic endoscopic evaluation of swallowing (FEES) was carried out using green-tinted ice chips, water, nectar-thickened liquid, and puree consistency (applesauce). All consistencies were presented to the right posterior lingual region using a 5-mL syringe. The SLP noted Patient C had difficulty containing the bolus in the oral cavity secondary to poor labial closure due to tongue protruding out of the mouth at rest. She triggered the swallow once the bolus entered the right pyriform sinus. Patient C demonstrated mild to moderate oropharyngeal dysphagia characterized by mild pooling in the right valleculae and pyriform sinus on nectar thickened liquid and puree consistencies. Secondary swallows were beneficial for clearing the residue. No penetration or aspiration was noted during the examination. Table 3–5 summarizes the FEES examination results.

Table 3–4. Oromotor Examination: Initial Evaluation

Parameter (cranial nerve involved)	Observations
Lingual ROM (CN XII)	Decreased forward/upward/downward/lateral, protrusion, Decreased base of tongue retraction
Lingual symmetry (CN XII)	Protrudes between lips at rest, edematous
Stimulation of gag reflex (CN X)	Intact bilaterally
Velar elevation/retraction (CN V_3)	Retraction noted, nasal gastric tubed noted on left
Hard palate contour/vault	Within functional limits
Dentition	Natural
Breathing	Diaphragmatic
Speech characteristics	Dysarthria
Vocal quality	Slightly raspy
Resonance	Slightly hypernasal
Hyolaryngeal excursion on palpation	Decreased
Mental status	Alert, cooperative
Other comments	Mild to moderate drooling secondary to tongue protrusion at rest and no lip closure, drooling increased during conversational speech

Table 3–5. FEES Examination: Initial Evaluation

Structure/Movement	Observations
Velopharyngeal competence on vocal tasks	Within functional limits, nasogastric tube inserted in the nares on the left
Base of tongue movement	Decreased secondary to edema
Pharyngeal and longitudinal constrictors on high-pitched /i/	Moderately decreased on left
True vocal fold adduction and abduction on alternate sniff-/i/ task	Left true vocal fold paralysis
Complete laryngeal adduction on breath hold	Incomplete on adduction secondary to left true vocal fold paralysis
Epiglottic inversion/retroversion on dry swallow	Absent
Secretions	Stasis/pooling/thin mucus in pyriforms
Laryngeal evaluation	Decreased
Other observations	Edema—base of tongue Lymphedema of jaw, submandibular, and left neck

RECOMMENDATIONS

Following FEES, it was recommended Patient C continue with the nasal gastric tube for caloric and nutritional intake. Dysphagia therapy was recommended with thin and nectar-thickened liquid consistencies administered using a 5-mL syringe in small bolus amounts presented to the right oral cavity. The goal was to complete oral intake to focus on improvement of glottal closure, develop labial closure to maintain oral containment, increase lingual range of motion and strength, and exercises to increase hyolaryngeal elevation. The following exercises were reviewed and a recommended home practice treatment plan of five repetitions of each exercise per set with five sets daily was provided to Patient C (Logemann, Pauloski, Rademaker, & Colangelo, 1997):

- supraglottic swallow;
- effortful swallow;
- tongue base retraction;
- lingual range of motion;
- suck swallow;
- articulation of hard /g/ syllables;
- pitch glides up on "e" from low to high pitch;
- manual lymphedema drainage therapy to reduce edema in the jaw and submandibular regions; and
- articulation exercises to improve speech intelligibility at the phoneme, syllable, word, phrase, sentence, paragraph, and discourse level to 90% accuracy.

POSTSWALLOWING EVALUATION: 14 DAYS AFTER INITIAL FEES

A repeat FEES examination was repeated 14 days after the initial assessment. Lingual edema was notably decreased with the natural tongue/flap staying in the oral cavity at rest. She was able to demonstrate a complete labial seal; however, at rest the labial seal was inconsistent. Base of tongue movement was mildly decreased for retraction to the left. A left true vocal fold paresis was noted with inconsistent adduction of the vocal folds during breath hold. The epiglottis was noted to invert and retrovert on dry

swallow. Pooling was noted in the valleculae prior to swallowing. Assessment of the swallow was tested with tinted ice chips, water, nectar-thickened liquid, and applesauce presented by cup and spoon. Slight pooling was noted in the valleculae and pyriform sinuses on all consistencies. Secondary swallows were useful at clearing the residue. No penetration or aspiration was noted during the examination. Sight drooling was present with thin liquids secondary to inconsistent labial seal. The NGT (present for a total of 35 days) was removed at this session.

Recommendations

1. Start Level 1 dysphagia diet with thin liquid and nectar-thickened consistencies (soup) using spoon and cup presentation in small bolus amounts with a therapeutic target of maintaining lip seal when swallowing.
2. Begin working on fine motor articulation exercises using syllable repetitions on vowels /a, e, o, u/ with dental, alveolar, palate-alveolar, velar, and palatal consonants.
3. Continue with swallowing exercises given at initial assessment.

FOLLOW-UP TREATMENT

After Patient C was discharged from the skilled nursing facility, she continued receiving outpatient dysphagia and speech therapy. Patient C reported softer foods tended to "stick to the roof of the mouth" and would have to use her finger to dislodge the food. As edema of the lingual, left facial, neck, and submandibular areas decreased, she was able to chew foods such as chicken and also taste sweet, salty, sour, bitter, and umami.

Articulation was challenging with the vocalic /r/ being the most difficult for Patient C in conversational speech. The vocalic /r/ continues to be the most challenging to articulate 1 year later as can be heard on the recordings (see Audio 3–1 to 3–5). Practice on articulation included syllable repetitions, words, short phrases, functional phrases, reading, and conversational speech. During home practices, Patient C recorded her speech in short segments for playback and critiquing.

SUMMARY

To date, Patient C is 10 years post operative treatment from ileocecal Stage I colon cancer and 1 year posthemiglossectomy. She is eating a normal diet but prefers foods that are moist. Patient C continues to have difficulty articulating the vocalic /r/ phoneme especially in rapid conversation; however, in spite of this, she is 100% intelligible in conversation with naïve listeners. Recent scans have come back clear with no evidence of disease.

REFLECTION AND ANALYSIS FOR FURTHER STUDY

1. Most head and neck cancer patients are male. Given your current understanding of head and neck cancer and patients affected by head and neck cancer, what are some gender-specific issues that you feel are clinically relevant? Why?
2. What strategies would you offer a patient who was experiencing difficulty with speech intelligibility? In your response contrast the demands of face-to-face familiar listener, face-to-face unfamiliar listener, and remove (e.g., telephone or Skype) communications.

REFERENCE

Logemann, J. A., Pauloski, B. R., Rademaker, A. W., & Colangelo, L. A. (1997). Speech and swallowing rehabilitation for head and neck cancer patients. *Oncology, 11*(5), 651–659.

4

Prolonged Dysphagia Following Chemoradiation of the Soft Palate and Tonsillar Fossa

Donna S. Lundy, Mario A. Landera, and Zoukaa B. Sargi

HISTORY

This case is referred to as Mr. J, a 69-year-old African American male. He is a retired bartender and accomplished tennis player. During his free time he enjoys reading books. He has been married to his wife for 35 years, and they do not have children.

Medical History

In August 2010, Mr. J sought care from his primary care physician regarding issues of nasal congestion, nasal regurgitation of liquids, throat discomfort, and changes in his speech. Mr. J began noticing these instances of speech changes and air leaking from the nose without change in the voice itself. Due to the complexity of these symptoms, he was referred to our otolaryngology practice. His medical history was significant for hypertension, hypercholesterolemia, emphysema, chronic obstructive pulmonary disorder, and glaucoma. He also had tuberculosis at age 15 years and was hospitalized for this for 5 months. Surgical history was significant for undergoing corneal transplant. Mr. J has a history of smoking at least one pack of cigarettes per day for more

than a 50-year period. He quit smoking tobacco in 2009. Mr. J also previously consumed alcoholic beverages on a social basis, though quit drinking alcohol in 2005. During his younger years, he also reported using cocaine recreationally.

DIAGNOSTIC WORKUP

Upon presentation to our otolaryngology practice, physical examination showed a well-developed, well-nourished, and healthy appearing gentleman. His voice was hypernasal. Head and neck examination was significant for an ulcerated lesion replacing the central portion of his soft palate and uvula that was indurated and tender on palpation. Fiberoptic evaluation revealed benign appearing hypertrophy of the base of tongue and minimal swelling of the pharyngeal walls.

A destructive lesion of the soft palate was suspected with the two most likely diagnoses considered being neoplastic and inflammatory conditions. Computed tomography (CT) scan with contrast was obtained, and this was relatively unremarkable, although the area of concern was difficult to evaluate because of dental streak artifacts. This being said, no bone erosion was appreciated, and there were no abnormal neck nodes on contrasted CT. Following CT, the recommendation was to proceed to the operating room for examination under anesthesia and biopsies of the lesion. At that point, a lesion involving the soft palate and extending to both tonsillar fossae, more so on the left side than on the right side, was noted. The lesion was biopsied and showed keratinizing squamous cell carcinoma on intraoperative frozen section exam. The nasopharyngeal surface of the soft palate was not involved, and the posterior pharyngeal wall as well as lateral pharyngeal walls were uninvolved with tumor. There was some swelling along the posterior tonsillar pillars. The base of tongue, vallecula, larynx, and hypopharynx were clear. The esophagus, trachea, and mainstem bronchi examination was within the normal limits.

Permanent pathology confirmed invasive keratinizing squamous cell carcinoma. Positron emission tomography (PET CT) was obtained ruling out metastatic disease. Based on intraoperative measurement of the tumor (slightly more than 4 cm) and the absence of bone erosion and metastatic disease, the tumor was staged as T3N0M0 stage 3 oropharyngeal (soft palate) squamous cell carcinoma.

Mr. J's case was reviewed at tumor board and recommendation was for definitive nonsurgical treatment. Medical oncology and radiation oncology consultations were obtained.

Pretreatment Speech and Swallowing Evaluation

Prior to starting his treatments, Mr. J underwent a pretreatment speech and swallowing evaluation with a speech-language pathologist. A comprehensive clinical speech and swallowing evaluation helped to capture this information. This included collection of a case history, completion of functional and quality of life scales, oral mechanism exam, and administration of swallow trials. The case history consisted of a review of pertinent medical history, current diet, speech intelligibility, swallowing complaints, speech complaints, and planned mode(s) of treatment. As previously stated above, clinicians knew that Mr. J had a long history of tobacco and alcohol use.

> Alcohol and tobacco use are known to increase the risk of developing cancer, particularly when consumed synergistically (Goldstein, Chang, Hashibe, La Vecchia, & Zhang, 2010; Saman, 2012; Sivasithamparam, Visk, Cohen, & King, 2013).

Mr. J was on a regular diet, though was having complaints of nasal regurgitation with liquids and also reported that his speech was nasal. His plan of treatment was to undergo induction chemotherapy followed by concurrent chemoradiation therapy (CRT).

An oral mechanism examination was performed to assess structure and function of the speech and swallowing mechanism. Significant findings included asymmetric soft palate elevation with weakness on the left side and mild hypernasal speech. He was also noted to be edentulous. His speech was rated as 95% intelligible. Functional and quality of life scales were administered to not only collect baseline information, but to also use for comparative purposes during and after the planned course of treatment. The Functional Oral Intake Scale (FOIS), the Eating Assessment Tool (EAT-10; Belafsky et al., 2008), and the University of Washington Quality of Life (UW-QOL) questionnaire were used as the assessment tools.

The FOIS was developed to document the functional oral intake of food and liquids in patients over time (Crary, Mann, & Groher, 2005). Ratings are made by clinicians on a 7-point scale with Level 1 corresponding to "nothing by mouth" and Level 7 corresponding to "total oral diet with no restriction." Mr. J's FOIS score will be discussed later in this chapter during his clinical swallow assessment. The EAT-10 is a symptom-specific outcome instrument for dysphagia that documents patient perceptions of dysphagia. There are a total of 10 items with 0 corresponding to no problem and 4 corresponding to severe problem. Scores of 3 or higher are considered abnormal on the EAT-10. Mr. J gave himself a rating of 5 on the EAT-10. The UW-QOL questionnaire was also given. This questionnaire consists of 12 domain-specific questions addressing the physical, functional, and emotional quality of life in patients with head and neck cancer. In addition, four generic questions are included. Each of the domain-specific items are scored from 0, corresponding to worst QOL to 100, corresponding to best QOL (Rogers et al., 2002). Mr. J achieved a composite score of 90.33% on the UW-QOL.

Swallow trials of water, applesauce, and a graham cracker were given as part of the clinical swallowing assessment. Laryngeal excursion was noted to be present with a timely swallow response during all trials given. No overt signs or symptoms of aspiration were noted. Specifically, no coughing, throat clearing, or changes in vocal quality were observed after all of his swallow trials. In addition, no nasal regurgitation was noted. This latter finding was interesting as nasal regurgitation was one of Mr. J's main complaints. Based on Mr. J's clinical swallow assessment, he achieved a FOIS Level 7 score.

At the time of this assessment, our protocol was to conduct instrumental assessments only if overt signs or symptoms of aspiration were noted. As Mr. J did not demonstrate any signs or symptoms of aspiration, an instrumental examination was not performed. Our protocol has since evolved, and we now routinely conduct instrumental swallow assessments on all patients with cancer involving the oral cavity, nasopharynx, oropharynx, larynx, or hypopharynx who will be receiving radiation therapy with or without chemotherapy.

> Numerous studies have shown that dysphagia may occur before treatment due to the presence of the tumor interfering with bolus flow or airway protection when swallowing (Pauloski et al., 2000; Rosen, Rhee, & Kaufman, 2001; Stenson et al., 2000; van der Molen et al., 2009). When considering the tumor site, patients with hypopharyngeal and laryngeal tumors were more likely to have symptoms related to dysphagia (Pauloski et al., 2000; Stenson et al., 2000). In addition, those with lower-stage tumors were less likely to state complaints related to their swallowing (Pauloski et al., 2000). Although aspiration is considered a consequence of reduced airway protection or reduced bolus control, pretreatment swallow studies have shown an incidence of aspiration occurring between 18% and 41% (Rosen et al., 2001; van der Molen et al., 2009).

After the swallowing assessment was completed, a counseling session was provided to Mr. J and his wife involving explanation of the anticipated changes in the speech and swallowing mechanism related to his upcoming chemotherapy and radiation therapy. Specifically, the development of mucositis, xerostomia, odynophagia, dysgeusia, nausea, emesis, and lethargy were explained with focus on how these changes might impact swallowing function (Gaziano, 2002; Kammer, Wiederholt, & Knigge, 2011; Logemann, 2006; Starmer, 2014). The importance of maintaining the maximally tolerated oral diet throughout treatment was also emphasized, as we know that patients who experience greater than 2 weeks of nonoral feeding status experience higher rates of post treatment dysphagia (Gillespie, Brodsky, Day, Lee, & Martin-Harris, 2004).

Our protocol has all patients receiving radiation, with or without chemotherapy, participating in routine appointments throughout treatment with a speech pathologist to ensure they are tolerating a least-restrictive diet, maintain safe swallowing status, and receive instruction on rehabilitative and prophylactic swallowing exercises, if indicated. Numerous studies have shown that administration of prophylactic swallowing exercises may be helpful in reducing the extent and severity of the acute toxicities impacting swallowing function (Carnaby-Mann, Crary, Schmalfuss, & Amdur, 2012; Carroll et al., 2008; Kotz et al., 2012; van der Molen et al., 2011). Patients deemed to be more at risk for developing complications or side effects related to their swallowing are scheduled once weekly throughout their treatment. Those with no baseline dysphagia or those at lower risk of developing dysphagia are scheduled once every 2 weeks.

TREATMENT

Plan of Care

Mr. J underwent induction chemotherapy (Cisplatin and Docetaxel) with excellent response noted after the first cycle of treatment. Percutaneous endoscopic gastrostomy (PEG) tube was placed to assist with nutrition. He then received a second cycle of Cisplatin/Docetaxel and 5FU and proceeded with definitive CRT with weekly Cisplatin and 70 Gy delivered in 35 fractions using intensity-modulated radiation therapy (IMRT). Treatment was completed in March 2011, and post treatment PET CT in June 2011 showed excellent response. Subsequent cancer surveillance follow-ups showed no evidence of recurrent cancer.

Swallow Intervention During Treatment

Mr. J attended only one swallowing therapy session approximately halfway into CRT. During that visit he described pain and discomfort when chewing and swallowing. He was also experiencing some dysgeusia. Due to these symptoms, he had downgraded his diet to swallowing only small amounts of puree foods and liquids. He began to supplement through his PEG tube, as he was losing weight. The speech-language pathologist emphasized the importance of continuing to maintain some portion of his nutrition by mouth. Discussion of timing his swallowing with his pain medication and anesthetics was emphasized to further encourage continued oral intake. This visit placed him on a FOIS Level 3 score (Crary et al., 2005), corresponding to "tube supplements with consistent oral intake."

POST TREATMENT

Mr. J was seen for his first post treatment speech-language pathology appointment 3 weeks after completion of CRT. At that point, he was 100% PEG dependent taking nothing by mouth, FOIS Level 1 (Crary et al., 2005). He complained of an inability to swallow, odynophagia, dysgeusia, and fatigue. He had lost about 25 pounds during the course of his treatment. As previously stated, he came for only one visit during his treatment, despite recommendation of participating in swallowing therapy biweekly during the course of his treatment.

First Visit

This first visit consisted of a clinical swallowing evaluation (CSE) and modified barium swallow (MBS), and QOL measures. At this first visit, Mr. J was noted to swallow his secretions. Speech was mildly hypernasal without nasal air emission, and overall intelligibility was judged to be fair to good (see Video 4–1).

The CSE included an oral peripheral mechanism examination that documented a mild degree of mucositis involving the oral mucosa and hard and soft palate but otherwise full range of motion of the lips and tongue. Asymmetric soft palate elevation was observed with increased weakness on the left side. Mr. J was edentulous and not wearing his dentures. Attempted swallow trials in the clinic yielded brisk coughing without apparent swallowing in a more fearful manner. It was then elected to discontinue the swallow trials and complete the MBS.

A MBS was performed according to standard procedure in both lateral and anterior to posterior views with a progression of barium consistencies from thin liquids, nectar, honey, pudding, and cookie-coated presentations (see Video 4–2). The first and most impressive finding was significant guarding of the entire swallow with holding of the bolus in the oral cavity prior to propelling accompanied by head shaking in a "no" gesture which was not captured on video. This resolved after the first two successful swallows. The overall interpretation from this first post treatment MBS was moderate weakness and reduced motion involving base of tongue retraction, hyolaryngeal excursion, epiglottic inversion, and cricopharyngeal relaxation. Significant edema could be visualized involving the epiglottis. A mild amount of nasal regurgitation was noted during the swallow that returned back to the posterior oral cavity with gravity, and no significant residual material was seen in the nasal cavity. Significant residue pooled postswallow in the vallecula and to a lesser degree in the bilateral pyriform sinuses which increased with denser barium boluses. Pooled material eventually cleared with multiple repeat swallows but was observed to be laborious. Trace laryngeal penetration and aspiration was observed on intermittent swallows after the swallow and was felt to be related to pooled material spilling into the unprotected larynx/airway after the swallow response had been completed. He was not sensate of the aspirated material but was able to eject it from his airway with directed coughing. Penetration Aspiration Score was 6 (Rosenbek, Robbins, Roecker, Coyle, & Woods, 1996). Questionable mild narrowing was noted in the postcricoid/upper cervical esophageal area, but due to lack of adequate barium to distend the area, this observation was not conclusive. Strategies and maneuvers were attempted during the study, and a combined chin down with a super-supraglottic swallow maneuver improved overall swallowing efficiency with less residual material after the repeat swallow.

The rationale for using the chin tuck after seeing its improved efficiency during the MBS is due to its benefit in maximizing base of tongue retraction (Welch, Logemann, Rademaker, & Kahrilas, 1993). Combining this with a super-supraglottic swallow maneuver was helpful in adding an extra layer of airway closure while helping to clear residual in the pharynx after the first swallow (Martin, Logemann, Shaker, & Dodds, 1993).

The recommendations at the end of the evaluation were for Mr. J to begin eating, focusing on liquids and thin pureed materials using the combined chin down posture with the super-supraglottic swallow maneuver. It was not felt to be realistic that he would be able to be immediately weaned from his PEG due to the laborious task of swallowing and would need to begin slowly and progress with feeding tube weaning as tolerated. Additionally, he was strongly encouraged to participate in an aggressive swallowing therapy program.

Comparison of pre- and post treatment QOL measures revealed a significant decline in all areas. Mr. J achieved a score of 8 on the EAT-10 and a composite score of 52% on the UW-QOL. It was interesting to note that his swallowing deficits as delineated on the MBS were specific to the oropharyngeal area and not to the primary tumor site of the palate (Logemann et al., 2006). Additionally, despite mildly hypernasal speech and asymmetrical palatal elevation on endoscopy, only modest nasal regurgitation was appreciated. This material returned to the oral cavity/oropharynx with gravity after the swallow.

In adults, hypernasal speech is typically iatrogenic (following surgery or other treatment impacting the muscles and functional integrity of velopharyngeal closure), as in this case, or neurologic in etiology, thereby prompting an appropriate referral (Dworkin, Marunick, & Krouse, 2014). Hypernasality does not always result in nasal regurgitation. It is important to remember that the two most common causes of nasal regurgitation are velopharyngeal insufficiency as evidenced by backflow during the swallow and esophageal and/or cricopharyngeal hypertonicity or obstruction as seen by backflow after the swallow (Logemann, 1983).

Swallowing Therapy

Mr. J returned for swallowing therapy on a weekly basis consisting of both traditional swallowing exercises and functional swallowing recommendations. The swallowing exercises focused on improving strength and motion in three primary areas: base of tongue retraction, hyolaryngeal excursion, and cricopharyngeal relaxation. Specific exercises to maximize tongue base retraction included voluntary, forceful, and sustained tongue retraction and the Masako maneuver (Fujiu & Logemann, 1996), which was modified (given that he was edentulous) to involve requiring him to swallow with his tongue fixed between his front dental arches. Exercises aimed at maximizing hyolaryngeal excursion included the Mendelsohn maneuver (Kahrilas, Logemann, Krugler, & Flanagan, 1991), falsetto drill work (Pauloski, 2008), and sliding glissandos (LaGorio, Carnaby-Mann, & Crary, 2008). Finally, emphasis was placed on improving cricopharyngeal relaxation to allow more efficient entry of the bolus into the esophagus through introduction and practice of the Shaker exercise (Shaker et al., 1997). A compensatory strategy consisting of a combined chin tuck with a super-supraglottic swallow maneuver was recommended for use with all attempted per oral (PO) trials. Guidelines were provided at each visit for advancing his oral diet. The therapeutic plan was for Mr. J to practice the above exercises during therapy sessions to determine compliance and readiness for advancement both with exercises and PO.

Progress was assessed at each session with modest improvement noted during the first month of therapy. Laryngeal elevation improved with exercises although not to a "normal" level. He was able to be advanced with the Shaker exercises from an initial 5 s head raise to 25 s and equivalent repetitions by the end of the first month. However, while Mr. J was compliant with exercises in therapy, he admitted to not practicing consistently at home. He continually offered rationales for not having time to practice. His progress with taking things by mouth initially progressed well with consistent intake of small amounts of liquids up to a honey-like consistency two to three times per day by the second week of therapy; however, this volume was not sufficient to make up the calories/nutrition provided by one can of supplement through his PEG. He seemed to plateau at this level despite denying difficulties tolerating PO. He blamed his resistance on a poor appetite, dysgeusia, and dissatisfaction with the consistency of the foods that were recommended. Repeated attention was given to the significance of gradually increasing his PO intake with the ultimate goal of weaning from the PEG. Despite this, he resisted progressing his diet. Consideration of his initial swallowing behavior when performing the MBS with regard to the apparent guarding and hesitation brought up the potential for some type of fear regarding swallowing/eating. It was elected to discuss his status with his otolaryngologist.

Discussion regarding Mr. J's progress was had with the treating otolaryngologist after which it was decided to repeat an MBS to determine the level of improvement with therapy as well as any other needs that might be impeding his progress (see Video 4–3). A repeat MBS demonstrated decreased overall swallowing efficiency compared to the first study relative to increased residue postswallow and more definitive narrowing in the upper cervical esophagus. However, persistent trace aspiration was now sensate and spontaneously cleared from the airway, resulting in a Penetration-Aspiration Scale score of 6. Base of tongue retraction and hyolaryngeal excursion were reduced, essentially unchanged

from the prior study. Persistent nasal regurgitation was seen. After further review with the otolaryngologist, it was elected to attempt esophageal dilation (EGD) to determine if this would assist with his progress in therapy.

> Esophageal strictures are not an uncommon finding in patients that have undergone combined chemoradiation therapy of the head and neck area. Multiple authors have studied this development, and the consensus is that the more common etiologies are related to prolonged nonoral feeding in an area that has undergone tissue changes with probable mucositis and possible ulcerations that can lead to scarring (Franzmann, Lundy, Abitbol, & Goodwin, 2006; Lawson, Otto, Grist, & Johnstone, 2006; Wang, Goldsmith, Holman, Cianchetti, & Chan, 2012). The importance of continuing anything by mouth throughout treatment is emphasized as well as returning patients to PO status as quickly as possible following treatment is critical.

Flexible fiberoptic videonasendoscopy was performed to better assess velopharyngeal closure and resultant speech hypernasality (see Video 4–4). This revealed a small central gap remaining with phonation and bubbling of secretions. This was felt to not be amenable to behavioral management, and prosthodontic consultation was arranged for consideration of an obturator. The timing of this was significant as Mr. J had dentures that he had not worn since midway through his treatment and was unable to comfortably wear them at present. Frequently, modifications need to be made to dental appliances after treatment due to tissue alterations. Thus, the intent was for the prosthodontist to modify, if possible, his dentures and add on an extension with a small obturator to improve velopharyngeal closure. Unfortunately, Mr. J was unable to tolerate any extension beyond the palatal portion of his upper denture due to gagging, rendering the obturator not feasible. However, his old dentures were able to be modified for continued wear.

Swallowing therapy was reinstated a few days after planned EGD with continuation of prior goals.

At this point, Mr. J claimed he was able to increase the amount of liquids and thin pureed foods by mouth but still not enough to begin weaning from the PEG. This was expected, as dilating the narrowed area of the cervical esophagus while improving transit into the esophagus would not impact the oropharyngeal issues above that level that were preventing more efficient overall bolus passage. Thus, continued therapy was determined to be vital to maximize oropharyngeal bolus control and maintain patency of the esophagus. Therapeutic exercises were similar to previous ones but with increased intensity. Significant attention was given to increasing PO while gradually weaning from the PEG. After a few more sessions, it became concerning that other reasons might be preventing his persistent resistance to progressing with his oral diet. Recall of his initial tentative swallows on the first MBS as well as long discussion with the patient revealed that he was fearful of choking. He denied choking in the past but nonetheless was fixated on this. He was subsequently referred to the Integrative Medicine Division at the Cancer Center for a more holistic approach to his swallowing recovery, and attention to the potential "phobic" behavior might be preventing further progress. He participated in meditation, and psychological counseling including desensitization. This treatment was conducted in coordination with his speech/swallowing and otolaryngologic management. After 4 months of active treatment with Integrative Medicine and continued, less frequent swallowing therapy, he was gradually weaned from full PEG dependency down to about 75% PO. However, he plateaued again at this level prompting another discussion between speech and otolaryngology. It was elected to repeat another MBS to determine whether the prior dilation was still effective.

Repeat MBS was performed and demonstrated improved overall swallowing efficiency (see Video 4–5). Persistent reduced base of tongue retraction and hyolaryngeal excursion was seen and felt to be modestly improved from his last study. Nasal regurgitation persisted with increased residue in the nasal cavity postswallow. This was felt to be related to increased quantity and density of barium given. Trace laryngeal penetration was again noted but no aspiration was visualized; Pen-Asp Score = 2. Persistent retention in the vallecula postswallow was noted and increased with denser consistencies. The postcricoid area was noted to be more open than seen in the last study but still somewhat restricted. At this point, Mr. J was 18 months post treatment and still PEG dependent for about 25% of his nutrition. It was elected to perform serial EGDs in hopes of maintaining the opening of the esophagus along with further swallowing therapy and psychological counseling. He underwent three more EGD on a monthly basis and participated in swallowing therapy, also on a monthly basis, with emphasis on reinforcing home practice and PEG tube weaning. He was finally able to have his PEG tube removed 2 years following completion of chemoradiation therapy for his palatal lesion.

He managed well without his PEG while on a restricted diet of liquids up to a puree consistency, FOIS Level 5, and was able to maintain his weight. He returned to his usual activities other than playing tennis which he felt he did not have enough energy to do. At this point, he was discharged from active swallowing therapy. However, he was strongly encouraged to continue with maintenance exercises at home for life.

Unfortunately, approximately 1 year later, Mr. J was diagnosed with prostate cancer with possible pulmonary metastasis. During the course of his workup, an area of high uptake on a PET scan was identified in the alveolar ridge that was suspicious for malignancy. Careful evaluation by the treating otolaryngologist demonstrated an area of edema and erythema under his upper denture that was more consistent with osteoradionecrosis (Figure 4–1). Of interest, Mr. J was asymptomatic for this lesion and thus continued wearing his denture. Typical treatment for this entails excision with or without hyperbaric oxygen (HBO) treatment. As the patient had current disease from his prostate, this was not possible as it could potentially impact growth potential of the tumor. Due to his lack of subjective symptoms, the otolaryngologist elected to treat him conservatively with antibiotics and close observation. He was advised to avoid wearing his denture until the area had improved and/or resolved. At his 1 month follow-up visit, the involved area was noted to be less edematous and erythematous. The plan was for continued monitoring.

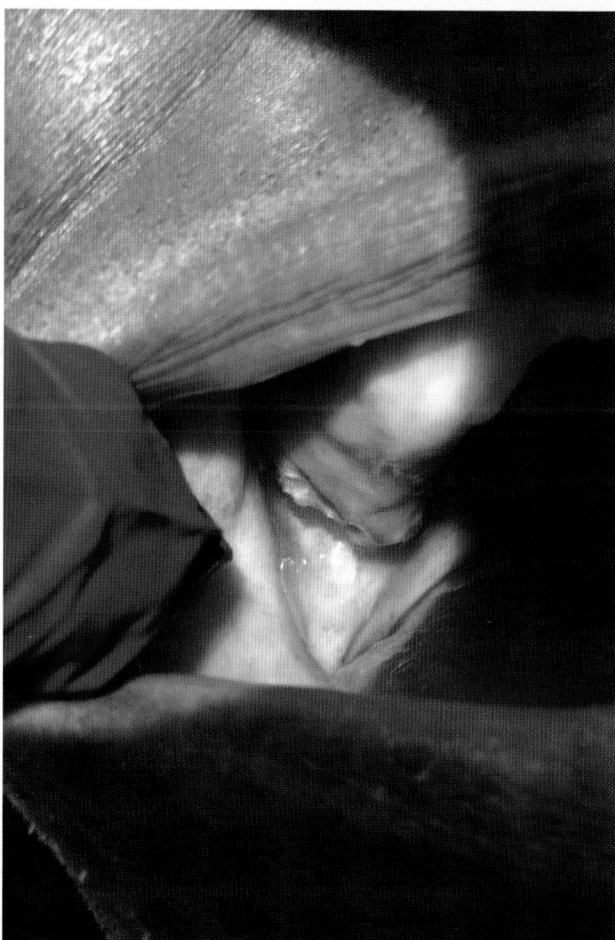

Figure 4–1. Osteoradionecrosis.

CONCLUSION

This case represents the complex scenario of a head and neck cancer patient who has undergone multimodality treatment. Rehabilitation for his swallowing was extremely challenging and represents the effectiveness of a well-coordinated multidisciplinary team approach. And, as it is known that late-onset dysphagia can occur at any time after radiation therapy (Hutcheson et al., 2012), particularly when combined with chemotherapy, his case will need to be monitored over time.

REFLECTION AND ANALYSIS FOR FURTHER STUDY

1. What medical professionals are most ideally qualified to deal with a patient's fear and how might these approaches vary by discipline? Why or why not?
2. Do you agree with the decision to not pursue a palatal prosthesis secondary to the patient's hyperactive gag reflex?
3. Can a hyperactive gag be remediated in some cases?

REFERENCES

Belafsky, P. C., Mouadeb, D. A., Rees, C. J., Pryor, J. C., Postma, G. N., Allen, J., & Leonard, R. J. (2008). Validity and reliability of the Eating Assessment Tool (EAT-10). *Annals of Otology, Rhinology, and Laryngology, 117,* 919–924.

Carnaby-Mann, G., Crary, M. A., Schmalfuss, I., & Amdur, R. (2012). "Pharyngocise": Randomized controlled trial of preventative exercises to maintain muscle structure and swallowing function during head and neck chemoradiotherapy. *International Journal of Radiation Oncology Biology Physics, 83,* 210–219.

Carroll, W. R., Locher, J. L., Canon, C. L., Bohannon, I. A., McColloch, N. L., & Magnuson, J. S. (2008). Pretreatment swallowing exercises improve swallow function after chemoradiation. *Laryngoscope, 118,* 39–43.

Crary, M. A., Mann, G. D., & Groher, M. E. (2005). Initial psychometric assessment of a functional oral intake scale for dysphagia in stroke patients. *Archives of Physical Medicine and Rehabilitation, 86,* 1516–1520.

Dworkin, J. P., Marunick, M. T., & Krouse, J. H. (2014). Velopharyngeal dysfunction: Speech characteristics, variable etiologies, evaluation techniques, and different treatments. *Language Speech and Hearing Services in the Schools, 35,* 333–352.

Franzmann, E. J., Lundy, D. S., Abitbol, A. A., & Goodwin, W. J. (2006). Complete hypopharyngeal obstruction by mucosal adhesions: A complication of intensive chemoradiation for advanced head and neck cancer. *Head & Neck, 28,* 663–670.

Fujiu, M., & Logemann, J. A. (1996). Effect of a tongue holding maneuver on posterior pharyngeal wall movement during deglutition. *American Journal of Speech-Language Pathology, 5,* 23–30.

Gaziano, J. E. (2002). Evaluation and management of oropharyngeal dysphagia in head and neck cancer. *Cancer Control, 9,* 400–409.

Gillespie, M. B., Brodsky, M. B., Day, T. A., Lee, F., & Martin-Harris, B. (2004). Swallowing-related quality of life after head and neck cancer treatment. *Laryngoscope, 114,* 1362–1367.

Goldstein, B. Y., Chang, S. C., Hashibe, M., La Vecchia, C., & Zhang, Z. (2010). Alcohol consumption and cancers of the oral cavity and pharynx from 1988 to 2009: An update. *European Journal of Cancer Prevention, 19,* 431–465.

Hutcheson, K. A., Lewin, J. S., Barringer, D. A., Lisec, A., Gunn, G. B., Moore, M. W. S., & Holsinger, F. C. (2012). Late dysphagia after radiotherapy-based treatment of head and neck cancer. *Cancer, 118,* 5793–5799.

Kahrilas, P. J., Logemann, J. A., Krugler, C., & Flanagan, E. (1991). Volitional augmentation of upper esophageal sphincter opening during swallowing. *American Journal of Physiology, 260,* 450–456.

Kammer, R., Wiederholt, P., & Knigge, M. (2011). Collaborative dysphagia care for chemoradiation patients. *The ASHA Leader,* October 11.

Kotz, T., Federman, A. D., Kao, J., Milman, L., Packer, S., Lopez-Prieto, C., . . . Genden, E. M. (2012). Prophylactic swallowing exercises in patients with head and neck cancer undergoing chemoradiation: A randomized trial. *Archives of Otolaryngology-Head and Neck Surgery, 138,* 376–382.

LaGorio, L. A., Carnaby-Mann, G. D., & Crary, M. A. (2008). Cross-system effects of dysphagia treatment on dysphonia: A case report. *Cases Journal, 1,* 1–6.

Lawson, J. D., Otto, K., Grist, W., & Johnstone, P. A. S. (2006). Frequency of esophageal stenosis after simultaneous modulated accelerated radiation therapy and chemotherapy for head and neck cancer. *American Journal of Otolaryngology-Head and Neck Surgery, 29,* 13–19.

Logemann, J. A. (1983). *Evaluation and treatment of swallowing disorders.* San Diego, CA: College-Hill Press.

Logemann, J. A. (2006). Protocol for swallowing management in patients treated for head and neck cancer. *Perspectives on Swallowing and Swallowing Disorders (Dysphagia), 15,* 22–26.

Logemann, J. A., Rademaker, A. W., Pauloski, B. R., Lazarus, C. L., Mittal, B. B., Brockstein, B., . . . Liu, D. (2006). Site of disease and treatment protocol as correlates of swallowing function in patients with head and neck cancer treated with chemoradiation. *Head & Neck, 28,* 64–73.

Martin, B. J. W., Logemann, J. A., Shaker, R., & Dodds, W. J. (1993). Normal laryngeal valving patterns during three breath hold maneuvers: A pilot investigation. *Dysphagia, 8,* 11–20.

Pauloski, B. R. (2008). Rehabilitation of dysphagia following head and neck cancer. *Physical Medicine and Rehabilitation Clinics of North America, 19,* 889–928.

Pauloski, B. R., Rademaker, A. W., Logemann, J. A., Stein, D., Beery, Q., Newman, L., . . . MacCracken, E. (2000). Pretreatment swallowing function in patients with head and neck cancer. *Head and Neck, 22,* 474–482.

Rogers, S. N., Gwanne, S., Lowe, D., Humphris, G., Yueh, B., & Weymuller, E. A. (2002). The addition of mood and anxiety domains to the University of Washington Quality of Life scale. *Head & Neck, 24,* 521–529.

Rosen, A., Rhee, T. H., & Kaufman, R. (2001). Prediction of aspiration in patients with newly diagnosed untreated advanced head and neck cancer. *Archives of Otolaryngology-Head and Neck Surgery, 127,* 975–979.

Rosenbek, J. C., Robbins, J., Roecker, E. V., Coyle, J. L., & Woods, J. L. (1996). A Penetration-Aspiration Scale. *Dysphagia, 11,* 93–98.

Saman, D. M. (2012). A review of the epidemiology of oral and pharyngeal carcinoma: Update. *Head and Neck Oncology, 4,* 1.

Shaker, R., Kern, M., Bardan, E., Taylor, A., Stewart, E. T., Hoffmann, R. G., . . . Bonnevier, J. (1997). Augmentation of deglutitive upper esophageal sphincter opening in the elderly by exercise. *American Journal of Physiology, 272,* 1518–1522.

Sivasithamparam, J., Visk, C. A., Cohen, E. E., & King, A. C. (2013). Modifiable risk behaviors in patients with head and neck cancer. *Cancer, 119,* 2419–2426.

Starmer, H. M. (2014). Dysphagia in head and neck cancer: Prevention and treatment. *Current Opinion in Otolaryngology and Head and Neck Surgery, 22,* 195–200.

Stenson, K. M., MacCrackern, E., List, M., Haraf, D. J., Brockstein, B., Weichselbaum, R., & Vokes, E. E. (2000). Swallowing function in patients with head and neck cancer prior to treatment. *Archives of Otolaryngology-Head and Neck Surgery, 126,* 371–377.

van der Molen, L., van Rossum, M. A., Ackerstaff, A. H., Smeele, L. E., Rasch, C. R., & Hilgers, F. J. (2009). Pretreatment organ function in patients with advanced head and neck cancer: Clinical outcome measures and patients' views. *BMC Ear, Nose and Throat Disorders, 9,* 1–9.

van der Molen, L., van Rossum, M. A., Burkhead, L. M., Smeele, L. E., Rasch, C. R., & Hilgers, F. J. (2011). A randomized preventative rehabilitation trial in advanced head and neck cancer patients treated with chemoradiotherapy: Feasibility, compliance, and short-term effects. *Dysphagia, 26,* 155–170.

Wang, J. J., Goldsmith, T. A., Holman, A. S., Cianchetti, M., & Chan, A. W. (2012). Pharyngoesophageal stricture after treatment for head and neck cancer. *Head & Neck, 34,* 967–973.

Welch, M. V., Logemann, J. A., Rademaker, A. W., & Kahrilas, P. J. (1993). Changes in pharyngeal dimensions effected by chin tuck. *Archives of Physical Medicine and Rehabilitation, 74,* 178–181.

PART III

Oropharyngeal Cases

5

Overview of Multidisciplinary Management for Oropharyngeal Cancer

Katherine A. Hutcheson, Kristen B. Pytynia, and G. Brandon Gunn

INTRODUCTION: OROPHARYNGEAL CANCER

Squamous cell carcinoma is by far the most common histology of oropharyngeal cancer, accounting for approximately 95% of oropharyngeal cancers. Oropharyngeal squamous cell carcinoma (OPSCC) was commonly linked to tobacco exposure. As the use of tobacco has decreased in the United States over the past few decades, there has been a concomitant decrease in the incidence of tobacco-related cancers. During this same time, however, incidence rates of oropharyngeal cancer have paradoxically increased (Chaturvedi et al., 2011). Investigations revealed this increase in OPSCC incidence to be due to oncogenic human papillomavirus (HPV) (Chaturvedi, Engels, Anderson, & Gillison, 2008; Mehta, Yu, & Schantz, 2010; Sturgis & Cinciripini, 2007). The incidence of OPSCC is now rising precipitously (namely in men) along with a change in the epidemiology of the disease, and the annual number of OPSCC cases in the United States is projected to almost double by the year 2030 (Chaturvedi et al., 2011).

There are two epidemiologically and molecularly distinct forms of OPSCC classified according to tumor HPV status. HPV-negative OPSCC is caused by long-term exposure to tobacco and alcohol and occurs usually in males over 55 years of age. HPV-positive OPSCC begins with exposure to high risk HPV, most often HPV type 16, and while the majority of those exposed to HPV will clear the infection, some exposed will have persistent infection that progresses to OPSCC after some latency period. HPV-positive OPSCC is more likely to affect middle-aged white men and can develop independent of tobacco or alcohol exposure (Gillison et al., 2000; Mork et al., 2001). Patients with HPV-positive OPSCC are more likely to present with small primary tumors and extensive nodal disease. Survival is significantly improved in patients with HPV-positive OPSCC compared to patients with HPV-negative OPSCC (82.4% versus 57.1% at 3 years, respectively) (Ang et al., 2010; Benoit and Lachapelle, 1990; Li et al., 2003; O'Sullivan et al., 2012). Patients with HPV-positive OPSCC have a 20% to 80% reduction in the overall risk of death compared to those with HPV-negative OPSCC (Ang et al., 2010; Fakhry et al., 2008; Posner et al., 2001). The epidemic of HPV-positive OPSCC is occurring among relatively younger patients who, with the associated improved prognosis, may live longer, making late side effects of therapy in a functionally critical region of the pharynx particularly concerning.

Surgical Management of OPSCC

The current standard of treatment for OPSCC is radiation with chemotherapy added for advanced disease. Surgery is usually reserved for persistent nodal disease after radiation (i.e., adjuvant neck dissection after radiation), although there is a growing trend toward primary transoral surgery of OPSCC followed by radiation, and centers with large volumes of transoral surgery have reported success with this approach (Adelstein et al., 2012; Haughey et al., 2011; Quon et al., 2013; Weinstein et al., 2012). Primary surgery to the oropharynx is difficult as the anatomical areas are not easy to access. Open surgery typically requires removing or splitting the mandible and was traditionally a morbid approach associated with long-term functional deficits. Transoral surgery was formerly limited by the ability to access deep parts of the oropharynx through the mouth. The advances in robotic surgery technology have improved access to certain areas of the oropharynx. The goal of transoral robotic surgery (TORS) is to achieve tumor removal while maintaining function by avoiding compromise of adjacent laryngopharyngeal architecture by pharyngotomy or mandibulectomy. The need for tracheostomy is also less for TORS compared to traditional open surgery. TORS may also allow dose reduction in radiotherapy for patients who require postoperative radiotherapy, since definitive radiotherapy dose is typically 66 to 72 Gy for OPSCC and postoperative doses can be delivered in range of 60 to 66 Gy. Postoperative radiotherapy is indicated for positive margins, multiple lymph node involvement, extracapsular spread in lymph nodes, and perineural or lymphovascular invasion. Collectively, published series suggest that 9% to 27% of patients treated with frontline TORS avoid radiotherapy altogether and as many as 40% avoid concurrent chemotherapy, although exact numbers depend on study design and further research needs to be done (de Almeida & Genden, 2012; Weinstein, Quon, O'Malley, Kim, & Cohen, 2010).

There is not yet sufficient prospective, randomized evidence for clinicians to change treatment of patients with HPV-positive OPSCC based on HPV status (Radiation Therapy Oncology Group, 2015). There are ongoing trials that address this question, but clinicians should not independently de-escalate treatment of protocol, and must await the long-term results of prospective randomized trials before determining any treatment change based on HPV status. A large prospective randomized trial (ECOG-3311) is currently enrolling and investigating de-escalated

postoperative radiotherapy after up-front TORS by credentialed and experienced TORS surgeons (Eastern Cooperative Oncology Group, 2015). Functional outcomes will be detailed in all patients enrolled.

Chemoradiation

Chemoradiation is widely considered the standard of care for locoregionally advanced OPSCC, with goals of cure and functional organ preservation. Modern-day RT treatment standards have been established through numerous seminal phase III clinical trials, which have led to improved overall disease control and survival rates, namely, through the combination of radiation therapy and systemic therapy, and reduced treatment-related toxicity through advances in RT planning and delivery.

Over the past decade or so, advances in intensity-modulated RT (IMRT) have led to the delivery of more accurate and desirable dose distributions. One of the main benefits of IMRT for OPSCC compared to traditional methods is the ability to conform the distributions to the targets with relative sparing of the parotid glands, which has translated into reduced xerostomia and improved quality of life outcomes. This clinical benefit has been reinforced in several prospective studies including the multi-institutional, randomized phase III trial PARSPORT trial (Nutting et al., 2011). Beyond its ability for salivary sparing, the safety and efficacy of IMRT have also been established. Garden and colleagues at the University of Texas MD Anderson Cancer Center reported excellent long-term clinical outcomes of IMRT for OPSCC (Garden, Kies, et al., 2013). In this study of more than 700 patients with OPSCC treated in the modern era, with a median follow-up of 54 months, rates of locoregional control, relapse-free survival, and overall survival were 90%, 82%, and 84% at 5 years (Garden, Kies, et al., 2013). As for acute and late toxicity, 47% of patients had a feeding tube placed during treatment, but only 18 (<5%) had a feeding tube in place at last assessment. Importantly, no patient had disease recurrence in or immediately adjacent to a spared parotid gland, further justifying the use of a parotid-sparing IMRT approach for patients with OPSCC (Garden, Kies, et al., 2013). Ongoing advances in proton therapy planning and delivery are providing new opportunities to investigate whether additional gains in toxicity reduction are achievable.

Concurrent systemic therapy can be added to RT with the intent of sensitizing malignant cells to the damaging effects of ionizing radiation. Calais and colleagues carried out an important trial in locally advanced OPSCC, comparing RT with or without concurrent 5-flourouracil and carboplatin. Substantial treatment-related reactions were observed; high-grade mucositis was experienced by ~70% of patients in the chemoradiation group versus ~40% in the RT-alone group (Calais et al., 1999). Nonetheless, long-term follow-up revealed a strong benefit for chemoradiation in terms of both locoregional control rates at 5 years (48% versus 25%) and long-term survival (22% versus 16%) (Denis et al., 2004). Pignon, le Maître, Maillard, Bourhis, and MACH-NC Collaborative Group reported updated results from their highly cited meta-analysis of more than 16,000 patients participating in randomized trials that incorporated chemotherapy along with local treatment. Overall, the addition of chemotherapy improved patient survival, and the largest benefit from chemotherapy was seen among those receiving chemotherapy concurrent with radiation therapy, with a 6.5% absolute benefit in 5-year survival. Interestingly, patients with OPSCC achieved the greatest benefit from the addition of concurrent chemotherapy relative to those with non-OPSCC head and neck cancer primaries (Pignon et al., 2009).

Given the importance of cancer-cell epidermal growth factor receptor (EGFR) expression in head and neck cancer, Bonner and colleagues conducted a phase III randomized clinical trial in patients with locally advanced head and neck cancer comparing RT with or without concurrent cetuximab, a monoclonal antibody inhibitor of EGFR. The majority of patients in this study had OPSCC. A greater number of acute reactions were observed for the cetuximab group, such as infusion reaction and acneiform-like rash. Yet the addition of cetuximab did not increase the peak RT-related mucosal reactions or clinically graded dysphagia per NCI's common toxicity criteria. The addition of cetuximab to RT improved tumor control and patient survival rates and extended the median overall survival time by 20 months (Bonner et al., 2006). This trial established RT and concurrent cetuximab as a popular combined modality standard treatment option for patients with locally advanced disease. The optimal concurrent systemic therapy agent and schedule for use along with RT is yet to be defined and is currently the subject of study in multiple ongoing cooperative group studies.

Radiotherapy Alone

It is notable that most patients who participated in the aforementioned trials that established the survival advantage for chemoradiation had locally advanced disease (i.e., higher T-category tumors), and patients with T1 primary tumors were often excluded from these trials. For example, more than 80% of the patients in the GORTEC study had T3 or T4 disease (Calais et al., 1999). Although RT with concurrent systemic therapy is the standard of care for patients with locally advanced tumors, excellent locoregional control rates can be achieved with RT alone (i.e., without systemic therapy), and this strategy may improve patient tolerance and reduce severity of treatment-related toxicity without compromise of ultimate disease control and survival outcomes. Garden, Dong, et al. (2013) reported excellent locoregional disease control rates for patients with T1 or T2 primary OPC tumors but who had Stage III through IVA disease (i.e., patients who had smaller primary tumors but an advanced AJCC stage group due to the presence of regional nodal disease). No outcome differences were observed for those receiving concurrent chemotherapy versus those receiving RT alone in this early T-category cohort. The authors' current approach is to consider both the local and regional extent of disease when considering patient-specific therapeutic strategies. In terms of local therapy, the authors generally select concurrent chemoradiation as a component of treatment for patients with locally advanced primary tumors, but often favor single modality RT alone for favorable, earlier T-category OPSCC (Garden, Kies, et al., 2013).

For carefully selected patients with well-lateralized carcinomas of the tonsillar fossa, the IMRT treatment volume can often be safely restricted to treatment of the primary site and ipsilateral cervical and ipsilateral lateral retropharyngeal lymph nodes, rather than the bilateral cervical nodal regions. This approach substantially reduces the dose to contralateral major salivary glands, nontarget mucosa-bearing surfaces, and a number of important swallowing structures. Chronowski and colleagues reported outcomes for 102 patients treated with primary site and ipsilateral neck-only radiation approach at the University of Texas MD Anderson Cancer Center. The ideal patients for this approach were those who had T2 or less primary site disease, no more than minimal soft palate invasion, no base of tongue invasion, no contralateral nodal disease (ideally assessed by two diagnostic imaging modalities), and preferably lesser ipsilateral nodal burden (i.e., smaller nodal volume). With a median follow-up time of over 3 years, only two patients had developed any contralateral disease recurrence. The acute and late toxicity profile was quite favorable, as only nine patients had placement of a feeding tube during therapy, and no patient experienced long-term feeding tube dependence (Chronowski et al., 2012).

Dysphagia Management After OPSCC: Prevention Through Late Effects

Dysphagia is the primary functional concern for head and neck cancer survivors (Wilson, Carding, & Patterson, 2011), drives perception of quality of life (QOL) after chemoradiation for OPSCC (Hunter et al., 2012), and significantly predicts for pneumonia in long-term survivorship (Hunter et al., 2013). In addition, for those treated with IMRT, objective measures of dysphagia per videofluoroscopy are a stronger predictor of long-term quality of life than xerostomia (Hunter et al., 2012). Thus, optimizing swallowing outcomes is a major focus of rehabilitation in oropharyngeal cancer survivorship.

Great strides have been made in delivery of chemoradiation. Highly conformal methods of radiotherapy (e.g., dysphagia-optimized IMRT and proton therapy) that minimize dose to nontarget swallowing critical structures and targeted agents show promise to lessen dysphagia. Yet even in modern practice, at least half of patients require a feeding tube during chemoradiation (Bhayani et al., 2013; Setton et al., 2015). More alarmingly, still up to 30% of survivors develop chronic aspiration, even after dysphagia-optimized IMRT incorporating dose

constraints to the pharyngeal constrictors and larynx (Feng et al., 2010).

Classically, radiation-associated dysphagia (RAD) develops during chemoradiation as an acute toxicity of treatment, but the majority of patients who develop acute RAD achieve partial recovery of swallowing function. That is, most regain an acceptable but not fully normal level of swallowing function (i.e., "the new normal"). A smaller minority suffer clinically significant levels of chronic dysphagia, which may be a consequential late effect of intensive local treatment. Although swallowing outcomes highly depend on tumor burden and baseline functionality, treatment intensity (radiation dose-volume parameters, systemic therapy) and supportive care, after primary radiotherapy or chemoradiation for OPSCC, it is estimated that 7% to 31% develop chronic aspiration (Feng et al., 2010; Hutcheson, Lewin, et al., 2014), 11% develop aspiration pneumonia (Hunter et al., 2013), and 4% are chronically feeding tube dependent after chemoradiation (Bhayani et al., 2013).

Pathophysiology of RAD

Normal tissue effects that drive RAD occur along a continuum, but features predominate in each phase of survivorship. In the early months after chemoradiation, the dysphagia-aspiration related structures (DARS, i.e., constrictors and larynx) in the field of radiotherapy become edematous but then stiffen over time as fibrosis evolves as chronic sequela of treatment. Acute and persistent RAD in the first year or so of survivorship has traditionally been thought to reflect varying degrees of muscle edema, subcutaneous fibrosis, and disuse atrophy. Neuropathic injury is also a noteworthy source of RAD. Delayed mono- or polyneuropathies of the lower cranial nerves, while rare, are a major contributor to late-onset radiation-associated dysphagia (late-RAD) (Awan et al., 2014; Hutcheson et al., 2012; Hutcheson, Yuk, Holsinger, Gunn, & Lewin, 2014). Regardless of the pathology, the end result of edema, fibrosis, atrophy, and/or neuropathy is reduced mobility of critical laryngeal and oropharyngeal structures (i.e., the DARS) that ultimately impairs supraglottic closure and pharyngeal propulsion.

It is a common misconception that stricture is the primary driver of dysphagia in this population. A recent meta-analysis reported a 7% summary risk estimate of stricture after head and neck radiotherapy, suggesting that stricture is the source of dysphagia in only a small minority of patients (Wang, Goldsmith, Holman, Cianchetti, & Chan, 2012). Notably, stricture was more common in the IMRT era (17%), possibly representing unintentional or unrecognized increase in dose to the esophageal inlet using IMRT over older methods of laryngeal dose sparing. Care must be taken to ensure adequate larynx and esophageal shielding or dosimetric constraints are applied at the time of IMRT treatment planning. Common symptoms of stricture include solid foods sticking in the distal pharynx or sternal region, inability to swallow pills, and difficulty belching or vomiting. Suspicion for stricture should be heighted in patients who had prolonged intervals (3 or more months) with high-grade mucositis or nothing by mouth (Best et al., 2011; Gillespie, Day, Sharma, Brodsky, & Martin-Harris, 2007).

Dysphagia After TORS

Mature dysphagia data are not yet published on patients treated with primary TORS. To date, surgical series have been published in highly selected cohorts, and functional outcomes have been explored primarily with questionnaire data (rarely with instrumental studies). Acknowledging these limitations, after primary TORS for OPSCC, it is estimated that 0% develop chronic aspiration (Genden, Park, Smith, & Kotz, 2011), 0% to 7% develop postoperative pneumonia, 20% to 40% require gastrostomy placement, and 0% to 7% are chronically feeding tube dependent after treatment (Hutcheson, Lewin, et al., 2014).

T-stage and need for adjuvant therapy are likely to impact post-TORS swallow outcomes. Extrapolating data from work in patients treated with primary transoral laser surgery, surgical outcomes are highly dependent on tumor size (T-stage) that dictates the volume of the resection (Hutcheson, Holsinger, Kupferman, & Lewin, 2014). It is suggested that more than 90% of patients treated with primary transoral surgery for T1-T2 and more than 80% treated for T3 tumors will have acceptable swallowing outcomes,

but almost half of patients treated with transoral surgery for T4 tumors never recovered acceptable swallowing (Rich, Liu, & Haughey, 2011). Adjuvant therapy after TORS may be required to secure local and regional disease control and is an equally important driver of swallowing outcomes. Dose-dependent effects are suggested in published series, whereby swallowing outcomes are best among those patients who get postoperative radiotherapy alone (avoiding chemotherapy) and among those who are treated with postoperative doses that are lower than those delivered for definitive treatment.

Preventive Swallowing Therapy During Head and Neck Radiotherapy—Eat and Exercise

Preventive swallowing therapy is best practice for patients treated with radiotherapy (whether definitive or postoperative) for OPSCC. Because of acute toxicities that make eating unpleasant during radiotherapy, at least half of patients require feeding tube placement during radiation, and the vast majority stop eating solid foods. It is suggested that this prompts varying degrees of disuse atrophy in the absence of the normal resistive load on pharyngeal musculature that accompanies a typical and complex oral diet. Thus, the central premise of proactive swallowing therapy is "Use It or Lose It" to mitigate muscular wasting and remodeling that occur after even brief intervals of disuse. Preventive or proactive swallowing therapy encourages maximal use of the swallowing musculature during treatment by (a) avoiding NPO intervals and (b) adhering to swallowing exercise. The benefits of these swallowing activities (eat and exercise) are reported by numerous investigators in randomized trials and observational studies and are shown to be independently beneficial. That is, patients who both eat and exercise throughout radiation do better than those who eat or exercise.

Three randomized trials have shown a benefit of preventive swallowing exercise during chemoradiation (Carnaby-Mann, Crary, Schmalfuss, & Amdur, 2012; Kotz et al., 2012; van der Molen et al., 2011). A sham-controlled trial found a 36% absolute risk reduction for loss of functional swallow ability in patients randomized to active swallow exercise during chemoradiation (Carnaby-Mann et al., 2012). Other favorable outcomes reported in association with preventive exercise include superior swallowing-related quality of life, better tongue base and epiglottic inversion, larger postchemoradiation muscle mass and T2 signal intensity on MRI of the genioglossus, mylohyoid, and hyoglossus muscles, shorter duration of gastrostomy, and greater return to normal oral diet levels.

Observational studies also suggest the benefit of maintaining any oral intake during chemoradiation (i.e., avoidance of NPO intervals). Even brief NPO intervals of just 2 weeks have been shown to significantly and independently predict lower swallowing-related quality of life scores in long-term survivorship after chemoradiation (median: 4.7 years; Hutcheson et al., 2013). Multidisciplinary management of acute chemoradiation toxicities including pain, mucositis, odynophagia, dysgeusia, weight loss, and dysphagia, is necessary to help patients safely maintain oral intake. Prophylactic neuropathic pain management has also been associated with lower pain scores, decreased PEG utilization, and decreased aspiration after chemoradiation, and prophylactic pain control was suggested by the authors of this study to allow to eat and exercise throughout treatment ultimately conferring a physiologic advantage in preserved swallowing function (Starmer et al., 2014).

A practical, evidence-based approach to implement preventive swallowing therapy includes

1. pretreatment referral to speech pathologist for baseline evaluation (preferably via instrumental examination) and training on swallow exercise;
2. on-treatment swallowing therapy with speech pathologist: at minimum, mid-RT and end-RT sessions to monitor swallowing function and adjust swallow exercise program as toxicities increase; and
3. speech-language pathology evaluation (preferably via instrumental examination) post treatment.

Swallowing Therapy After Primary Surgery

The degree of immediate postoperative dysphagia after primary oropharyngeal surgery varies sub-stantially depending on the volume of resection and reconstruction. Even after robotic surgery where it is possible to begin oral intake within days of surgery, most patients experience significant odynophagia limiting their oral intake. Postsurgical swallowing rehabilitation follows these steps:

1. Saliva management: Saliva swallows are functional swallows. Patients should be encouraged to start swallowing their saliva (rather than exclusively suctioning) immediately postoperatively and minimize dependence on oral suction. Even those who require a temporary NPO period in the setting of flap reconstruction can benefit from this practice.
2. Reintroduce oral intake: In the setting of primary closure or healing by secondary intention, patients are ready for oral intake as soon as pain allows and the oropharyngeal swallow is safe. Bedside examination by the speech pathologist is recommended as early as POD#1 when there is no pharyngeal or intraoral flap. After flap reconstruction, oral intake is delayed until (a) the surgical anastomosis has healed and (b) the oropharyngeal swallow is safe (for at least some textures). Videofluoroscopy is ideal to test both these factors in the postreconstruction setting (i.e., to simultaneously rule out leak and rule out aspiration) and thereby to determine a patient's readiness for oral intake after major oral resection. In addition to imaging the postsurgical bed with contrast to rule out leak (as indicated by abnormal extravasation of contrast into oral soft tissues), modified barium swallow (MBS) allows the clinician to test in real time the efficacy of swallow therapies (such as head rotations, supraglottic swallow strategies, adaptive equipment, or thickener) to identify any means by which oral intake can be safely delivered when aspiration is detected. Most patients are ready for their first MBS by 10 days postsurgically, with studies delayed 4 to 6 weeks in patients with prior radiotherapy to the head and neck. Although some patients may have oropharyngeal dysphagia sufficient to require ongoing feeding tube support, the goal of the first MBS is to find something that they can safely begin swallowing for practice.

3. Increase volume then complexity of oral intake: Surgically treated patients typically resume oral intake of a quite limited range of textures (e.g., only liquids, or very runny pureed foods), and often in quite limited amounts. The end goal is to normalize the oral diet as much as possible. Normalizing the diet is not simply getting back to solid foods, but also normalizing how much ("volume") and how fast one can eat. After reintroducing oral intake, the first goal is to increase the volume of oral intake of the most successful PO consistencies to ensure adequate nutritional intake. Next follows increasing the complexity of intake. This may include advancing the patient to chewable foods or (if once restricted from liquids) moving back to thin liquids (if previously aspirated). The length of this stage of rehabilitation varies, but one should strive to advance oral intake, both volume and complexity, as much as possible before the patient begins adjuvant radiation. Mass practice of functional swallows is the hallmark of this phase.

4. Preventive swallow therapy during adjuvant radiotherapy: Two goals take focus during adjuvant therapy: eat and exercise. The approach to preventive swallowing therapy during adjuvant radiotherapy is no different than the approach previously described for patients receiving definitive (chemo)radiotherapy. Two goals are outlined: (a) eat—maintain oral intake throughout radiotherapy, and (b) exercise—adhere to swallowing-specific exercises. The obvious caveat is that these goals are carried out in the context of any preexisting postsurgical dysphagia.

5. Post treatment swallowing therapy: Persistent dysphagia after surgery and adjuvant treatment can vary significantly in its severity and presentation. Rehabilitation needs are driven by the functional profile of the patient and findings of the post treatment MBS study. Methods and principles of swallowing therapy in this interval of care follow those outlined in the next section.

Reactive Swallowing Therapy After Head and Neck Radiotherapy or Surgery

Persistent post treatment dysphagia is a challenging clinical problem. To some degree irreversible, intensive swallowing therapy has been shown to optimize functional status and quality of life of the patient with persistent dysphagia (Carnaby-Mann & Crary, 2010; Crary, Carnaby, LaGorio, & Carvajal, 2012; Martin-Harris et al., 2015). Primary therapy options include (a) compensatory strategies to help minimize or clear aspiration and/or to improve swallowing efficiency, and (b) targeted exercise regimens with or without biofeedback or resistive devices. Because aspiration is extremely common in patients with moderate to severe persistent RAD or postsurgical dysphagia, a major therapeutic goal is to maximize quality of life while simultaneously minimizing the risk of life-threatening aspiration pneumonia.

Patients experiencing persistent post treatment dysphagia need a thorough multidimensional functional evaluation (including instrumental examination) once the acute toxicities of treatment have started to reasonably abate. Therapeutic targets must be clearly delineated and driven by understanding the pathophysiology of the dysphagia from the instrumental testing. Although many disorders may be evident on videofluoroscopy or endosocopy, clinicians must strive to seek out targets using these primary questions:

- What is the primary source of persistent dysphagia?
- What is changeable about the swallow?
- What is trainable?

In addition, patients' goals and priorities must be incorporated into the treatment plan. Data from the standardized interview and patient-reported outcome inventories (questionnaires) are helpful to understand the patient's perception of the problem and high-burden or high-concern areas. Post treatment swallowing therapy may incorporate

- swallowing exercise (without bolus);
- bolus-driven or device-driven exercise (i.e., a progressive resistance paradigm);
- training on compensatory strategies to minimize aspiration or improve bolus clearance (i.e., improve safety and efficiency of transport); and/or
- esophageal dilation.

Published literature offers no comparative studies to define the best approach to dysphagia therapy for persistent post treatment dysphagia. In current practice, dysphagia therapy remains highly individualized, and in the absence of dysphagia rehabilitation trials, best practice dictates beginning with a comprehensive evaluation and adhering to established exercise principles.

OROPHARYNGEAL CANCER:
A MULTIDISCIPLINARY APPROACH
TO TREATING HPV-POSITIVE
BASE OF TONGUE CANCER WITH
DEFINITIVE CHEMORADIATION

History

A 57-year-old gentleman, lifetime nonsmoker, with no significant past medical history initially pre-sented with a 4-month history of an asymptomatic left upper neck mass. He first noticed the mass while shaving. He sought medical attention and was pre-scribed antibiotics, which failed to resolve the mass.

Diagnostic Workup

The patient was subsequently evaluated by an oto-laryngologist who upon palpation, observed left upper jugular territory lymphadenopathy, which was mobile, nontender, and felt to likely represent a conglomerate of lymph nodes, measuring 4 cm in the greatest dimension. Indirect (mirror) pharyngos-copy revealed prominent lingual lymphoid tissue at the left tongue base. The remainder of the examina-tion was unremarkable.

Diagnostic computerized tomography (CT) scan of the neck with intravenous contrast was completed and revealed multiple heterogeneous, enlarged, and enhancing lymph nodes and asymmetric enhance-ment at the left tongue base (Figure 5–1A).

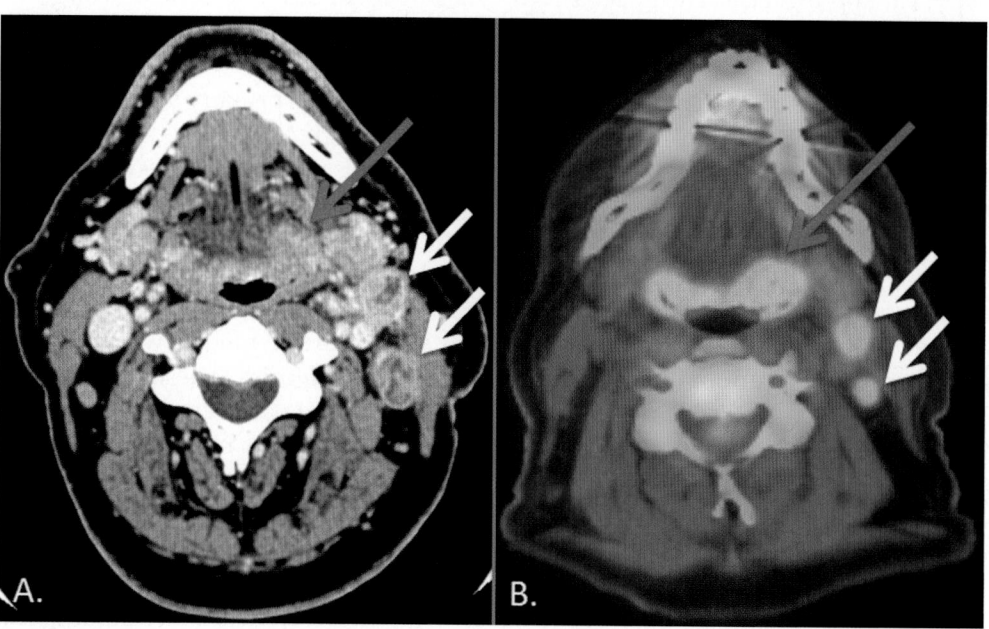

Figure 5–1. A. Axial image from initial pretreatment diagnostic CT neck with contrast showing enhancing mass in left base of tongue (*red arrow*) and multiple, enlarged, and heterogeneously enhancing lymph nodes in left Level II (*white arrows*). **B.** Corresponding FGD-PET-CT with asym-metric and increased FDG avidity in left base of tongue (*red arrow*) and multiple avid left Level II lymph nodes (*white arrows*).

Key point: Human papillomavirus (HPV)–associated oropharyngeal squamous cell carcinoma (OPSCC) commonly presents with an asymptomatic neck mass and can feature a small or clinically subtle primary tumor with advanced regional lymph node involvement. The lymph nodes often have heterogeneous nodal imaging characteristics with a variety of morphologic features including what can be a large dominant cystic component or necrotic appearing elements (Cantrell et al., 2013).

Fine-needle aspiration biopsy of the abnormal appearing left jugulodigastric lymph node revealed squamous cell carcinoma. Whole-body F-fluorodeoxyglucose (FDG)-positron emission tomography (PET)/computed tomography (CT) was done to (a) assess for primary site of origin, (b) stage regional lymph nodes, (c) rule out distant metastases, (d) guide anticipated examination under anesthesia biopsies, and (e) review for potential (radiation) treatment planning purposes. This imaging showed increased FDG avidity in the left base of tongue, left greater than right, with a maximum standard uptake value of 5.5 at the left base of tongue, and multiple FDG avid lymph nodes in the left upper neck, with maximum standardized uptake values (SUVs) of 8.5. There were no definite contralateral or distant metastases. Please refer to Figure 5–1B.

Key point: Equivocal lymph nodes seen on CT or PET-CT could be further assessed via ultrasonography and/or ultrasound-guided fine-needle aspiration biopsy if the results would impact treatment decisions, such as significant changes in radiation therapy volumes. Treating physicians should seek to further evaluate or confirm sites of suspected distant metastatic disease seen on PET before declaring a patient to have incurable or Stage IVC disease. A number of traumatic, inflammatory, or granulomatous disease findings could mimic distant metastases on PET.

To confirm the suspected primary site of disease at the left base of the tongue, for tumor mapping, and to rule out carcinoma at the right base of tongue, the patient was taken for direct laryngoscopic examination under anesthesia (EUA) with biopsies of the left and right base of tongue. At the time of EUA, there was friable, indurated mucosa at the left base of tongue and left glossopharyngeal sulcus tracking down toward the vallecula epiglottica. Biopsy of left base of tongue lesion confirmed invasive squamous carcinoma. The right base of tongue was normal to inspection and palpation. Biopsy of right base of tongue tissue was negative for tumor. The remainder of the examination was normal without other lesions seen in the upper aerodigestive tract mucosa.

The left base of tongue tumor tissue was positive for p16 by immunohistochemistry and high-risk HPV DNA type 16 by in situ hybridization.

Key point: HPV is both a causative agent and strong positive prognostic factor in oropharyngeal cancer (OPC); and p16 serves as a surrogate for HPV-association in OPC (Ang, *NEJM*, 2010).

Final diagnosis: Left base of tongue, squamous carcinoma, clinical Stage T2N2bM0 (IVA), HPV associated in an individual with no history of smoking, with excellent physical reserve, and Eastern Cooperative Oncology Group (ECOG) performance status of 0.

The patient underwent multidisciplinary oncologic specialty evaluations with head and neck surgery, medical oncology, and radiation oncology. The patient's case was presented and discussed at a head and neck cancer–specific multidisciplinary tumor board where final treatment recommendations, with the largest body of supporting medical evidence, were for the current standard of care: definitive concurrent chemoradiation, with concurrent chemotherapy (Cisplatin), with surgery reserved for residual disease following chemoradiation.

Additional Routine Pretherapy Evaluations

Laboratory and Audiology

To ensure candidacy for Cisplatin, a potentially nepthro- and ototoxic agent, baseline blood work was completed and showed good renal function and hematologic reserve; baseline audiometry showed age-appropriate hearing function. Carboplatin or cetuximab is often considered as alternative concurrent systemic therapy agents for individuals who are not candidates for Cisplatin treatment.

Dental Oncology

The patient was referred to dental oncology to ensure oral health was optimized before initiation of therapy, with restoration of restorable teeth, preradiotherapy extraction of nonrestorable teeth (preferably would be coordinated to be done at the time of EUA), fabrication of custom fluoride carriers for lifelong dental fortification, and creation of a custom mouth-opening and tongue-depressing oral stent to be used during RT simulation and treatment delivery. This stent immobilizes the tongue for more reliable targeting and delivery of radiation to the target. The stent is also used to minimize the toxic side effects of treatment by displacing the tongue away from other nontarget mucosal structures, such as the palate. Postradiation therapy tooth extractions are associated with high rates of osteonecrosis and should be avoided. If absolutely necessary, postradiotherapy extractions are best completed by an oral surgeon, using an atraumatic technique, prophylactic antibiotics, and pre- and postextraction hyperbaric oxygen to reduce the risk of nonhealing and/or osteonecrosis.

Speech-Language Pathology

For baseline evaluation and to establish proactive and preventative swallowing rehabilitation strategies during and after RT, baseline MBS evaluation with SLP revealed acceptable clinical swallowing function without clinical signs of dysphagia or aspiration. The MBS is the preferred method for objective documentation of swallow status in this patient group (see Video 5–1).

Gastroenterology and Nutrition

Our preferred strategy has been to place a feeding tube on an as-needed basis. When needed, percutaneous endoscopic gastrostomy (PEG) tubes are placed, but oftentimes a smaller-caliber nasogastric feeding (Dobhoff [DHT]) tube is considered in select cases, such as when tube feeds are anticipated to only be necessary for a short period of time. Given tumor location and treatment program, the probability of this patient requiring a feeding tube during or shortly after therapy was approximately 50% to 75%.

Smoking Cessation: Individualized

Cancer Prevention/Screening. Age and sex appropriate; noting HPV exposure risks.

> Key point: Early integration of supportive care and pretreatment implementation of rehabilitation services optimizes functional outcomes and quality of life.

Treatment: The patient underwent CT-based simulation for radiation therapy planning. With previously fabricated custom oral stent in place, he was immobilized using a custom thermoplastic mask, which was secured over his head, neck, and shoulders, which were displaced inferiorly. Figure 5–2 provides an illustration of patient positioning. Isocenter was placed just about the arytenoid cartilages. The gross disease within the left tongue base and left upper neck was delineated along with equivocal nodes in the right upper neck. The high-risk clinical target volume was then delineated to encompass the gross disease plus customized margin to coverage areas at highest-risk microscopic disease (CTV 70 Gy). The equivocal lymph nodes in the right upper neck were targeted likewise using intermediate-risk clinical target volume (CTV 66 Gy). The surrounding soft tissue regions and remainder of the regional lymph nodes at risk of harboring subclinical/microscopic disease were included in the standard risk clinical target volumes (CTV 57 Gy) (Figure 5–3A). The bilateral cervical lymph node levels including levels Ib through V and the bilateral lateral retropharyngeal lymph nodes were treated in this case. A geometric expansion of 3 mm was added to all clinical target volumes to create planning target volumes, which account for daily patient setup uncertainty. The critical organ and normal tissue

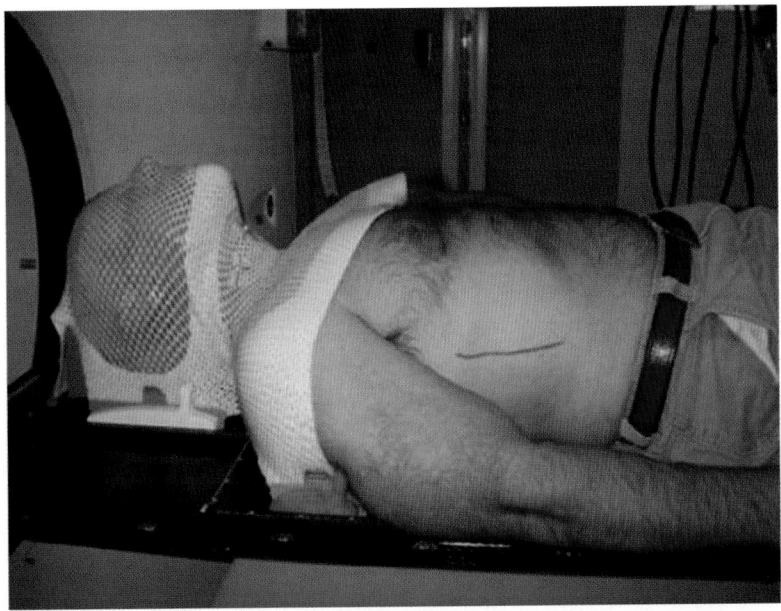

Figure 5–2. Representation of patient positioning and immobilization used for CT simulation and IMRT treatment delivery.

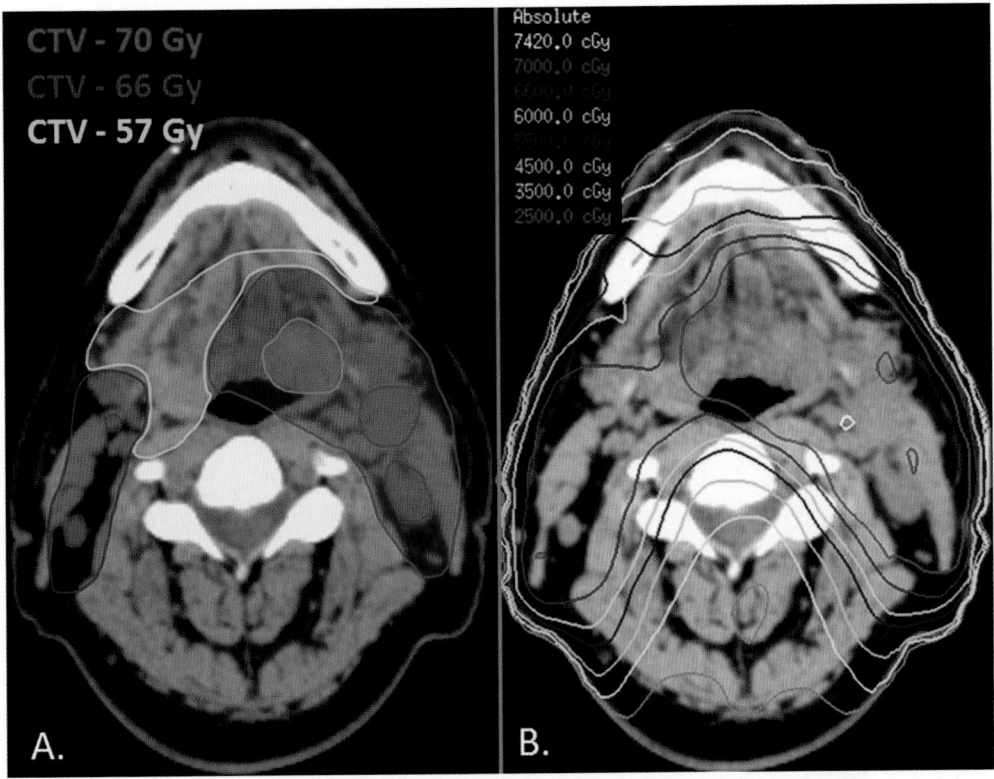

Figure 5–3. A. Representative axial image of planning CT showing delineation of the gross tumor volume (GTV) of both the primary tumor in the base of tongue (*light green*) and lymph nodes (*dark green*) with corresponding clinical target volumes (CTV) and accompanying dose levels. **B.** Axial image of planning CT showing IMRT isodose distributions, which were delivered over 33 daily fractions in 6.5 weeks.

avoidance structures were delineated and included brainstem, spinal cord, bilateral cochleas, bilateral parotid glands, mandible larynx, esophagus, and other nontarget upper aerodigestive tract mucosa. IMRT planning priorities were set to include (a) sparing of primary critical structures (typically central and peripheral nervous system structures); (b) coverage of both clinical and planning target volumes; and (c) sparing of secondary avoidance normal structures (which include parotid glands and key swallowing structures).

The high-, intermediate-, and standard-risk target volumes were treated to 70, 66, and 57 Gy, respectively, in 33 daily fractions over 6.5 weeks using split-field IMRT technique, where IMRT was used to the upper aspect of the treatment volume (Figure 5–3B), which was matched to a lower anterior neck fields utilizing a physical larynx block to maximize shielding of key swallowing structures (inferior pharyngeal constrictors, cricoarytenoid unit, and esophageal inlet) (Figure 5–4).

Concurrent Chemotherapy

The patient received concurrent chemotherapy with radiation: five weekly cycles of Cisplatin at 40 mg/m^2 along with IV supplemental hydration and antiemetics. Even though he experienced the anticipated in-field grade 2 to 3 mucocutaneous reactions, he completed the radiation therapy course without interruption or delays. For treatment, he met weekly with the radiation oncologist and clinical dietitian, and met every 3 weeks with the SLP.

Week 3 of chemoradiation (CRT), he returned to speech-language pathology for a mid-CRT swallow therapy session. He did not have a feeding tube and was maintaining oral intake of liquids and very soft foods. He reported fluctuating adherence to preventive swallowing exercises owing to growing pain from mucositis, but also nausea. Clinical swallow evaluation revealed no concerning signs of aspiration.

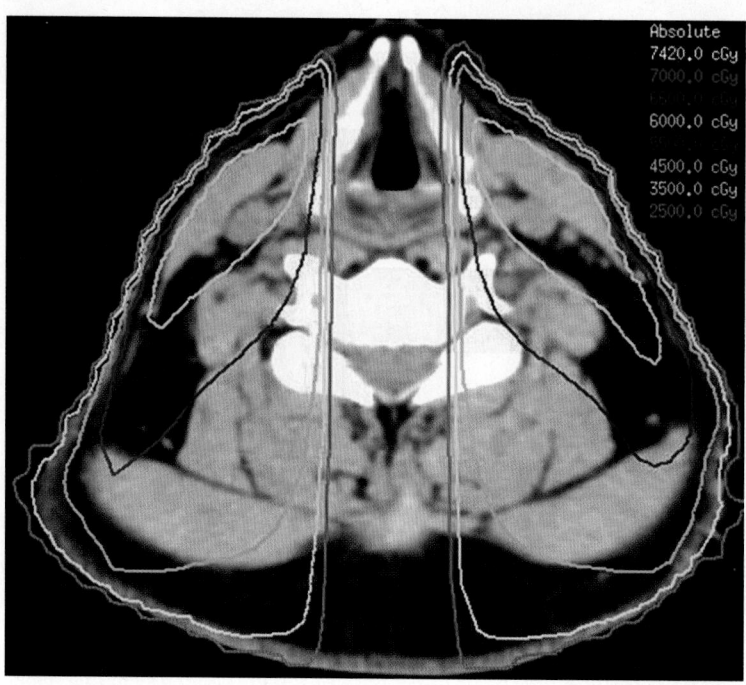

Figure 5–4. Axial image from planning CT at the level of the arytenoid cartilages demonstrating larynx shielding ability of split-field IMRT approach used in this case.

Week 4 of CRT, he underwent PEG placement without interruption of his treatment. On recommendation of the SLP, he continued daily oral intake of liquids and blended foods in addition to tube feedings.

After Treatment

Follow-up clinical examination with CT scan done 8 weeks after completion of CRT revealed no evidence of residual tumor at the base of tongue with regressing and now centimeter postradiation nodal remnants (Figure 5–5A). PET-CT was done at 12 weeks after completion of CRT revealed no evidence of residual tumor at the base of tongue with faint residual FDG avidity in left upper neck nodal remnants (Figure 5–5B). He then underwent left selective neck dissection of Level II, which showed treatment effect with no residual viable tumor cells on final pathology.

Swallow Follow-Up

Eight weeks after completing CRT, the patient was tolerating a soft oral diet. Clinical swallow evaluation revealed no overt signs of aspiration, and his PEG tube was removed after sustaining full oral nutrition for 2 weeks. A maintenance schedule of daily swallow exercise was encouraged in hopes of mediating the development of fibrosis during early postradiation healing. He reported limited exercise adherence.

Six months after CRT, he was consuming a regular diet but reported increasing dysphagia. MBS revealed moderate dysphagia with trace, compensated aspiration and residue of less than 50% in the pharyngeal recesses (see Video 5–2). Soft tissue thickness and edema were evident on MBS, resulting in inadequate pharyngeal propulsion and incomplete supraglottic closure. Swallow strategies were trained, and he was instructed on a home program of swallowing exercise. He performed swallowing

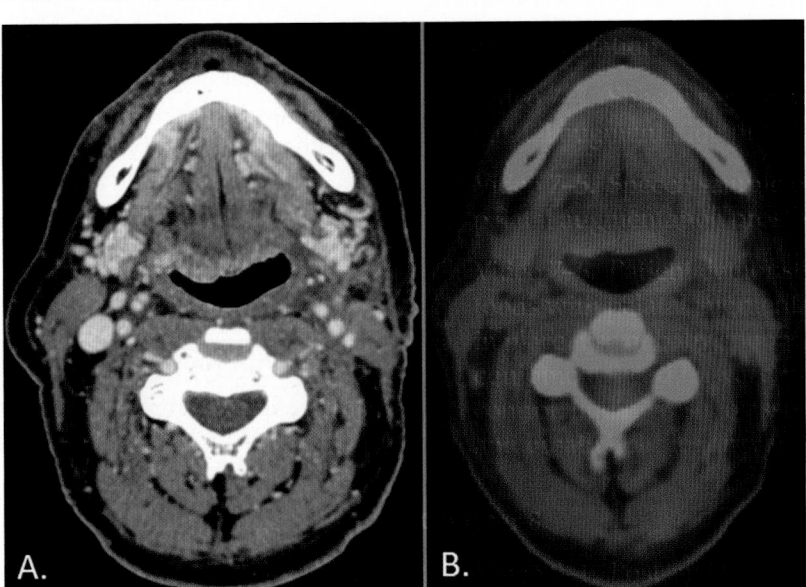

Figure 5–5. A. Axial image from post treatment diagnostic CT neck with contrast done at 8 weeks after treatment completion showing resolution of left base of tongue mass with regressing nodal remnants. **B.** Corresponding FGD-PET-CT axial image done 12 weeks after treatment completion with no evidence of FDG avid disease at tongue base and only slight avidity seen in left upper neck nodal remnants.

exercises routinely for 1 year and reported gradual improvement of his swallow. MBS completed 2 years after CRT found subtle improvements but persistent trace, compensated aspiration.

Routine Post treatment Surveillance

Clinical examination and neck CT were completed every 3 months for first year after CRT, every 4 months in the second year after CRT, every 6 months in years 3 to 5 after CRT, and annually from that point forward. Chest imaging, usually chest x-ray (CXR), were done on an annual basis. Measurement of thyroid and thyroid-stimulating hormone are done at every visit, with replacement thyroid hormone prescribed as needed.

Other post treatment evaluations and procedures include continued dental care and prophylaxis with cleanings at least twice a year and continue fluoride prophylaxis for life. Preventative measures such as routine jaw and neck stretching may mitigate neck fibrosis and trismus. Other survivorship issues include management of cancer and treatment-related fatigue and cancer prevention strategies and cardiovascular surveillance and risk reduction, noting potential for increased risk for treatment-related carotid artery atherosclerosis.

Five years after completing CRT, he presented to his annual survivorship visit with new onset of a unilateral hypoglossal palsy ipsilateral to his index oropharyngeal tumor. He noted also treatment for an interval "walking pneumonia" at a hospital closer to home, and had begun to complain of progressive dysphagia and slurred speech. MBS found severe dysphagia with repeated aspiration and significant inefficiency of pharyngeal transit (see Video 5–3). Intensive, "boot camp"–style swallowing therapy was offered. He participated in McNeil Dysphagia Therapy daily for 3 weeks with modest gains in swallow efficiency but persistent aspiration. He elected to continue oral intake adhering to swallow strategies and thickening some liquids he drinks, and remains pneumonia free 2 years later. A trial of pentoxyfyllene and vitamin E therapy was initiated in hopes of slowing the progression of fibrosis and atrophy.

> Key point: Postradiation dysphagia is an evolving target. Early manageable levels of dysphagia thought of as the "new normal" may progress into clinically significant levels of dysfunction with high risk of secondary pneumonia. Late radiation-associated dysphagia (RAD) is commonly precipitated by lower cranial neuropathies.

The patient has remained free of disease now 7 years after treatment completion.

Reflection and Analysis for Further Study

1. As is typical in many cases of head and neck cancer patients, the patient presented above demonstrated fluctuating levels of compliance with the SLP-recommended home dysphagia treatment program. Brainstorm factors that might contribute to poor patient compliance. When you are done, generate one to two strategies that might be used clinically to mitigate these factors.
2. How have methods of targeted delivery of radiation therapy changed the types of and severity of expected treatment side effects?
3. What are the advantages and disadvantages to "boot camp"–style dysphagia rehab programs? Which patients would likely benefit most from such procedures, and why?

OROPHARYNGEAL CANCER: A MULTIDISCIPLINARY APPROACH TO TREATING HPV-POSITIVE TONSIL CANCER WITH TRANSORAL ROBOTIC SURGERY (TORS)

History

A 66-year-old previously healthy male presented to his primary care provider with a 3-month history of a neck mass. He did not have any symptoms referable to the neck mass, in particular, no pain, dysphagia, or odynophagia. On exam he was noted to have tonsil mass and a palpable neck mass. Tonsil biopsy was performed and positive for squamous cell carcinoma. The tonsil tumor was tested for HPV and was positive both by in situ hybridization and by p16 immunohistochemistry. He was a former smoker (quit over 2 decades ago) with a cumulative exposure of approximately 30 pack-years.

Diagnostic Workup

The patient was referred to a head and neck surgeon. Imaging included CXR, CT scan, and a MBS study. CT revealed an enlarged right palatine tonsil (2.2 × 1.9 cm) with multiple ipsilateral metastatic lymph nodes (Figure 5–6). CXR was negative for lung metastasis. Final staging according to (tumor, node, metastasis) TNM criteria was T1 N2b M0 SCCA tonsil, representing Stage III according to American Joint Committee on Cancer (AJCC) summary staging. Multidisciplinary workup included consultations with head and neck surgery, radiation oncology, and medical oncology. Allied health referrals included speech-language pathology (SLP) and clinical nutrition. Preoperative endoscopy confirmed lesion in the right palatine tonsil with minor extension to the adjacent tongue base and glossopharyngeal sulcus (see Video 5–4). Baseline MBS confirmed well-preserved oropharyngeal swallow safety and efficiency (see Video 5–5).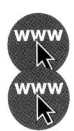

The case was presented at multidisciplinary tumor board with review of relevant imaging, histopathology, and physical examination findings. Tumor board consensus was chemoradiation as standard therapy or alternatively primary robotic surgery (TORS) with adjuvant radiotherapy. The proposed advantage of primary TORS was to remove the tumor and neck disease in one surgery in minimally invasive fashion. The patient was deemed a good candidate for TORS as his cancer was small and well localized, and he was otherwise healthy. Although it was anticipated he would need radiation therapy (RT) due to multiple involved lymph nodes, it could be offered at a postoperative dose and chemotherapy might be avoided if no adverse pathologic features were identified. Pretreatment functional counseling was provided during baseline SLP evaluations in which normal anatomy and physiology of structures central to speech and swallowing were discussed along with potential acute and chronic impairments related to primary TORS versus CRT. Limited comparative data for primary TORS versus CRT were acknowledged by the multidisciplinary team.

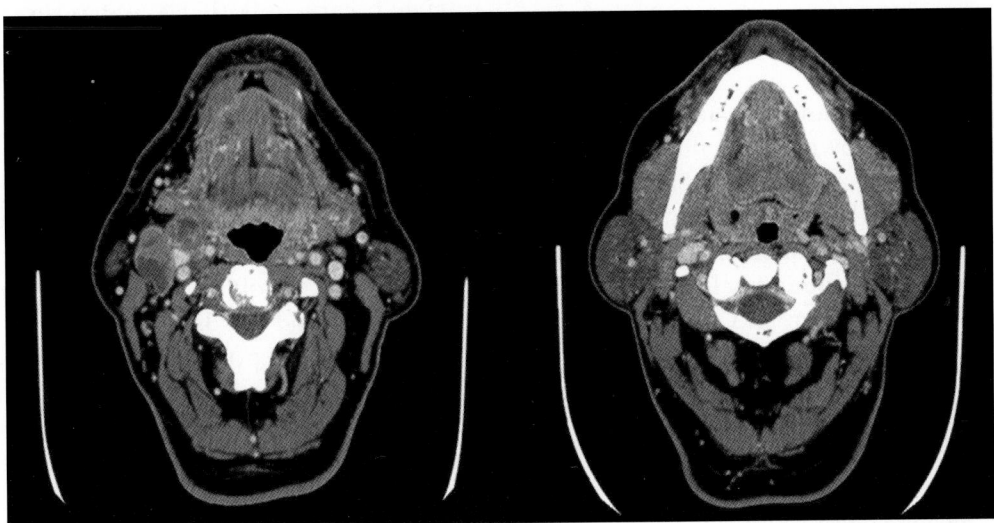

Figure 5–6. Axial image from initial pretreatment diagnostic CT neck showing enlarged right palatine tonsil with multiple ipsilateral metastatic lymph nodes.

Additional Routine Pretherapy Evaluations

Laboratory and Audiology

To ensure candidacy for Cisplatin, a potentially nephro- and ototoxic agent, baseline blood work was completed that showed good renal function and hematologic reserve; baseline audiometry showed age-appropriate hearing function. Carboplatin or cetuximab is often considered as alternative concurrent systemic therapy agents for noncisplatin candidates.

Dental Oncology

The patient was referred to dental oncology to ensure oral health was optimized before initiation of therapy, with restoration of restorable teeth, preradiotherapy extraction of nonrestorable teeth (preferably would be coordinated to be done at the time of TORS), with fabrication of custom fluoride carriers for lifelong dental fortification, and custom mouth-opening, tongue-depressing oral stent to be used during RT simulation and treatment delivery. This stent was used to immobilize the tongue for more reliable targeting and radiation delivery to the target and to reduce toxicities of treatment by displacing the tongue away for other nontarget mucosal structures, such as the palate.

Speech-Language Pathology

For baseline evaluation and to establish proactive and preventative swallowing rehabilitation strategy after TORS and during and after RT, baseline evaluation with SLP showed acceptable clinical swallowing function without clinical signs of dysphagia or aspiration. Modified barium swallow is preferred for objective documentation and safe and efficient baseline swallow function (see Video 5–6).

Gastroenterology and Nutrition

Our preferred strategy has been to place a feeding tube on an as-needed basis. TORS patients often benefit from a short-term placement of a Dobhoff tube (DHT) at the time of surgery, and most are able to have the DHT removed prior to hospital discharge.

Anesthesia Evaluation

All patients who undergo extensive surgery have preoperative evaluation to assess cardiopulmonary risk factors, as well as determine the likelihood of any potential medical complications that may affect surgical intervention and healing.

Smoking Cessation: Individualized

Cancer Prevention/Screening. Age and sex appropriate; noting HPV exposure risks.

Treatment

The patient elected to pursue primary surgery with TORS and neck dissection. He underwent successful TORS with selective unilateral neck dissection (Levels II–IV). Pathologic assessment revealed negative margins and 5 of 65 nodes positive. He did not require tracheostomy. An intraoperative DHT was placed. Given adverse features of extracapsular extension in several nodes, adjuvant chemoradiation was recommended. He completed postoperative chemoradiation with concurrent Cisplatin (weekly 30 mg/m^2).

Post Treatment: He was hospitalized 3 days after surgery. He did not require admission to the intensive care unit (ICU). On postoperative day (POD) 2, a SLP consultation was ordered. Bedside examination found mild tongue swelling, rhinolalia, odynophagia, and suspected, well-compensated oropharyngeal dysphagia on clinical swallow examination. A right head turn (ipsilateral to primary tumor resection) appeared to aid swallow efficiency. He started a liquid diet and his DHT was removed. He advanced to soft foods per os (PO) before discharge home on POD 3.

Three weeks postoperatively, he returned for multidisciplinary evaluation. Final pathology was reviewed, and he was dispositioned to receive adjuvant CRT. Radiation plans were rendered. Clinical swallow evaluation with the speech pathologist found persistent abnormality with suspected oropharyngeal dysphagia without overt indicators of aspiration. He felt he no longer required the right head turn to facilitate bolus clearance. He was eating a soft diet but continued to self-report nasal regurgitation, and nasal emissions were audible during PO trials. A postoperative MBS was ordered for the purpose of tailoring dysphagia rehabilitation before starting adjuvant chemoradiation (see Video 5–7).

Four weeks postoperatively, he underwent MBS finding minimal oropharyngeal dysphagia. Airway protection was intact with infrequent flash laryngeal penetration (Penetration-Aspiration Scale score [PAS] max = 2]. Pharyngeal bolus clearance was efficient despite right-sided pharyngeal paresis and mild nasal reflux (see Video 5–8).

A regular diet was recommended without restrictions or strategies. He was trained in preventive swallow exercise and encouraged to maintain PO intake through adjuvant chemoradiation. Postoperative laryngoscopy shows a well-healed, mucosalized postsurgical defect.

Five weeks postoperatively, he started adjuvant CRT. On treatment, he met weekly with the radiation oncologist and clinical dietitian, and met every 3 weeks with the SLP.

Week 3 of CRT (8 weeks postoperatively), he returned to SLP for a mid-RT swallow therapy session. He did not have a feeding tube. He was maintaining oral intake of liquids and semiliquid blended foods. He reported partial adherence (2×/day) to swallow exercises. Confluent oropharyngeal mucositis (Grade 3) was noted in the postsurgical target volume with associated odynophagia. Pain was well controlled with opioids. Clinical swallow evaluation found no new indicators of aspiration. He independently, accurately demonstrated swallow exercises. The patient's exercise and PO goals were subsequently adjusted in order to account for his acute toxicity profile.

One month post CRT, he returned for multidisciplinary assessment. Physical examination and laryngoscopy found no evidence of residual disease, with healing patchy mucositis. Clinical swallow evaluation was stable with no new signs of aspiration. He did not have a feeding tube, but oral intake remained limited to mostly liquids due to significant odynophagia. He reported partial adherence to swallow exercises (<1×/day). SLP adjusted his home swallow therapy goals to include (a) PO goals to gradually reintroduce masticated solids along a food hierarchy and (b) daily exercise adherence. A repeat MBS was not completed due to the extent of persistent pain and mucositis.

Three months after CRT, physical examination and CT found no evidence of disease. Mucositis was resolved on visible inspection. He reported improving oral intake, now eating two to three small portions of soft solid foods each day. He had no feeding tube but continued to drink by mouth more than three cans of nutritional supplements each day. Primary complaints included altered taste, thick saliva, and solid foods sticking in the pharynx. He reported partial adherence to swallow exercises (<1×/day). MBS was completed finding mild to moderate impairment. Swallow remained safe (PAS max = 2) without aspiration, but swallow efficiency was notably worse when comparing to his pre-CRT study. With solids, he now retained more than half the bolus in the pharyngeal recesses after the initial swallow attempt. Effortful, sequential swallows were recommended with an occasional liquid wash. Exercises promoting pharyngeal propulsion were recommended on a maintenance schedule indefinitely. Over the course of 1 year, oral intake gradually improved. By 1 year, he reported eating a regular diet with only occasional need for a liquid wash.

Routine surveillance included clinical examination with CT scan q3 months for the first year and q4months for the second year. He is now more than 2 years posttherapy with no evidence of disease, and no new late effects of therapy.

Reflection and Analysis for Further Study

1. For patients receiving radiation therapy, how would you explain why the size of the radiation field has been chosen? Additionally, how would you explain how the dosage will potentially affect the function of the remaining head and neck structures following completion of treatment?

2. In the case of this patient, was "partial" adherence to the home swallow program sufficient? Why or why not? As a clinician, how would you go about determining what exercises to recommend, as well as how frequently and with how many repetitions those exercises should be completed?

3. Suppose this patient was only willing or able to complete a full set of a single exercise daily. Given his individual profile, what exercise would you suggest and why?

REFERENCES

Adelstein, D. J., Ridge, J. A., Brizel, D. M., Holsinger, F. C., Haughey, B. H., O'Sullivan, B., . . . Ullmann, C. D. (2012). Transoral resection of pharyngeal cancer: Summary of a National Cancer Institute Head and Neck Cancer Steering Committee Clinical Trials Planning Meeting, November 6–7, 2011, Arlington, Virginia. *Head & Neck, 34*(12), 1681–1703. doi:10.1002/hed.23136

Ang, K. K., Harris, J., Wheeler, R., Weber, R., Rosenthal, D. I., Nguyen-Tan, P. F., . . . Gillison, M. L. (2010). Human papillomavirus and survival of patients with oropharyngeal cancer. *New England Journal of Medicine, 363*(1), 24–35. doi:NEJMoa0912217 [pii]. doi:10.1056/NEJMoa0912217

Ang, K. K., & Sturgis, E. M. (2012). Human papillomavirus as a marker of the natural history and response to therapy of head and neck squamous cell carcinoma. *Seminars in Radiation Oncology, 22*(2), 128–142. doi:10.1016/j.semradonc.2011.12.004

Awan, M. J., Mohamed, A. S., Lewin, J. S., Baron, C. A., Gunn, G. B., Rosenthal, D. I., . . . Hutcheson, K. A. (2014). Late radiation-associated dysphagia (late-RAD) with lower cranial neuropathy after oropharyngeal radiotherapy: A preliminary dosimetric comparison. *Oral Oncology, 50*(8), 746–752. doi:10.1016/j.oraloncology.2014.05.003

Benoit, J., & Lachapelle, P. (1990). Temporal relationship between ERG components and geniculate unit activity in rabbit. *Vision Research, 30*(6), 797–806. Retrieved from http://www.ncbi.nlm.nih.gov/pubmed/2385920

Best, S. R., Ha, P. K., Blanco, R. G., Saunders, J. R., Jr., Zinreich, E. S., Levine, M. A., . . . Messing, B. P. (2011). Factors associated with pharyngoesophageal stricture in patients treated with concurrent chemotherapy and radiation therapy for oropharyngeal squamous cell carcinoma. *Head & Neck, 33*(12), 1727–1734. doi:10.1002/hed.21657

Bhayani, M. K., Hutcheson, K. A., Barringer, D. A., Lisec, A., Alvarez, C. P., Roberts, D. B., . . . Lewin, J. S. (2013). Gastrostomy tube placement in patients with oropharyngeal carcinoma treated with radiotherapy or chemoradiotherapy: Factors affecting placement and dependence. *Head & Neck, 35*(11), 1634–1640. doi:10.1002/hed.23200

Bonner, J. A., Harari, P. M., Giralt, J., Azarnia, N., Shin, D. M., Cohen, R. B., . . . Ang, K. K. (2006). Radiotherapy plus cetuximab for squamous-cell carcinoma of the head and neck. *New England Journal of Medicine, 354*(6), 567–578. doi:10.1056/NEJMoa053422

Calais, G., Alfonsi, M., Bardet, E., Sire, C., Germain, T., Bergerot, P., . . . Bertrand, P. (1999). Randomized trial of radiation therapy versus concomitant chemotherapy and radiation therapy for advanced-stage oropharynx carcinoma. *Journal of the National Cancer Institute, 91*(24), 2081–2086. Retrieved from http://www.ncbi.nlm.nih.gov/pubmed/10601378

Cantrell, S. C., Peck, B. W., Li, G., Wei, Q., Sturgis, E. M., & Ginsberg, L. E. (2013). Differences in imaging characteristics of HPV-positive and HPV-negative oropharyngeal cancers: A blinded matched-pair analysis. *American Journal of Neuroradiology, 34*(10), 2005–2009. doi:10.3174/ajnr.A3524

Carnaby-Mann, G. D., & Crary, M. A. (2010). McNeill dysphagia therapy program: A case-control study. *Archives of Physical Medicine and Rehabilitation, 91*(5), 743–749. doi:10.1016/j.apmr.2010.01.013

Carnaby-Mann, G., Crary, M. A., Schmalfuss, I., & Amdur, R. (2012). "Pharyngocise": Randomized controlled trial of preventative exercises to maintain muscle structure and swallowing function during head-and-neck chemoradiotherapy. *International Journal of Radiation Oncology, Biology, Physics, 83*(1), 210–219. doi:10.1016/j.ijrobp.2011.06.1954

Chaturvedi, A. K., Engels, E. A., Anderson, W. F., & Gillison, M. L. (2008). Incidence trends for human papillomavirus-related and -unrelated oral squamous cell carcinomas in the United States. *Journal of Clinical Oncology, 26*(4), 612–619. doi:10.1200/JCO.2007.14.1713

Chaturvedi, A. K., Engels, E. A., Pfeiffer, R. M., Hernandez, B. Y., Xiao, W., Kim, E., . . . Gillison, M. L. (2011). Human papillomavirus and rising oropharyngeal cancer incidence in the United States. *Journal of Clinical Oncology, 29*(32), 4292–4301. doi:10.1200/JCO.2011.36.4596

Chronowski, G. M., Garden, A. S., Morrison, W. H., Frank, S. J., Schwartz, D. L., Shah, S. J., . . . Rosenthal, D. I. (2012). Unilateral radiotherapy for the treatment of tonsil cancer. *International Journal of Radiation Oncology, Biology, Physics, 83*(1), 204–209. doi:10.1016/j.ijrobp.2011.06.1975

Crary, M. A., Carnaby, G. D., LaGorio, L. A., & Carvajal, P. J. (2012). Functional and physiological outcomes from an exercise-based dysphagia therapy: A pilot investigation of the McNeill Dysphagia Therapy Program. *Archives of Physical Medicine and Rehabilitation, 93*(7), 1173–1178. doi:10.1016/j.apmr.2011.11.008

de Almeida, J. R., & Genden, E. M. (2012). Robotic surgery for oropharynx cancer: Promise, challenges, and future directions. *Current Oncology Reports, 14*(2), 148–157. doi:10.1007/s11912-012-0219-y

Denis, F., Garaud, P., Bardet, E., Alfonsi, M., Sire, C., Germain, T., . . . Calais, G. (2004). Final results of the 94-01 French Head and Neck Oncology and Radiotherapy Group randomized trial comparing radiotherapy alone with concomitant radiochemotherapy in advanced-stage oropharynx carcinoma. *Journal of Clinical Oncology, 22*(1), 69–76. doi:10.1200/JCO.2004.08.021

Eastern Cooperative Oncology Group (Philadelphia, PA). (2013). *Transoral surgery followed by low-dose or standard-dose radiation therapy with or without chemotherapy in treating patients with HPV positive Stage III-IVA oropharyngeal cancer*. Retrieved from ClinicalTrials.gov (cited June 22, 2015), https://clinicaltrials.gov/ct2/show/NCT01898494; NLM Identifier: NCT01898494

Fakhry, C., Westra, W. H., Li, S., Cmelak, A., Ridge, J. A., Pinto, H., . . . Gillison, M. L. (2008). Improved survival of patients with human papillomavirus-positive head and neck squamous cell carcinoma in a prospective clinical trial. *Journal of the National Cancer Institute, 100*(4), 261–269. doi:djn011 [pii]. doi: 10.1093/jnci/djn011

Feng, F. Y., Kim, H. M., Lyden, T. H., Haxer, M. J., Worden, F. P., Feng, M., . . . Eisbruch, A. (2010). Intensity-modulated chemoradiotherapy aiming to reduce dysphagia in patients with oropharyngeal cancer: Clinical and functional results. *Journal of Clinical Oncology, 28*(16), 2732–2738. doi:JCO.2009.24.6199 [pii]. doi:10.1200/JCO.2009.24.6199

Garden, A. S., Dong, L., Morrison, W. H., Stugis, E. M., Glisson, B. S., Frank, S. J., . . . Rosenthal, D. I. (2013). Patterns of disease recurrence following treatment of oropharyngeal cancer with intensity modulated radiation therapy. *International Journal of Radiation Oncology, Biology, Physics, 85*(4), 941–947. doi:10.1016/j.ijrobp.2012.08.004

Garden, A. S., Kies, M. S., Morrison, W. H., Weber, R. S., Frank, S. J., Glisson, B. S., . . . Sturgis, E. M. (2013). Outcomes and patterns of care of patients with locally advanced oropharyngeal carcinoma treated in the early 21st century. *Radiation Oncology, 8*, 21. doi:10.1186/1748-717X-8-21

Genden, E. M., Park, R., Smith, C., & Kotz, T. (2011). The role of reconstruction for transoral robotic pharyngectomy and concomitant neck dissection. *Archives of Otolaryngology-Head and Neck Surgery, 137*(2), 151–156. Retrieved from http://ovidsp.ovid.com/ovidweb.cgi?T=JS&CSC=Y&NEWS=N&PAGE=fulltext&D=medl&AN=21339401

Gillespie, M. B., Day, T. A., Sharma, A. K., Brodsky, M. B., & Martin-Harris, B. (2007). Role of mitomycin in upper digestive tract stricture. *Head & Neck, 29*(1), 12–17. doi:10.1002/hed.20476

Gillison, M. L., Koch, W. M., Capone, R. B., Spafford, M., Westra, W. H., Wu, L., . . . Sidransky, D. (2000). Evidence for a causal association between human papillomavirus and a subset of head and neck cancers. *Journal of the National Cancer Institute, 92*(9), 709–720. Retrieved from http://www.ncbi.nlm.nih.gov/entrez/query.fcgi?cmd=Retrieve&db=PubMed&dopt=Citation&list_uids=10793107

Haughey, B. H., Hinni, M. L., Salassa, J. R., Hayden, R. E., Grant, D. G., Rich, J. T., . . . Krishna, M. (2011). Transoral laser microsurgery as primary treatment for advanced-stage oropharyngeal cancer: A United States multicenter study. *Head & Neck, 33*(12), 1683–1694. doi:10.1002/hed.21669

Hunter, K. U., Lee, O. E., Lyden, T. H., Haxer, M. J., Feng, F. Y., Schipper, M., . . . Eisbruch, A. (2013). Aspiration pneumonia after chemo-intensity-modulated radiation therapy of oropharyngeal carcinoma and its clinical and dysphagia-related predictors. *Head and Neck, 36*(1), 120–125. doi:10.1002/hed.23275

Hunter, K. U., Schipper, M., Feng, F. Y., Lyden, T., Haxer, M., Murdoch-Kinch, C. A., . . . Eisbruch, A. (2012). Toxicities affecting quality of life after chemo-IMRT of oropharyngeal cancer: Prospective study of patient-reported, observer-rated, and objective outcomes. *International Journal of Radiation Oncology, Biology, Physics.* doi:S0360-3016(12)03450-5 [pii]. doi:10.1016/j.ijrobp.2012.08.030

Hutcheson, K. A., Bhayani, M. K., Beadle, B. M., Gold, K. A., Shinn, E. H., Lai, S. Y., & Lewin, J. (2014). Eat and exercise during radiotherapy or chemoradiotherapy for pharyngeal cancers: Use it or lose it. *JAMA Otolaryngology-Head & Neck Surgery, 11*, 1127.

Hutcheson, K. A., Holsinger, F. C., Kupferman, M. E., & Lewin, J. S. (2014). Functional outcomes after TORS for oropharyngeal cancer: A systematic review. *European Archives of Otorhinolaryngology, 272*, 463–471. doi:10.1007/s00405-014-2985-7

Hutcheson, K. A., Lewin, J. S., Barringer, D. A., Lisec, A., Gunn, G. B., Moore, M. W., & Holsinger, F. C. (2012). Late dysphagia after radiotherapy-based treatment of head and neck cancer. *Cancer, 118*(23), 5793–5799. doi:10.1002/cncr.27631

Hutcheson, K. A., Lewin, J. S., Holsinger, F. C., Steinhaus, G., Lisec, A., Barringer, D. A., . . . Kies, M. S. (2014). Long-term functional and survival outcomes after induction chemotherapy and risk-based definitive therapy for locally advanced squamous cell carcinoma of the head and neck. *Head & Neck, 36*(4), 474–480. doi:10.1002/hed.23330

Hutcheson, K. A., Yuk, M. M., Holsinger, F. C., Gunn, G. B., & Lewin, J. S. (2014). Late radiation-associated dysphagia (late-RAD) with lower cranial neuropathy in long-term oropharyngeal cancer survivors: Video case reports. *Head and Neck, 37*(4), E56–E62. doi:10.1002/hed.23840

Kotz, T., Federman, A. D., Kao, J., Milman, L., Packer, S., Lopez-Prieto, C., . . . Genden, E. M. (2012). Prophylactic swallowing exercises in patients with head and neck cancer undergoing chemoradiation: A randomized trial. *Archives of Otolaryngology-Head and Neck Surgery, 138*(4), 376–382. doi:10.1001/archoto.2012.187

Li, W., Thompson, C. H., O'Brien, C. J., McNeil, E. B., Scolyer, R. A., Cossart, Y. E., . . . Rose, B. R. (2003). Human papillomavirus positivity predicts favourable outcome for squamous carcinoma of the tonsil. *International Journal of Cancer, 106*(4), 553–558. doi:10.1002/ijc.11261

Martin-Harris, B., McFarland, D., Hill, E. G., Strange, C. B., Focht, K. L., Wan, Z., . . . McGrattan, K. (2015). Respiratory-swallow training in patients with head and neck cancer. *Archives of Physical Medicine and Rehabilitation, 96*(5), 885–893. doi:10.1016/j.apmr.2014.11.022

Mehta, V., Yu, G. P., & Schantz, S. P. (2010). Population-based analysis of oral and oropharyngeal carcinoma: Changing trends of histopathologic differentiation, survival and patient demographics. *Laryngoscope, 120*(11), 2203–2212. doi:10.1002/lary.21129

Mork, J., Lie, A. K., Glattre, E., Hallmans, G., Jellum, E., Koskela, P., . . . Dillner, J. (2001). Human papillomavirus infection as a risk factor for squamous-cell carcinoma of the head and neck. *New England Journal of Medicine, 344*(15), 1125–1131. Retrieved from http://www.ncbi.nlm.nih.gov/entrez/query.fcgi?cmd=Retrieve&db=PubMed&dopt=Citation&list_uids=11297703

Nutting, C. M., Morden, J. P., Harrington, K. J., Urbano, T. G., Bhide, S. A., Clark, C., . . . group, P. t. m. (2011). Parotid-sparing intensity modulated versus conventional radiotherapy in head and neck cancer (PARSPORT): A phase 3 multicentre randomised controlled trial. *Lancet Oncology, 12*(2), 127–136. doi:10.1016/S1470-2045(10)70290-4

O'Sullivan, B., Huang, S. H., Perez-Ordonez, B., Massey, C., Siu, L. L., Weinreb, I., . . . Xu, W. (2012). Outcomes of HPV-related oropharyngeal cancer patients treated by radiotherapy alone using altered fractionation. *Radiotherapy and Oncology, 103*(1), 49–56. doi:10.1016/j.radonc.2012.02.009

Pignon, J. P., le Maitre, A., Maillard, E., Bourhis, J., & Group, M.-N. C. (2009). Meta-analysis of chemotherapy in head and neck cancer (MACH-NC): An update on 93 randomised trials and 17,346 patients. *Radiotherapy and Oncology, 92*(1), 4–14. doi:10.1016/j.radonc.2009.04.014

Posner, M. R., Glisson, B., Frenette, G., Al-Sarraf, M., Colevas, A. D., Norris, C. M., . . . Garay, C. A. (2001). Multicenter phase I-II trial of docetaxel, cisplatin, and fluorouracil induction chemotherapy for patients with locally advanced squamous cell cancer of the head and neck. *Journal of Clinical Oncology, 19*(4), 1096–1104. Retrieved from http://www.ncbi.nlm.nih.gov/pubmed/11181674

Quon, H., Cohen, M. A., Montone, K. T., Ziober, A. F., Wang, L. P., Weinstein, G. S., & O'Malley, B. W., Jr. (2013). Transoral robotic surgery and adjuvant therapy for oropharyngeal carcinomas and the influence of p16 INK4a on treatment outcomes. *Laryngoscope, 123*(3), 635–640. doi:10.1002/lary.22172

Radiation Therapy Oncology Group (Philadelphia, PA). (2011). *Radiation therapy with cisplatin or cetuximab in treating patients with oropharyngeal cancer.* Retrieved from ClinicalTrails.gov (cited June 22, 2015), https://clinicaltrials.gov/ct2/show/NCT01302834 NLM Identifier: NCT 01302834

Rich, J. T., Liu, J., & Haughey, B. H. (2011). Swallowing function after transoral laser microsurgery (TLM) +/– adjuvant therapy for advanced-stage oropharyngeal cancer. *Laryngoscope, 121*(11), 2381–2390. doi:10.1002/lary.21406

Setton, J., Lee, N. Y., Riaz, N., Huang, S. H., Waldron, J., O'Sullivan, B., . . . Garden, A. S. (2015). A multi-institution pooled analysis of gastrostomy tube dependence in patients with oropharyngeal cancer treated with definitive intensity-modulated radiotherapy. *Cancer, 121*(2), 294–301. doi:10.1002/cncr.29022

Starmer, H. M., Yang, W., Raval, R., Gourin, C. G., Richardson, M., Kumar, R....Quon, H. (2014). Effect of gabapentin on swallowing during and after chemoradiation for oropharyngeal squamous cell cancer. *Dysphagia, 29*(3), 396–402. doi:10.1007/s00455-014-9521-1

Sturgis, E. M., & Cinciripini, P. M. (2007). Trends in head and neck cancer incidence in relation to smoking prevalence: An emerging epidemic of human papillomavirus-associated cancers? *Cancer, 110*(7), 1429–1435. doi:10.1002/cncr.22963

van der Molen, L., van Rossum, M. A., Burkhead, L. M., Smeele, L. E., Rasch, C. R., & Hilgers, F. J. (2011). A randomized preventive rehabilitation trial in advanced head and neck cancer patients treated with chemoradiotherapy: Feasibility, compliance, and short-term effects. *Dysphagia, 26*(2), 155–170. doi:10.1007/s00455-010-9288-y

Wang, J. J., Goldsmith, T. A., Holman, A. S., Cianchetti, M., & Chan, A. W. (2012). Pharyngoesophageal stricture after treatment for head and neck cancer. *Head & Neck, 34*(7), 967–973. doi:10.1002/hed.21842

Weinstein, G. S., Quon, H., Newman, H. J., Chalian, J. A., Malloy, K., Lin, A., . . . O'Malley, B. W. (2012). Transoral robotic surgery alone for oropharyngeal cancer: An analysis of local control. *Archives of Otolaryngology-Head and Neck Surgery, 138*(7), 628–634. doi:10.1001/archoto.2012.1166

Weinstein, G. S., Quon, H., O'Malley, B. W., Jr., Kim, G. G., & Cohen, M. A. (2010). Selective neck dissection and deintensified postoperative radiation and chemotherapy for oropharyngeal cancer: A subset analysis of the University of Pennsylvania transoral robotic surgery trial. *Laryngoscope, 120*(9), 1749–1755. doi:10.1002/lary.21021

Wilson, J. A., Carding, P. N., & Patterson, J. M. (2011). Dysphagia after nonsurgical head and neck cancer treatment: Patients' perspectives. *Otolaryngology-Head and Neck Surgery, 145*(5), 767–771. doi:10.1177/0194599811414506

6

An Interdisciplinary Approach to the Management of a Patient With Base of Tongue Carcinoma

Vrushali Angadi, Thomas J. Gal, and Joseph C. Stemple

HISTORY

Patient A is a 56-year-old female referred on October 1, 2012, by her otolaryngologist (ENT) to the multidisciplinary clinic at the Markey Cancer Center, University of Kentucky (UK).

Medical History

Patient A presented with a 4-month history of left-sided neck pain that she attributed to a muscle pull. She soon noticed two enlarged "lumps" in her neck and subsequently consulted an ENT. Laryngeal and oropharyngeal examination identified a suspicious mass in the left tongue base region, extending to the left tonsil. On physical examination, two left-sided Level II enlarged lymph nodes were appreciated. An outpatient fine-needle aspiration of one of the two lymph nodes was performed at the ENT's office. A week later, the pathology report revealed poorly differentiated metastatic squamous cell carcinoma. Patient A's consultant ENT advised her that she would be best served in a multidisciplinary cancer care center and referred her to the Markey Cancer Clinic (MCC).

Social History

Patient A presented as a generally healthy individual who exercised regularly and ate a well-balanced, healthy diet. She worked as a fitness instructor for 12 years and noted that being in the gym with her clients was the best part of her day. She reported being happily married with two daughters, both of whom are married. She consumed close to 60 oz of water per day and 1 cup of coffee every morning. She did not consume any carbonated beverages or alcohol. She has always been a nonsmoker and was not exposed to secondhand smoke at home or at work. She reported no history of illicit drug use.

Risk Factors

Based on the patient's social history, no conventional environmental risk factors for head and neck cancers were self-reported.

Past Medical History

Patient A's medical history was significant for gastroesophageal reflux disorder (GERD) since 2008, hiatal hernia since 2010, hypertension since 2000, and seasonal allergies. Patient A was on medication for GERD and hypertension and was regular and attentive in taking her medication as advised.

Past Surgical History

Past surgical history was significant only for a hysterectomy in 1999.

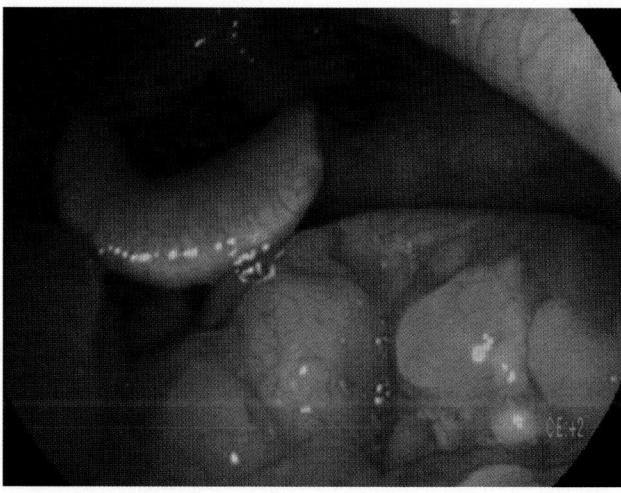

Figure 6–1. Suspicious lesion involving the left base of tongue.

DIAGNOSTIC WORKUP

Visual Examination

A visual examination including laryngeal stroboscopy using a flexible distal chip endoscope was conducted by the speech-language pathologist (SLP) in conjunction with the head and neck surgeon. Gross assessment of the oropharyngeal and laryngeal structures confirmed presence of the suspicious mass lesion involving the left base of tongue and tonsillar region (Figure 6–1 and Video 6–1). The right tongue base region, right tonsil, vallecula, larynx, and hypopharynx were free of mass lesions. Arytenoid mobility was symmetric bilaterally. Stroboscopic examination revealed stroboscopic parameters within normal limits.

Imaging Studies

Patient A underwent a full-body PET (positron emission tomography) scan on October 3, 2012, The scan showed focal tracer accumulation in left base of tongue with a peak SUV of 9.0. Two lymph nodes were noted at the level of the submandibular gland and left jugular chain with an SUV of 10.2 and 14.4 measuring 1.5 cm in size. No suspicious uptake was noted in the chest, abdomen, or pelvis.

Direct Laryngoscopy With Biopsies (Performed October 7, 2012)

An approximately 2-cm ulcerative lesion was noted on the left base of the tongue region. Biopsies were taken from the site of ulceration in the base of the tongue and the left pharyngeal wall. The remainder of the oropharyngeal and laryngeal structures did not show any evidence of mass lesions.

Pathology Reports

Pathology reports from the outside facility were reexamined. The diagnosis remained unchanged. The patient's fine-needle aspiration (FNA) from one left-sided Level II lymph node showed metastatic, poorly differentiated, squamous cell carcinoma. The most recent biopsies from the left base of tongue region showed poorly differentiated squamous cell carcinoma. In addition, p16 immunohistochemistry of the biopsied material was performed with the results being positive for human papillomavirus (HPV)–related tumor.

HPV-related tumors (also referred to as p16-positive tumors) are considered a unique group. In the past 30 years, the overall incidence of non-HPV related oropharyngeal squamous cell carcinoma

(OPSCC) has reduced in the United States; however, the incidence of HPV-related OPSCC has been rising during this same time period (Lewis et al., 2010). Patients with HPV-related OPSCC do not fit the traditional head and neck cancer patient profile. Often these cancers occur in younger patients with no discernible risk factors such as tobacco or alcohol consumption. This was the case with Patient A (Lewis et al., 2010). Studies show that HPV-positive tumors respond favorably to postoperative radiation therapy (Bhayani, Holsinger, & Lai, 2010; Iseli et al., 2009; Kaplan & Damrose, 2010). Depending on the stage of the disease and postsurgical pathology reports, chemotherapy may or may not be required.

Tumor Board Discussion and Staging

Staging of the primary tumor was based on the oropharyngeal and laryngeal exam, PET-CT scans, and biopsies. On clinical examination, the patient's primary tumor was restricted to the left base of the tongue and was less than or equal to 2 cm, the patient had two palpable cervical lymph nodes less than 6 cm in dimension, and there was no evidence of distant metastasis on the PET-CT scans. Based on the clinical examination, imaging studies, laryngeal examination, and biopsies, Patient A's base of tongue cancer was staged as T1N2bM0 based on current American Joint Committee on Cancer guidelines (Greene, 2002).

TREATMENT PLAN

Based on the results of her diagnostic tests, it was decided that Patient A would benefit from primary surgery followed by adjuvant radiation and chemotherapy as indicated by pathologic staging. The surgery entailed removal of the primary tongue base tumor via transoral robotic surgery (TORS) as well as a modified neck dissection for removal of the metastatic lymph nodes. The benefits of surgery include not only complete removal of the tumor, but also pathologic staging that allows for determining and potentially deescalating adjuvant chemoradiation. Patient A's treatment details are described below.

Surgical Management

Based on Patient A's recent PET-CT scans, biopsy results, and oropharyngeal and laryngeal examination, it was decided that she would undergo surgical resection. This entails a neck dissection as well as TORS. These procedures are frequently staged for numerous technical and logistical reasons. In this patient's instance, they were performed a week apart. Patient A was an ideal candidate for TORS because she had a well-localized lesion and neck disease that was amenable to a modified neck dissection. The intent of performing a TORS and neck dissection in Patient A's case was to perform adjuvant chemoradiation in a more directed manner, reducing therapy as indicated by the disease. Due to anticipated perioperative swallowing complications, Patient A was scheduled to have a percutaneous endoscopic gastrostomy (PEG) feeding tube placed at the time of the TORS. Important details from the two surgical procedures are as follows:

1. Modified radical neck dissection performed October 20, 2012: Neck dissection was performed from Levels I, Ia, IIa, IIb, III, IV, and V, and tissues were sent for pathologic analysis. Cranial nerves 7, 10, 11, and 12, sternocleidomastoid muscle, jugular vein, and carotid artery were all preserved.

2. TORS and PEG placement performed October 27, 2012: PEG placement was performed by a gastrointestinal surgeon prior to initiation of the TORS resection. PEG placement was performed intraoperatively without difficulty. TORS was performed utilizing the da Vinci surgical system (Figure 6–2) (Bhayani et al., 2010; Iseli et al., 2009; Kaplan & Damrose, 2010). A 2-cm left base of tongue mass was excised with negative margins per frozen section pathology reports. The primary tumor was resected using the da Vinci robot. The tumor involved the lateral tongue base including the inferior portion of the tonsillar fossa. Negative margins were obtained. Dissection included the ipsilateral tonsil laterally, which included the superior pharyngeal constrictor as a margin, extended posteriorly to the vallecula and medially to the midline of the tongue. The deep margin extended to the

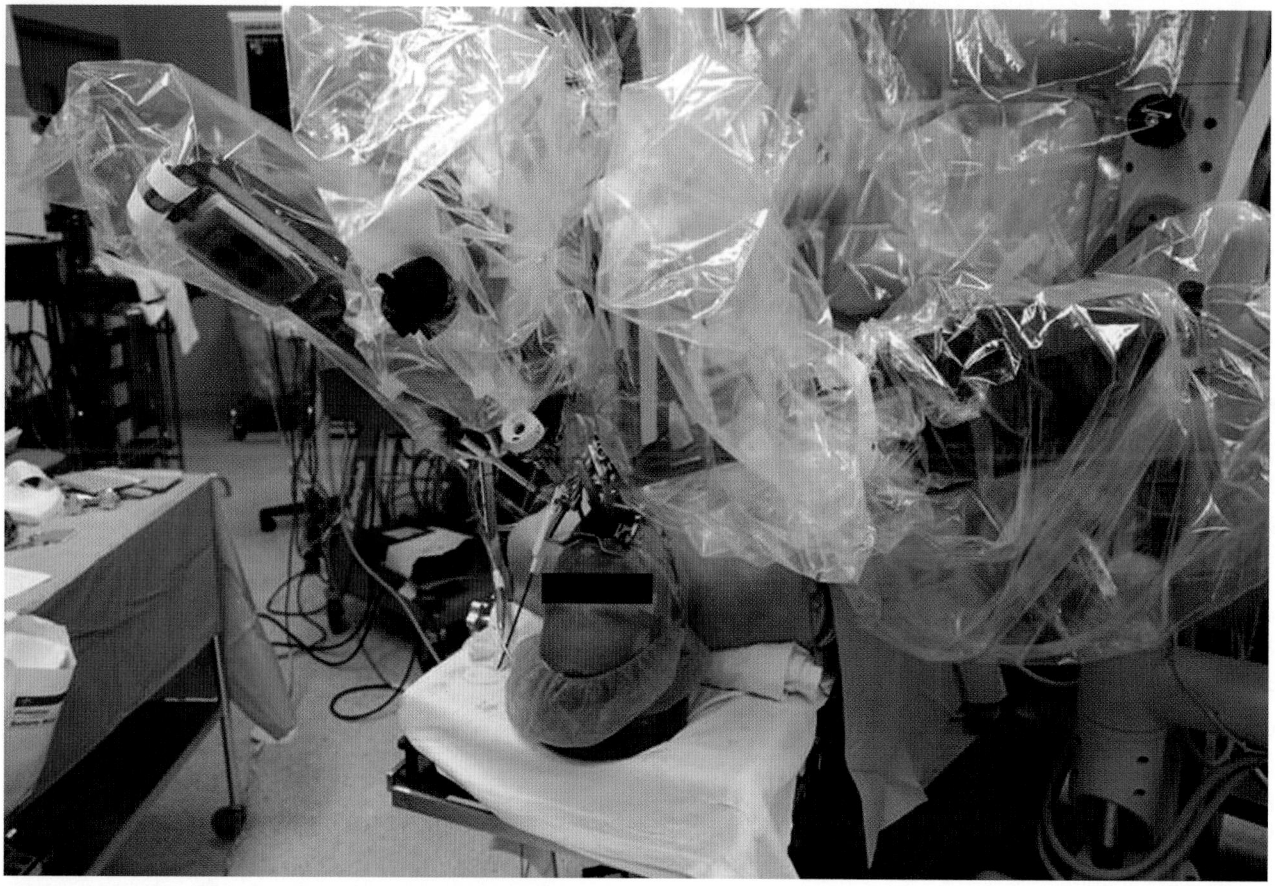

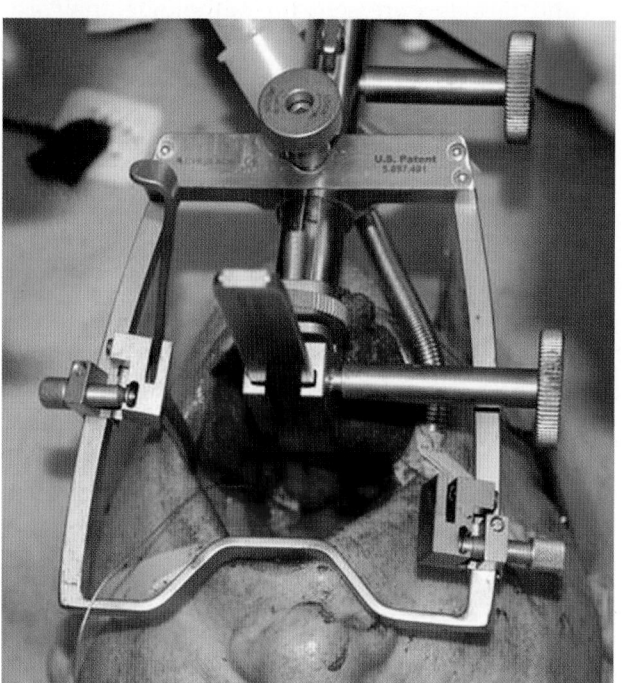

A

B

Figure 6–2. A. Surgical setup for transoral robotic surgery (TORS): Positioning of robotic arms. B. Surgical setup for transoral robotic surgery (TORS): Positioning of patient.

hyoid bone with exposure of the preepiglottic space as well as identification and ligation of the ipsilateral lingual artery. The lingual artery was sacrificed. No serious complications or adverse events occurred during the operative procedure (Figure 6–3 and Video 6–2).

Postoperative Swallowing Evaluation and Management

Patient A was seen at the UK Voice and Swallow clinic 2 weeks after surgery. At that time, Patient A had a PEG tube in place and was completely PEG dependent. She had been recommended five cans of tube feeds by the hospital dietician; a recommendation that she had diligently followed during her postoperative period. Her PEG intake had been calculated by the hospital dietitian based on her height and weight and postoperative nutritional needs. Her total recommended caloric intake with tube feeds was between 2000 and 2200 calories. She was also recommended to flush her PEG tube with water after every feed. During her visit, her main complaint was odynophagia with secretions.

A fiberoptic endoscopic evaluation of swallowing (FEES) was performed by the SLP during this visit with the following results: pooling of secretions was noted in the left tongue base region, in the left vallecula, and in the left piriform sinus. Base of tongue elevation was restricted on the left, and reduced left-sided pharyngeal squeeze was noted. On presentation of thin liquids, the patient showed one instance of penetration. Pooling was noted in the left piriform sinus and vallecula with presentation of nectar and pureed consistencies; this was eliminated with a liquid wash and effortful swallow. Patient A was reluctant to try cracker consistencies. We respected her wishes for the same. No instances of aspiration were noted on the examination. Based on the examination, patient was advised a mechanical soft diet with thin liquids.

Adjuvant Treatment

Prior to planning adjuvant treatment, Patient A's clinical, surgical, imaging, and pathology findings were presented and re-reviewed at the multidisciplinary head and neck tumor board conference. The patient had negative margins on the resection of the primary, with no unfavorable features such as lymphvascular or perineural invasion. As a result, she did not require any additional radiation to the base of tongue. The multiple lymph nodes in the neck did necessitate radiation to the neck. However, no evidence of extranodal extension of tumor was noted in the lymph nodes, and there was no oncologic indication for chemotherapy. RT was planned about 4 to 6 weeks after TORS. Based on pathology and surgical findings, her tumor was staged as pT2N2bM0. The patient underwent a course of adjuvant radiation therapy from December 8, 2012, to January 12, 2013. Patient A received a total dose of 60 (grey) Gy in 30 fractions at 2 Gy per fraction followed by 54 Gy to the low-risk areas. No complications were reported during treatment.

SLP Consultation

Prior to beginning radiation therapy (RT), the patient was referred to the SLP for preradiation counseling and initiation of swallowing exercises. Often

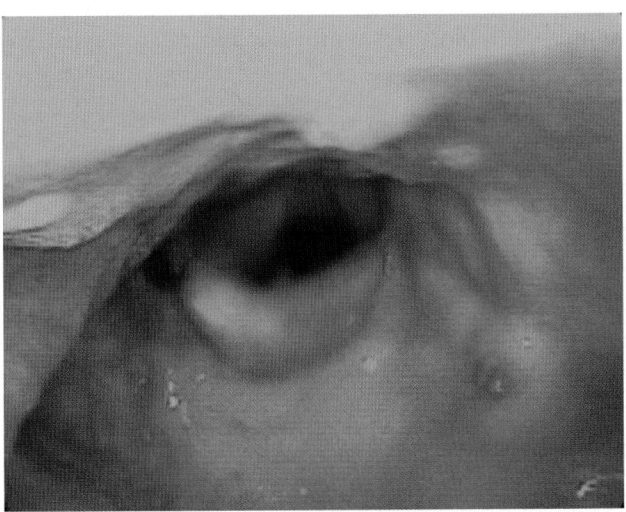

Figure 6–3. Postoperative oropharyngeal and laryngeal examination.

patients initiate RT without realizing the severity of swallowing and voice changes that can occur as a result of RT. It is important to prepare patients for postradiation sequelae, mainly to help them process the nature of the radiation-associated side effects. Patient A was counseled vigorously on the importance of performing swallowing exercises through RT. Patient A was explained that swallowing exercises during the RT period are aimed at reducing/preventing swallowing impairments by improving and maintaining the mobility of vital swallowing structures even after treatment is completed. The exercises prescribed for Patient A included the effortful swallow, Masako or tongue hold maneuver, Mendelsohn maneuver (Lazarus, Logemann, & Gibbons, 1993; Lazarus, Logemann, Song, Rademaker, & Kahrilas, 2002; Logemann, 1998), and jaw stretch exercises with a Therabite (Kamstra, Roodenburg, Beurskens, Reintsema, & Dijkstra, 2013). Patient A was scheduled for weekly dysphagia therapy sessions with the SLP during the period that she received RT. Patient A was also counseled on the signs and symptoms of aspiration and was advised to consult the SLP or head and neck surgeon if the symptoms were noted. Should the symptoms and signs occur, she was advised to switch to a completely PEG-dependent diet until a swallow study was completed to determine the safety of her swallow status.

PATIENT A's POST TREATMENT STATUS

Patient A attended all of her RT sessions and no complications were reported during this period. Her main complaint was xerostomia and frequent soreness of the oral cavity tissues. She was aware that these are common RT-related complications. She managed to maintain an oral diet through RT. She maintained her PEG tube by flushing it with water four to five times per day. As a fitness instructor, she was familiar with calorie counting and maintained a food diary through treatment. Her caloric intake through treatment ranged from 2000 to 2200 calories, which was the intake advised by the dietitian. Patient A lost a total of 20 pounds through RT.

Head and Neck Surgical Consultation

On her post treatment follow-up that was scheduled 8 weeks after RT, Patient A underwent a whole-body PET-CT scan and a clinical examination. Patient A's post treatment scans were favorable and did not show evidence of persistent or residual disease. Patient A's oropharyngeal and laryngeal examination showed healthy appearing mucosa in the tongue base region, tonsil and around the supraglottic, glottic, and hypopharyngeal region. Patient A's only complaint was stiffness in the left neck region around the site of the neck dissection. She revealed this stiffness had become worse through RT and was now causing pain. This stiffness was explained as a common complication after a neck dissection and RT to the neck region. She was referred to a physical therapist with expertise in post-RT complications to manage her neck problems.

Based on her diagnostic workup, Patient A was presently in remission. Of course, she and her family were visibly happy with her test results, and the importance of regular follow-ups was emphasized by her physician. At the visit, it was explained to Patient A that she will continue to undergo periodic surveillance for disease recurrence. She was also advised to carry out self-examinations and watch out for any "lumps or bumps" or pain in the head and neck region. Should any changes occur, she was advised to consult with the head and neck surgeon immediately and not wait until her next scheduled follow-up.

SLP Consultation

Patient A had maintained an oral diet through treatment without any instances of chest infection and pneumonia. She had maintained her weight since completion of RT and had been diligent with her swallowing exercises. Her only complaint was "food getting stuck" when she swallowed. The SLP completed a modified barium swallow study (MBS) to rule out any structural or physiological causes for the swallowing impairment. An esophageal screen was also performed in conjunction with the radiologist to rule out any esophageal stenosis or stricture which is a common RT-related complication. The MBS showed adequate swallowing physiology with the exception of reduced tongue base to posterior pharyngeal wall contact. This is understandable considering her postoperative status. Her esophageal screen was within functional limits. Her score on the Penetration-Aspiration scale (PAS) was 1, which indicated that material did not enter the airway (Rosenbek, Robbins, Roecker, Coyle, & Wood, 1996). She was deemed safe for a regular diet with thin liquids based on the results from her MBS.

After Patient A's disease remission was confirmed and swallow status was evaluated, she was asked to report back in 3 months for ongoing surveillance. Patient A's PEG tube was not removed during this current visit. It was explained to her that the removal of her PEG tube would be dependent on the following factors. For the next 3 months she would have to be solely on an oral diet, maintain her weight, and have no episodes of pneumonia, recurrent chest infections, or fevers. She would also need to have normal clinical and imaging findings as assessed by her head and neck surgeon on her 3-month follow-up. If she fulfilled the above criteria related to swallowing and disease status, a recommendation would be made for the PEG tube to be removed. Because she was on an oral diet during the current examination, she was advised to maintain the patency of the PEG tube by continuing to flush the tube with clear water periodically.

Three-Month Follow-Up Status

Patient A followed up with her head and neck surgeon as scheduled, for her 3-month follow-up. Her detailed head and neck clinical examination did not show any evidence of recurrent disease. She underwent a computed topography (CT) scan of the head, neck, and chest 1 week prior to her follow-up. CT scan results did not show any evidence of recurrent disease. The patient was reevaluated for her swallowing status by the SLP. The patient had gained 15 pounds since her last follow-up. She had maintained a completely oral diet through this period. She had no chest infections or pneumonia during this period of maintaining an oral diet. A clinical

evaluation of swallow function was performed by the SLP. Patient could tolerate all bolus consistencies presented during the evaluation without any signs of aspiration. Patient A continued to complain of xerostomia and needed a liquid wash with dryer consistencies. She did not have any instances of immediate or delayed cough with bolus presentations during the clinical evaluation of swallow function. Due to favorable results on her scans, clinical examination, and clinical swallow examination, removal of the PEG tube was recommended. A referral to the gastrointestinal surgeon was subsequently made for PEG tube removal.

SUMMARY OF CARE

Patient A had an ideal outcome from a disease and rehabilitative perspective. A major determinant in her favorable postoperative outcome was that Patient A was a candidate for TORS. Transoral robotic surgery for oropharyngeal squamous cell carcinoma (OPSCC) has been gaining popularity in the past few years. Advantages of TORS over traditional open surgery include less blood loss during surgery, fewer incidences of tracheostomy placement, faster return to functional swallowing, and less need for adjuvant therapy, depending on the stage of the tumor (Bhayani et al., 2010; Iseli et al., 2009). Studies have shown that TORS is effective in achieving locoregional control which can reduce the required postradiation dose or negate the need for adjuvant therapy altogether (Bhayani et al., 2010). The long-term effects of high-dose radiation therapy on swallow function are well established in the literature, and the possibility of avoiding adjuvant therapy has significant positive effects on swallowing-related quality of life. (Murphy & Gilbert, 2009; Rosenthal, Lewin, & Eisbruch, 2006).

Another determinant in Patient A's maintenance of swallowing function was her commitment to postoperative and peri-RT rehabilitation. Common post-RT swallowing deficits include decreased base of tongue retraction resulting in reduced bolus propulsion into the pharynx, and decreased laryngeal elevation resulting in residue in the valleculae and the pyriform sinus after the swallow. Patients also show decreased pharyngeal contraction that results in bolus residue in the pharynx after the swallow, which consequently reduces the effectiveness of bolus propulsion into the esophagus (Kotz et al., 2012). Swallowing exercises are started with the intent to improve range of motion of the swallowing structures, resulting in maintenance of oral feeding and discontinuation of feeding via PEG tubes at the earliest (Kotz et al., 2012; Lazarus et al., 1993; Lazarus et al., 2002; Logemann, Pauloski, Rademaker, & Colangelo, 1997). Patient A did not miss a single session of dysphagia therapy and maintained a log of her daily exercise performance. Patient A was intrinsically motivated to maintain her nutritional and swallow status that in the end proved effective. Maintaining a near-normal swallow status has significant positive implications on one's quality of life, especially when patients are coping and struggling with not just the diagnosis of cancer, but treatment-related morbidity as well.

REFLECTION AND ANALYSIS FOR FURTHER STUDY

1. What clinical indicators may provide insight into which patients will be compliant with swallow therapy versus patients who will not?
2. Create a brief description of less invasive (e.g., TORS) versus traditional surgical approaches for head and neck cancer including overview of the procedures, risks, benefits, and so on?
3. What questions would you offer to a patient in order to gain a comprehensive understanding of his or her ability to make an informed decision pertaining to the treatment plan?

REFERENCES

Bhayani, M. K., Holsinger, F. C., & Lai, S. Y. (2010). A shifting paradigm for patients with head and neck cancer: Trans-oral robotic surgery (TORS). *Oncology (Williston Park), 24*(11), 1010–1015.

Greene, F. L. (2002). *AJCC cancer staging manual* (Vol. 1). Berlin, Germany: Springer Science & Business Media.

Iseli, T. A., Kulbersh, B. D., Iseli, C. E., Carroll, W. R., Rosenthal, E. L., & Magnuson, J. S. (2009). Functional outcomes after transoral robotic surgery for head and neck cancer. *Otolaryngology-Head and Neck Surgery, 141*(2), 166–171. doi:10.1016/j.otohns.2009.05.014

Kamstra, J. I., Roodenburg, J. L. N., Beurskens, C. H. G., Reintsema, H., & Dijkstra, P. U. (2013). TheraBite exercises to treat trismus secondary to head and neck cancer. *Supportive Care in Cancer, 21*(4), 951–957.

Kaplan, M. J., & Damrose, E. J. (2010). Transoral robotic surgery (TORS): The natural evolution of endoscopic head and neck surgery. *Oncology (Williston Park), 24*(11), 1022, 1025, 1030.

Kotz, T., Federman, A. D., Kao, J., Milman, L., Packer, S., Lopez-Prieto, C., & Genden, E. M. (2012). Prophylactic swallowing exercises in patients with head and neck cancer undergoing chemoradiation: A randomized trial. *Archives of Otolaryngology-Head and Neck Surgery, 138*(4), 376–382.

Lazarus, C., Logemann, J. A., & Gibbons, P. (1993). Effects of maneuvers on swallowing function in a dysphagic oral cancer patient. *Head & Neck, 15*(5), 419–424.

Lazarus, C., Logemann, J. A., Song, C. W., Rademaker, A. W., & Kahrilas, P. J. (2002). Effects of voluntary maneuvers on tongue base function for swallowing. *Folia Phoniatrica et Logopaedica, 54*(4), 171–176. doi:10.1159/000063192

Lewis, Jr., J. S., Thorstad, W. L., Chernock, R. D., Haughey, B. H., Yip, J. H., Zhang, Q., & El-Mofty, S. K. (2010). p16 positive oropharyngeal squamous cell carcinoma: An entity with a favorable prognosis regardless of tumor HPV status. *American Journal of Surgical Pathology, 34*(8), 1088–1096.

Logemann, J. A. (1998). The evaluation and treatment of swallowing disorders. *Current Opinion in Otolaryngology and Head and Neck Surgery, 6*(6), 395–400.

Logemann, J. A., Pauloski, B. R., Rademaker, A. W., & Colangelo, L. A. (1997). Super-supraglottic swallow in irradiated head and neck cancer patients. *Head & Neck, 19*(6), 535–540.

Murphy, B. A., & Gilbert, J. (2009). Dysphagia in head and neck cancer patients treated with radiation: Assessment, sequelae, and rehabilitation. *Seminars In Radiation Oncology, 19*(Head and Neck Cancer), 35–42. doi:10.1016/j.semradonc.2008.09.007

Rosenbek, J. C., Robbins, J. A., Roecker, E. B., Coyle, J. L., & Wood, J. L. (1996). A penetration-aspiration scale. *Dysphagia, 11*(2), 93–98.

Rosenthal, D. I., Lewin, J. S., & Eisbruch, A. (2006). Prevention and treatment of dysphagia and aspiration after chemoradiation for head and neck cancer. *Journal of Clinical Oncology, 24*(17), 2636–2643.

7

Adenoid Cystic Carcinoma of the Base of Tongue

Annette H. May and Elizabeth Feldman

INTRODUCTION

Mr. D was 51 years of age at the time of diagnosis of T4N2c adenoid cystic carcinoma of the left base of tongue. Adenoid cystic carcinoma is a rare epithelial tumor of salivary gland origin. It accounts for 1% to 4% of all head and neck area malignancies. Adenoid cystic carcinoma presents a widespread age distribution but is most common in those over 55 years of age and more common among women than men with little known regarding etiology. It is typically a slow-growing malignancy but often with perineural invasion, local recurrence, and delayed onset of distant metastasis (Li, Xu, Zhao, El-Naggar, & Sturgis, 2012; Soares, Carreiro Filho, Costa, Vieira, & Alves, 2008).

HISTORY AT PRESENTATION

The patient was working full time as a vice president of information technology and services at a bank. He had a remote history of smoking tobacco for approximately 1 year, 12 years prior to diagnosis. He reported consuming one to two alcoholic beverages per week which consisted of wine and beer. He reported a family history of lung cancer (father), breast cancer (paternal aunt), and pancreatic can-

cer (maternal uncle). He also reported exposure to the air pollution in the aftermath of the 9/11 World Trade Center attacks.

The patient reported complaints of sore throat, dysphagia, odynophagia, hoarseness in the morning, globus sensation, and chronic fatigue for approximately 4 years prior to the cancer diagnosis. He was initially treated with proton pump inhibitors for gastroesophageal reflux, antibiotics for presumed sinusitis, and was prescribed a continuous positive airway pressure (CPAP) mask due to suspected obstructive sleep apnea. At the time of diagnosis, he reported pain as 4/10. He denied epistaxis, otalgia, trismus, hemoptysis, airway obstruction, facial paresthesia, dysarthria, or visual changes at the time of initial presentation. However, he began to experience bilateral otalgia, dysarthria, and weight loss of 10 pounds in the 3-month period between initial presentation and start of treatment.

Reported other past medical and surgical history included Barrett's esophagus, hypertension, obstructive sleep apnea, and correction of a deviated septum.

DIAGNOSTIC WORKUP

The patient was initially evaluated by an otolaryngologist who noted a lesion at the tongue base on endoscopic exam. A noncontrast computed tomography (CT) scan of the neck was ordered, revealing a 2.7 × 2.2 cm low-density soft tissue lesion of the tongue. He was referred to a tertiary care cancer center for further workup that included positron emission tomography (PET)/IV contrast CT, magnetic resonance imaging (MRI), and direct laryngoscopy with biopsy. Direct laryngoscopy noted only fullness in the left base of tongue. Multiple biopsies were taken in this area, revealing adenoid cystic carcinoma with perineural invasion. PET/CT (Figure 7–1) demonstrated a 3.34 × 2.04 cm mass in the left base of tongue with standardized uptake value (SUV) of 3.64, intermediate adenopathy in the left neck at Level IIA with the largest lymph node measuring 2.8 cm with only minimal fluorodeoxyglucose (FDG) uptake, maximum SUV of 1.8. An additional left Level IB lymph node was seen measuring 2.4 × 1.3 with relatively low FDG uptake, maximum SUV of 2.5. A right-sided lymph node was also noted measuring 2.4 × 1.5 with a maximum SUV of 2.7. MRI of the brain, face, orbits, and neck demonstrated a large lobulated mass involving the base of tongue, narrowing the airway, 5.9 cm width, up to 5.7 cm cephalad caudad dimension, and 5.9 cm anterior-posterior dimension. Irregular lobulated margins were noted with the mass bulging eccentrically inferiorly on the left. The mass was noted to course from the anterior to posterior aspect of the tongue. Bilateral Level IIA lymph nodes were noted measuring 17 mm cross section on the right and 16 mm on the left. Scattered subcentimeter nonspecific Level III and Level IV lymph nodes were noted. Normal thyroid, salivary, and larynx were found. No intracranial disease was found. A solitary 9 mm indeterminate lung nodule in the left lower lobe was noted on chest CT. This was not FDG avid on PET.

Once the diagnosis was confirmed, the patient was referred for multidisciplinary consults, which included radiation oncology, medical oncology, speech pathology, dental oncology/maxillofacial prosthodontics, and the dietitian. Multidisciplinary cancer conference recommendation for treatment was for surgery followed by adjuvant radiation therapy with or without chemotherapy. The lung nodule was not biopsied prior to treatment, and a decision was made instead to monitor the node as results would not alter the treatment plan for the primary tumor. The patient was not found to have any significant comorbidities that would present as potential barriers to the recommended treatment plan.

Additional Pretreatment Evaluation

The patient was evaluated by speech pathology at time of diagnosis. Speech and voice were grossly within normal limits with 100% intelligibility. The patient reported dysphagia mainly restricted to solid foods, complaining of a sticking sensation high in the throat. He denied coughing with liquids. He was tolerating a regular diet despite dysphagia complaints without weight loss and no reported difficulty swallowing pills. Modified barium swallow (Video 7–1) was performed and noted functional oral preparatory and oral phases of the swallow and moderate pharyngeal dysphagia. The patient was noted to have fullness at the base of tongue consistent with his lesion site, significantly reduced base of tongue propulsion, incomplete epiglottic deflection, and reduced anterior hyolaryngeal excursion. Deficits yielded trace laryngeal penetration of thin liquids during the swallow, overall moderate residue in the right vallecula, greater with thicker consistencies, and trace-mild residue in the pyriform sinuses. Laryngeal penetration ultimately cleared with multiple independent swallows without aspiration. Postural strategies, including a right head turn and chin tuck were ineffective in reducing pharyngeal residue. Left head turn reduced pharyngeal residue slightly. Liquid wash was effective to clear most residue. Despite increasing pharyngeal residue with solids versus liquids, the barium tablet passed through the pharynx and cervical esophagus without delay. Recommendations included continuation of a regular diet with liquid wash to follow purees/solids and use of a left head turn to assist in clearance of residue.

The patient was also referred for pretreatment dental and nutrition evaluations. However, he opted to be seen for a second opinion at another tertiary care cancer center before these evaluations could be performed. Recommendations from the site of the second opinion also were for surgery followed by adjuvant radiation with or without chemotherapy.

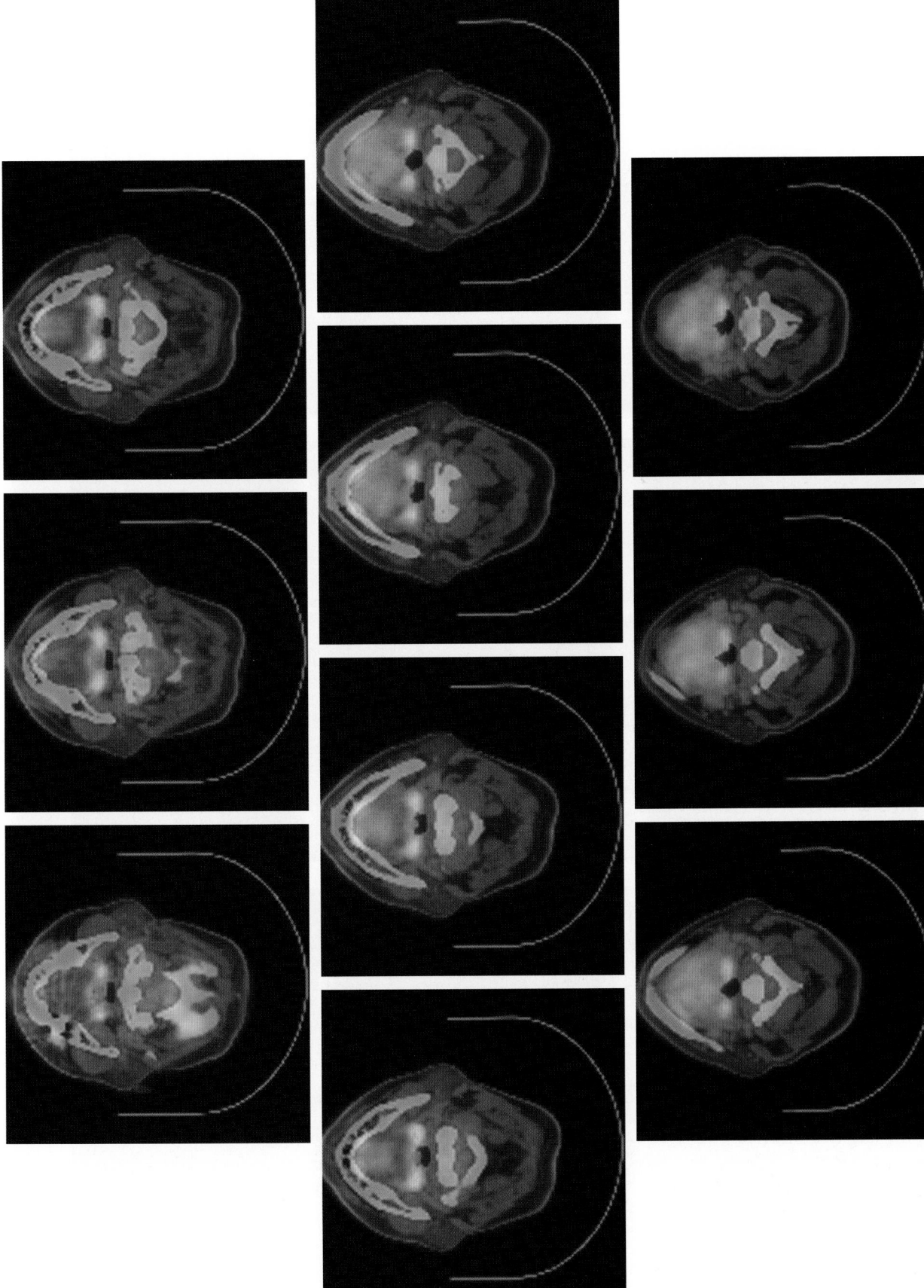

A

Figure 7–1. A. Pretreatment PET/CT fused axial images. *continues*

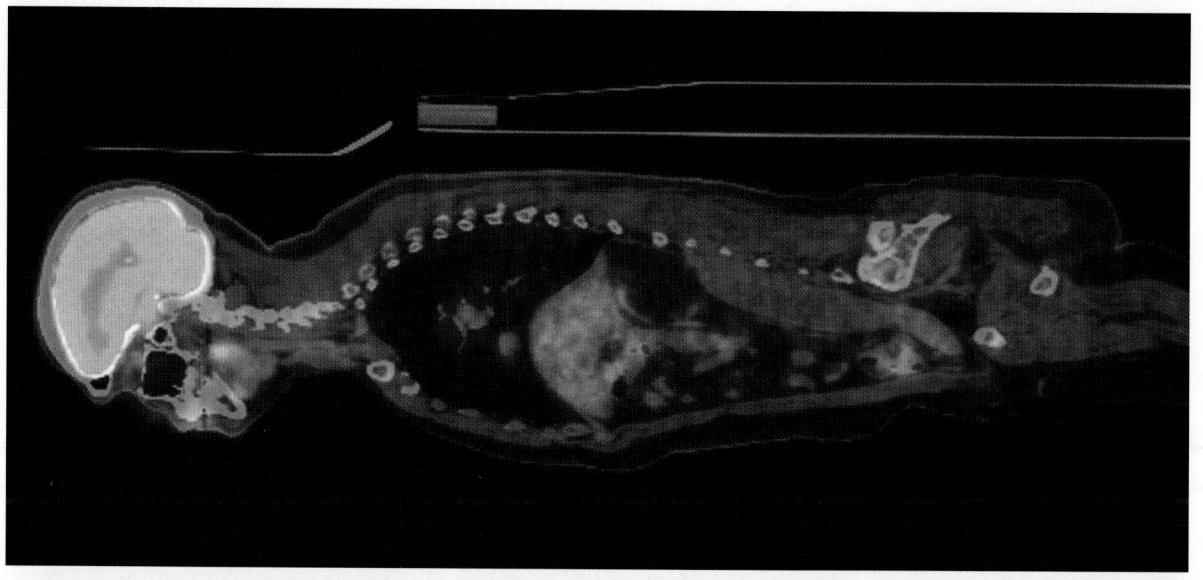

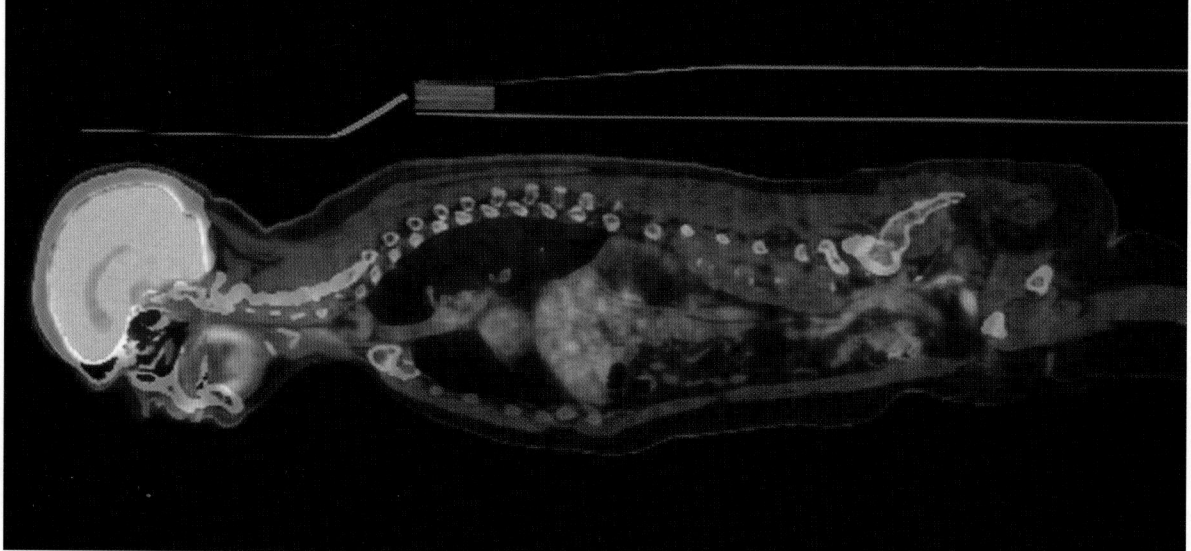

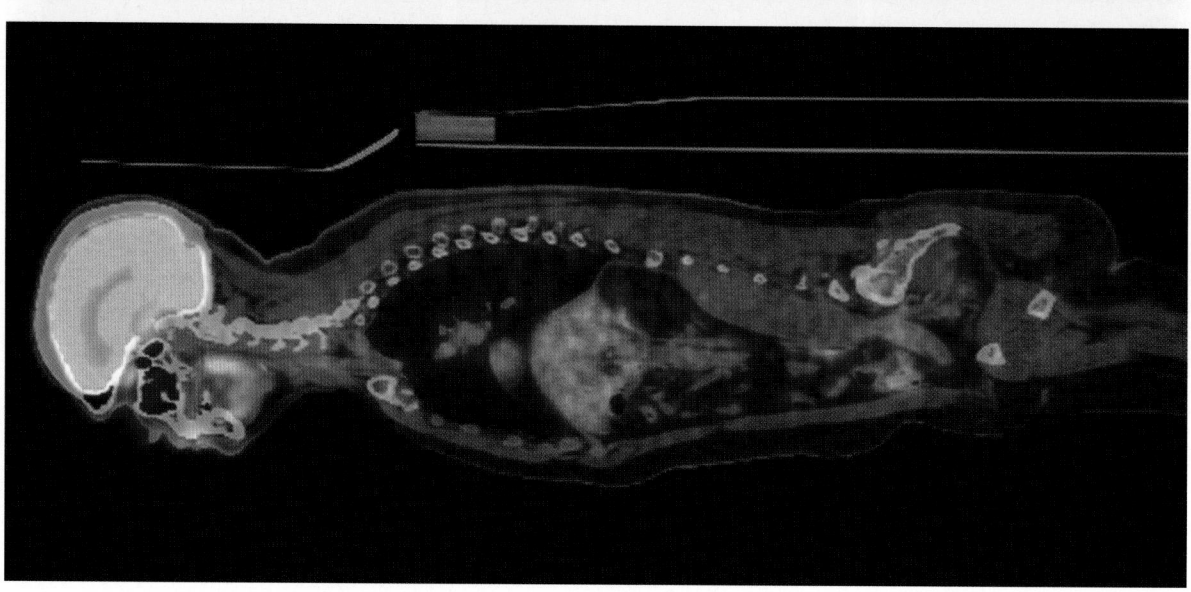

B

Figure 7–1. *continued* **B.** Pretreatment PET/CT fused sagittal images.

He opted to have surgery at the site of his second opinion and return to the initial site for adjuvant treatment, at which point the remaining consults were carried out postoperatively.

TREATMENT

Surgery

Surgical resection included total glossectomy, bilateral neck dissections Levels I, II, and III, rectus abdominis myocutaneous free tissue transfer to the neck, pharyngoesophageal repair, anterior and lateral vestibuloplasty, tracheostomy, and nasogastric tube placement. Surgical findings reported a large base of tongue tumor involving the entire base of tongue to the lateral edges, grossly free of the hyoid and mandible, bilateral hypoglossal nerves identified and involved with tumor and sacrificed, bilateral lingual nerves sacrificed for tumor resection, and grossly suspicious lymph nodes in Level II bilaterally. Final pathology reported adenoid cystic carcinoma with predominant cribriform pattern of minor salivary glands. The tumor measured 5.8 cm in greatest dimension, invading the skeletal muscle of the tongue with extensive perineural invasion and suspected vascular invasion with 2/17 lymph nodes containing metastatic disease. Initial margins were positive for adenoid cystic carcinoma with additional excision of margins ultimately showing no residual tumor.

Acute Postoperative Course

The patient was hospitalized for approximately 3 weeks postoperatively. He underwent placement of a percutaneous endoscopic gastrostomy (PEG) tube prior to discharge from the hospital as he was initially only able to take small amounts of water orally (2 ounces per day) for therapeutic purposes with use of a supraglottic swallow after initial clinical swallow evaluation by a speech pathologist once cleared by his surgeon for oral intake. The tracheostomy was removed prior to discharge from the hospital. The patient was healing well and taking 100% nutrition via PEG.

Dental Diagnostic Workup

The patient was seen for a preradiation therapy evaluation postoperatively. The extraoral examination revealed a patient who had lymphedema at the chin and neck levels. His maximum vertical oral opening (VO) was 25 mm measured from tooth #9 to #24. The patient's saliva was frothy and thick at the time of the initial examination. He had a full complement of teeth. The native tongue was absent and reconstructed with a flap. The patient's oral hygiene was acceptable. He had multiple dental fillings and crowns. There was no decay noted. The patient had erupted wisdom teeth in sites #16 and #17. The panoramic radiograph revealed an impacted wisdom tooth in site #32. No pathology was noted on the panorex imaging. Bitewing radiographs were taken of the posterior premolars and molars with no decay noted. The patient reported that he saw his dentist on a regular basis.

The patient was recommended to have his wisdom teeth extracted due to high risk of dental decay leading to future extractions after radiation therapy which may pose the complication of osteoradionecrosis (Toth, Chambers, & Fleming, 1996). The patient also had trismus, and this was a concern for the inability of proper oral care coupled with high caries risk after radiation therapy. The patient was recommended to have trismus therapy. He was placed on a fluoride protocol that consisted of fluoride carriers and the use of 1.1% neutral sodium fluoride daily. The patient was also referred for lymphedema therapy. He was prescribed Caphosol oral rinse for use during chemoradiation therapy. The radiation oncologist had also prescribed the use of a mouth-opening tongue-depressing radiation stent to be used during radiation therapy that was customized and fabricated for the patient.

Postoperative Counseling

The patient was referred to the patient/family counselor due to the nature of surgery, upcoming adjuvant treatment, and multidisciplinary approach to patient care. He was seen in conjunction with his significant other. His significant other reported that the patient became frustrated at times with being unable to eat and drink normally, especially when he was around other people doing so. His significant other also reported that it appeared the patient became frustrated when people were unable to understand him. The patient reported some anxiety on days of doctor's appointments, but reported sleeping well and feeling that he was coping well. The patient was provided with supportive and psychoeducational counseling regarding common emotional and psychological responses to being diagnosed with head and neck cancer.

Postoperative Speech Pathology Intervention

Clinical examination by speech pathology postoperatively was notable for moderate trismus at 25-mm VO (Stubblefield, 2011), moderate submandibular lymphedema, bilateral marginal mandibular nerve palsy, well-healed intraoral flap, symmetric soft palate elevation, bilateral contraction of visible lateral pharyngeal walls upon forceful voicing, and severe dysarthria consistent with total glossectomy defect. Despite level of dysarthria, the patient was independently using a slower rate of speech and exaggerated articulatory compensations with fair intelligibility. He was noted to have an aggressive cough with small volumes of water. He was initially instructed on passive jaw range of motion exercises as well as gentle stretching with tongue blades and then provided a prescription from the dental oncologist/maxillofacial prosthodontist for a Dynasplint to address trismus (Buchbinder, Currivan, Kaplan, & Urken, 1993; Cohen, Deschler, Walsh, & Hayden, 2005; Dijkstra, Sterken, Pater, Spijkervet, & Roodenburg, 2007. He was reinstructed on the supraglottic swallow and demonstrated no overt clinical indicators of aspiration with small trials of water after practice. He was referred to a lymphedema therapist to evaluate and treat submandibular lymphedema but was only able to tolerate this treatment for a limited amount of time prior to onset of acute radiation side effects. It was felt that the patient may benefit from a palatal augmentation prosthesis, but with his level of trismus and anticipation of acute radiation effects, this was deferred initially.

 Modified barium swallow (Video 7–2) was performed 1 week following the clinical exam and was notable for severe oral dysphagia and moderate pharyngeal dysphagia. The patient was noted to have poor oral control/manipulation due to absence of the tongue. This resulted in premature spillage to the pharynx. Additionally, the patient's flap reconstruction was still quite bulky at the level of the oropharynx, filling the valleculae, so that premature spillage was directly into the laryngeal vestibule. The patient was noted to have reduced anterior hyolaryngeal elevation with reduced upper esophageal sphincter (UES) opening. He was unable to use adaptive equipment effectively to bypass the oral phase due to a hyperactive gag reflex. Deficits yielded penetration of liquids prior to and during the swallow as well as moderate to gross residue in the pyriform sinuses following the swallow. Deficits also yielded significant oral residue, especially with pureed consistencies. Despite this, the patient effectively used an airway protection strategy with liquids and in combination with a left head turn, he was able to clear the pharynx of the majority of residue and avoid aspiration as long as liquids were in isolation. Dysphagia therapy was recommended with a short-term goal to initiate at least partial oral nutrition of liquids with effective airway protection strategies prior to beginning adjuvant radiation treatment due to the concern that the patient may have greater difficulty with recovery of function if gains were not made prior to onset of acute radiation effects. Long-term goal of the patient was to resume full oral nutrition. Goals were targeted initially as follows.

Initiating Oral Trials

Oral trials were initiated with repetitive practice of thin and thick liquids. Trials started with small volumes (5–10 cc) focusing on consistent use of a breath hold, throat clear/cough, and re-swallow (modified supraglottic swallow) for airway protection. He was instructed to use a slight posterior head tilt to assist in bolus transit. Multiple swallows per bolus while using a left head turn was implemented to clear residue through the pharynx. He learned to clear oral residue by using a "slurp/swallow" after all swallows to clear pharyngeal residue. Once the patient demonstrated these techniques consistently and without overt indicators of aspiration, we slowly advanced the volume per trial until he was able to take large consecutive swallows of both thin and thick liquid, thereby increasing efficiency of oral intake and allowing him to increase oral nutrition. In addition to taking liquid nutritional supplements, he was provided a recipe book for ideas to increase variety of oral nutrition on a liquid diet. Puree trials were also introduced once he was consistently using airway protection strategies with liquids, as he required a liquid wash to clear puree residue from the oral cavity and pharynx. Prior to initiating adjuvant oncologic treatment, the patient was able to transition from taking only therapeutic trials of liquid to taking liquids in public, taking approximately 20% of his nutrition orally on a liquid diet, and taking therapeutic trials of purees consistently.

Desensitization of Gag Reflex

Those who have required surgical resection of more than 50% of the tongue most often require adaptive equipment to assist in bolus manipulation and transfer of solid foods to improve both oral control and efficiency of the oral preparatory and oral phases of the swallow. Solid foods that are not well masticated or the adaptive tools used to assist in bolus manipulation can often trigger a gag reflex. Initially a 20-cc syringe coupled with a shortened 20 French red rubber catheter (Figure 7–2) was used to place purees to the entrance of the oropharynx to bypass the oral cavity. The catheter alone without a bolus trial was slowly advanced posteriorly until the patient could tolerate the device in the oropharynx without a gag reflex before introducing any bolus trials. Once this

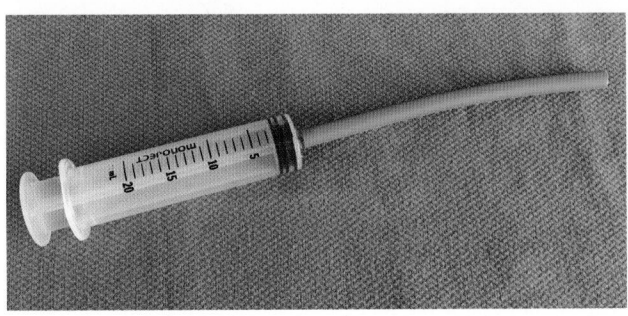

Figure 7–2. Example of 20-cc syringe coupled with a shortened 20 French red rubber catheter to assist in bypassing oral cavity for oral intake postglossectomy.

was accomplished, bolus trials began with small volumes of only 1 to 3 cc. Bolus size was slowly advanced as trials were tolerated without a gag reflex. Although the patient was also able to begin to take pureed trials using a liquid wash to clear the oral cavity instead of using the more cumbersome and socially awkward syringe/catheter, this technique was continued to focus on control of the gag reflex in anticipation of future solid food intake.

Swallowing Exercises

The patient was instructed on the Shaker exercise (Ohba, Yokoyama, Kojima, Fujimaki, Anzai, Komatsu, & Ikeda, 2014; Shaker et al., 1997), Mendelsohn maneuver repetitions (Hoffman et al., 2012; Lazarus, Logemann, Song, Rademaker, & Kahrilas, 2002), and effortful swallow repetitions (Hoffman et al., 2012; Lazarus et al., 2002). An exercise regimen was recommended three times daily at least 5 days per week. He demonstrated independent technique and maintained consistent compliance with this regimen prior to onset of adjuvant oncologic treatment.

Trismus

The patient began with passive jaw range of motion exercises and gentle stretching with tongue blades (Figure 7–3) working up to 30 min of stretching, three times daily. He was able to increase VO from his postoperative baseline of 25 mm, to 35 mm with 4 weeks of exercise. He was able to obtain the Dynasplint (Figure 7–4) after this period and transitioned to using this device in lieu of the tongue blades for 30 min, three times daily and was able to increase VO to 40 mm in an additional 2 weeks.

Speech

Direct intervention to improve speech intelligibility was not initially targeted during this period as the patient was independently using a slower rate of speech and exaggerated articulatory compensations with fair intelligibility without the need for augmentative communication methods. Speech goals were deferred initially in lieu of concentrating heavily on dysphagia and trismus rehabilitation (Duarte, Chhetri, Liu, Erman, & Wang, 2013).

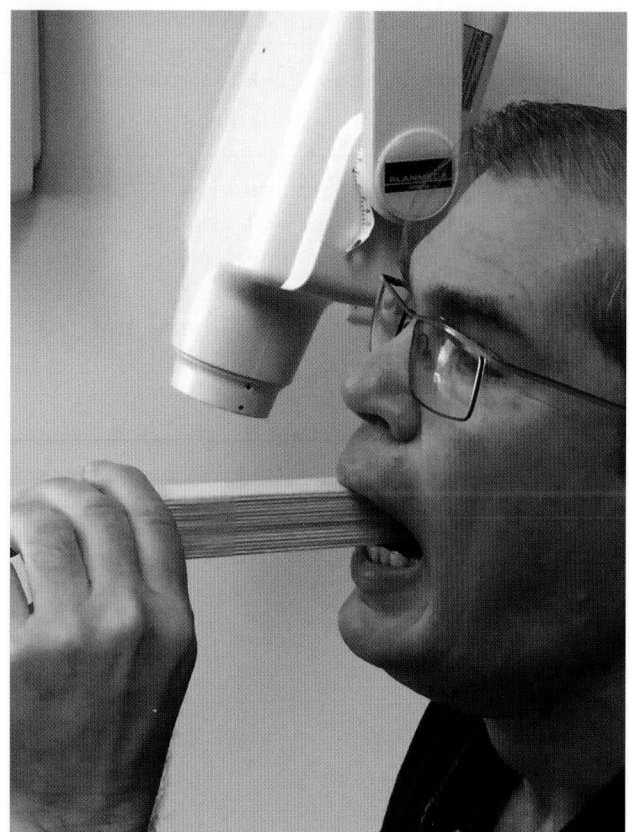
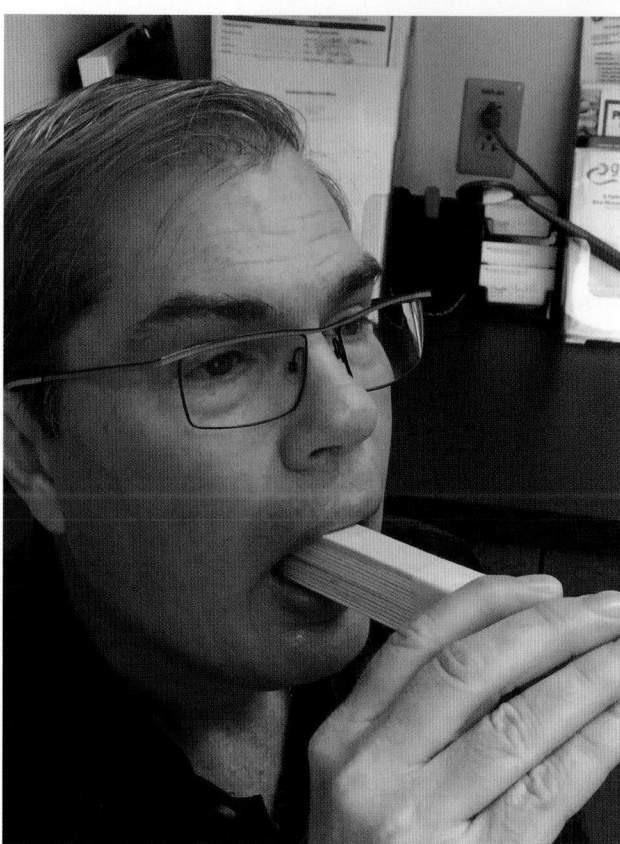

Figure 7–3. Example of patient using stacked tongue blades to address trismus.

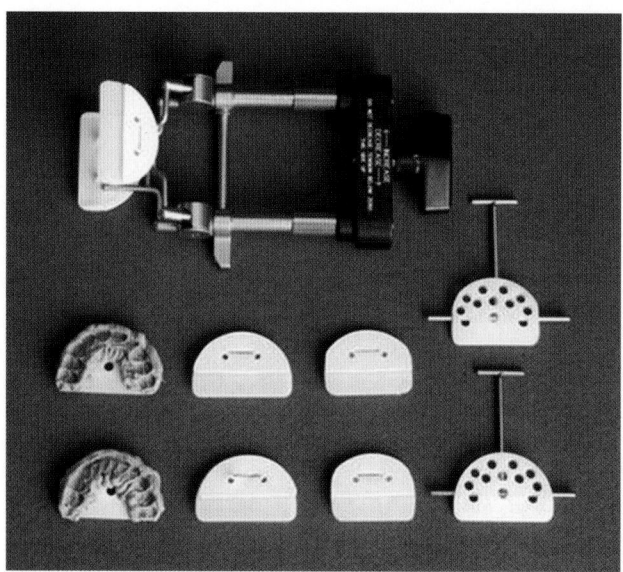

A

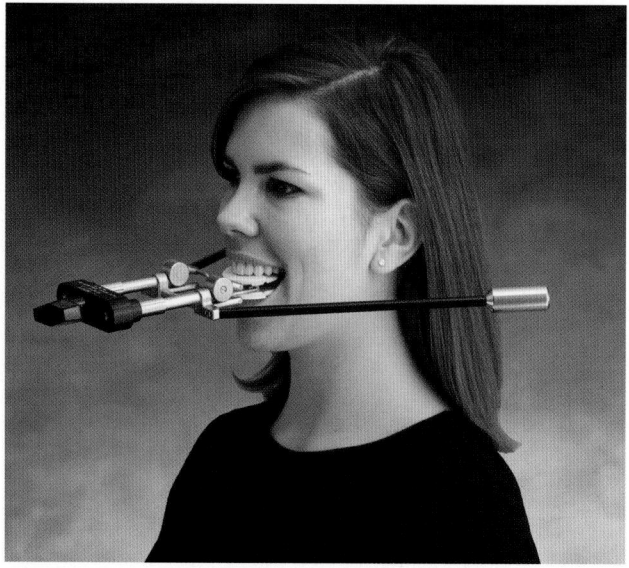

B

Figure 7–4. A. Dynasplint Trismus/TMD System; Jaw Dynasplint System with assorted mouthpieces. **B.** Dynasplint Treatment Positions; Jaw Dynsplint System with Counterbalance Bars. Dynasplint and Dynasplint Systems are registered trademarks of Dynasplint Systems, Inc. Reprinted with permission.

Adjuvant Chemotherapy and Radiation

Postoperatively, the patient's case was discussed again at a multidisciplinary cancer conference with review of final surgical pathology as well as presurgical diagnostics. The group recommendation was ultimately to offer the patient systemic adjuvant chemotherapy in conjunction with radiation therapy. Surgical resection is considered the standard of care for primary treatment of adenoid cystic carcinoma. Additionally, there is evidence to support adjuvant radiation therapy in the presence of perineural and vascular invasion. However, the role of chemotherapy for adenoid cystic carcinoma in adjuvant settings is not well defined. Recommendations were based on the data for squamous cell carcinoma, the patient's extensive disease, and younger age. Information on treatment options and evidence to support such options was discussed in detail with the patient and his significant other. Ultimately, the patient decided to proceed with chemotherapy concurrently with radiation. Chemotherapy consisted of weekly low-dose cisplatin (63 mg; 30 mg/m^2) with a recommendation for six cycles. Intensity-modulated radiation therapy was employed on a tomotherapy platform to spare adjacent at-risk normal structures including, but not limited to the salivary glands and spinal cord. All treatment was delivered using 6 MV photons. The patient was initially treated to a total dose of 60 Gy in 2 Gy daily fractions to the high-risk area that included the operative bed and pathologically involved lymph node basins. The lower-risk neck was treated concurrently to a total dose of 54 Gy in 30 fractions. Following the initial phase of treatment, the patient underwent a 6 Gy boost in three fractions using intensity-modulated radiation delivered to the area of margin positivity from the main tumor specimen in the base of tongue.

Overall, the patient tolerated the treatment well with anticipated acute side effects. He was prophylactically treated for nausea with IV fluids and antiemetics prior to each cisplatin infusion and additionally as needed. He reported mild nausea, dysgeusia, xerostomia, thick secretions, moderate fatigue, and neck stiffness and swelling. Toward the end of treatment, when the patient reached 60 Gy of radiation, he began to develop mucositis with associated oral and oropharyngeal pain. This was treated with Magic Mouthwash (lidocaine viscous/Benadryl elixir/Mylanta topical rinse) and an extended-release opioid. There was no compromise to the airway. The patient had diffuse dry desquamation of the skin throughout the treatment field for which he used a fragrance-free, glycerin-based topical ointment to reduce discomfort and promote healing. The patient opted to have his last dose of chemotherapy held due to mild tinnitus. The patient was reevaluated by dental oncology and found to have Grade 3 mucositis. He was encouraged to continue frequent use of Caphosol (a supersaturated calcium phosphate rinse), baking soda/salt rinses, as well as frequent oral care for the next 2 months of recovery.

Speech Pathology Intervention/ Goals During Chemoradiation

Goal #1: *Maintain Airway Protection Strategies*

- The use of an airway protection strategy was evaluated at each follow-up session during adjuvant treatment with whatever consistency the patient was still able to tolerate.
- Re-instruction on supraglottic swallow was required toward end of radiation.

Goal #2: *Maintain at Least Therapeutic Oral Intake of Liquids*

- Therapeutic purees and thicker liquids were discontinued midway through adjuvant treatment due to pain.
- Via PEG, 100% nutrition resumed.
- Between 30 and 60 ounces of thin liquid daily were continued for therapeutic purposes (Krisciunas, Sokoloff, Stepas, & Langmore, 2012) and for partial relief of xerostomia.

Goal #3: *Reinforce Exercise Program*

- The patient was still compliant and used adequate technique, but with reduced frequency. The patient required encouragement at each session to continue (Duarte et al., 2013).

- A 3-mm decrease in VO was noted midway through adjuvant treatment and an overall 6-mm decline was noted by treatment completion (34-mm VO).

Goal #4: Secretion Management

- The patient had difficulty expectorating thickened secretions due to surgically absent tongue.
- Warm liquids were used to assist in mobilizing secretions.
- Oral care (brushing, flossing, fluoride, salt/baking soda rinses, Caphosol) was reinforced.

Goal #5: More Active Focus on Speech

- No decline in speech was noted during adjuvant treatment, but the initial focus in therapy was swallowing to attempt to maximize function prior to the onset of radiation effects.
- Once swallowing was limited due to radiation effects, therapy goals targeted speech function.
- Intelligibility testing in preparation for palatal augmentation prosthesis was 50% in an unknown context with an unfamiliar listener with an audio-only recorded speech sample (Yorkston, Beukelman, & Traynor, 1984).
- Compensatory strategies were implemented.
- Plosive/fricative approximation was demonstrated.

POST TREATMENT

Lymphedema Therapy

The patient had moderate lymphedema throughout the jaw line, submandibular area, and into the neck with decreased range of motion in the neck and increased tightness after completion of adjuvant chemoradiation therapy. He received manual therapy that included manual lymph drainage to the head and neck area concentrating on the submandibular area and around the temporomandibular joint area. He was also seen for therapeutic exercise in the neck area to decrease fibrosis. He was prescribed a compression device for complete decongestive lymphedema therapy (Smith et al., 2015; Tacani et al., 2014). The patient achieved good initial response to therapy with a decrease in volume of lymphedema, decrease in neck stiffness, and increase in neck range of motion. He continued to perform home exercises with independent manual lymph drainage and range of motion exercises as well as ongoing use of the compression garment. He began to experience an increase in lymphedema again approximately 3 years following oncologic treatment (Figure 7–5) with decreased ability to control it on his own with his home program which began to affect his ability to turn his head while driving as well as ability to sustain a head-forward posture required for com-

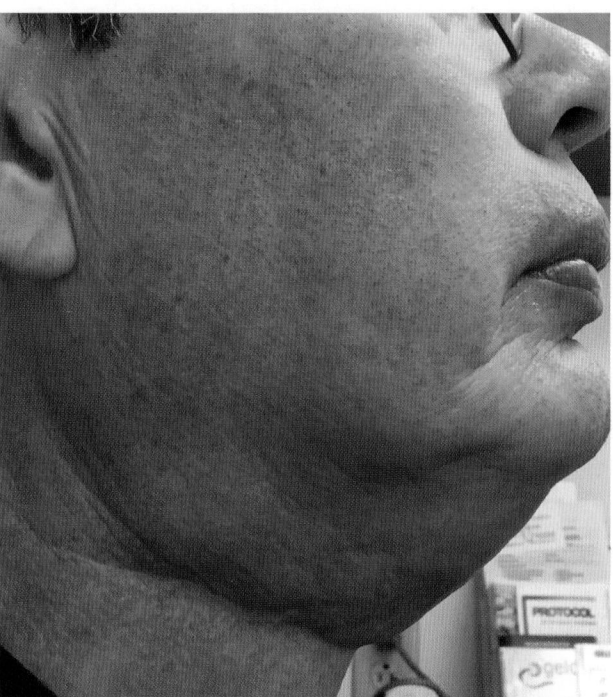

Figure 7–5. Residual chronic submental lymphedema.

puter work (career is in Information Technology). He returned for therapy approximately 1 year ago and continues to work with the lymphedema therapist to date on a more active maintenance program.

Speech Pathology Intervention

As acute side effects of chemoradiation began to subside (odynophagia, fatigue, dysgeusia, and thick secretions), the patient was able to resume regular dysphagia therapy approximately 1-month post treatment. He was also referred back to the maxillofacial prosthodontist for a palatal augmentation prosthesis to assist in both speech and swallow rehabilitation.

Goal #1: Regain Swallowing Status Prior to Onset of Adjuvant Treatment

- The patient resumed partial liquid nutrition.
- The patient resumed therapeutic puree trials.
- The patient advanced to three small meals of liquid/puree (50% of nutrition) and most hydration orally within 1 month of resuming more aggressive dysphagia therapy.

Goal #2: Wean From PEG

- The patient increased oral liquid nutrition (most efficient means of oral intake).
- The patient maintained oral nutrition/hydration on a full liquid diet without weight loss or respiratory complications by 4 months post treatment; PEG was removed.

Goal #3: Palatal Augmentation Prosthesis to Improve Speech/Swallowing

- Device was fit 3 months post treatment (see "Forming a Palatal Augmentation Prosthesis" below).
- Immediate improvements in resonance and articulatory approximations were noted with 80% on intelligibility testing (Yorkston et al., 1984), an increase of 30%.

- The patient noted a gag reflex with prosthesis in place when attempting to swallow.
- Desensitization to the prosthesis during swallowing was attempted with
  ○ dry swallows;
  ○ water trials, slowing increasing volume per bolus
  ○ thick liquids and purees.

Goal #4: Oral Intake of Solids

- Repeat modified barium swallow (Video 7–3) results
  ○ moderate/severe oral dysphagia and severe pharyngeal dysphagia;
  ○ more effective and efficient use of compensatory strategies for liquids and purees;
  ○ stable airway protection (intermittent trace aspiration, but effective throat clear/cough to clear);
  ○ improved pharyngeal contraction;
  ○ ability to protect the airway during "swishing"; technique in future therapy to assist in oral residue clearance; and
  ○ limited pharyngeal recesses with bulk of flap and postradiation pharyngeal/laryngeal edema; concern for obstruction of solids if not well masticated.
- Therapy-targeted oral manipulation/mastication of solids with adaptive equipment and liquid wash with strict compliance with airway protection strategy as follows:
  ○ slight head-forward posture during mastication and anterior mastication to prevent early posterior spillage;
  ○ plastic chopstick or baby spoon (Figure 7–6) to sweep food to teeth when lost to flap and to push bolus posteriorly after mastication;
  ○ liquid wash with airway protection strategy to clear oral cavity of residue; and
  ○ palatal augmentation prosthesis to assist in bolus formation and oral transfer.

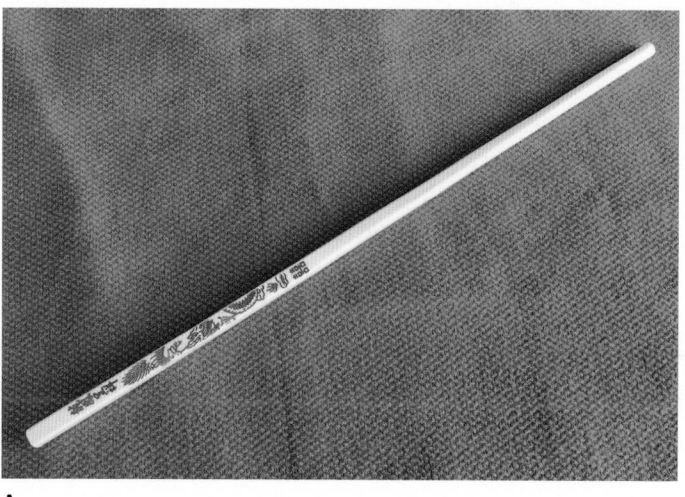
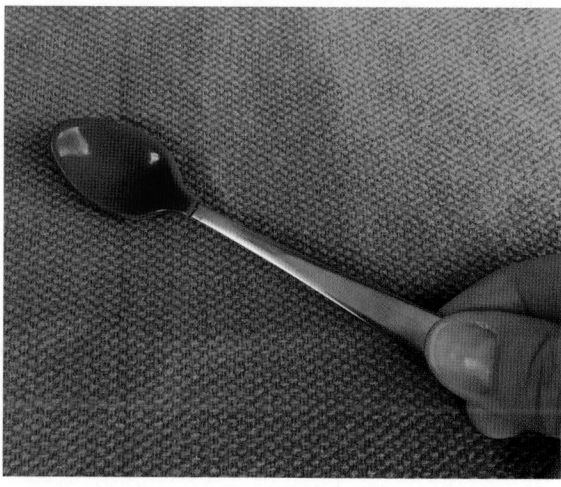

A   **B**

Figure 7–6. A. Plastic chopstick used to assist in bolus manipulation and oral transfer of solid foods postglossectomy. **B.** Rubber-coated baby spoon used to assist in bolus manipulation and oral transfer of solid foods postglossectomy.

Forming a Palatal Augmentation Prosthesis (Figure 7–7)

The palatal augmentation prosthesis was contoured to accommodate the acquired range of motion of the reconstructed tongue flap. The prosthesis consisted of a dental baseplate that clasped onto natural teeth, similar to a dental retainer. This was to be worn in the maxillary arch. After fitting the baseplate, the prosthodontist added dental wax to the palatal portion of the baseplate to conform to the flap during speech while being simultaneously evaluated by the speech pathologist. Depending on the sounds articulated with more or less clarity, the prosthesis was contoured and shaped to achieve the optimal flap to prosthesis contact and control of air escape. A pressure-indicating paste was also used to reveal areas of the flap contact and its absence during speaking and swallowing to assist in adjustment. Speed with which the patient initiated the swallow, decrease in extraneous head movements during the swallow, pooling of bolus material in the mouth, and decrease in indicators of aspiration were all factors considered during simultaneous clinical swallow evaluation by the speech pathologist for evaluation of the palatal augmentation prosthesis.

Once the wax augmentation was complete and the prosthesis was considered optimal by the speech pathologist and the prosthodontist, the wax was changed by the dental laboratory procedures to a prosthesis made of acrylic material and later delivered to the patient. The palatal augmentation prosthesis can become quite bulky and heavy, and these effects were lessened by hollowing out the prosthesis. This reduced stress to the dentition, providing more comfort for the patient. After the prosthesis was delivered to the patient, the patient initiated speech and swallowing therapy to maximize effectiveness of the prosthesis (Marunick & Tselios, 2004; Robbins, Bowman, & Jacob, 1987).

Long-Term Speech Pathology Intervention

Solid food intake was a long-term goal for the patient. He initially demonstrated a significant gag reflex with the posterior transfer of solids using either a chopstick or liquid wash. Upon oral exam, it was noted that his intraoral flap was less bulky on the right side. This prompted consideration of transferring the bolus to the right side of the oral cavity before transferring to the pharynx to allow

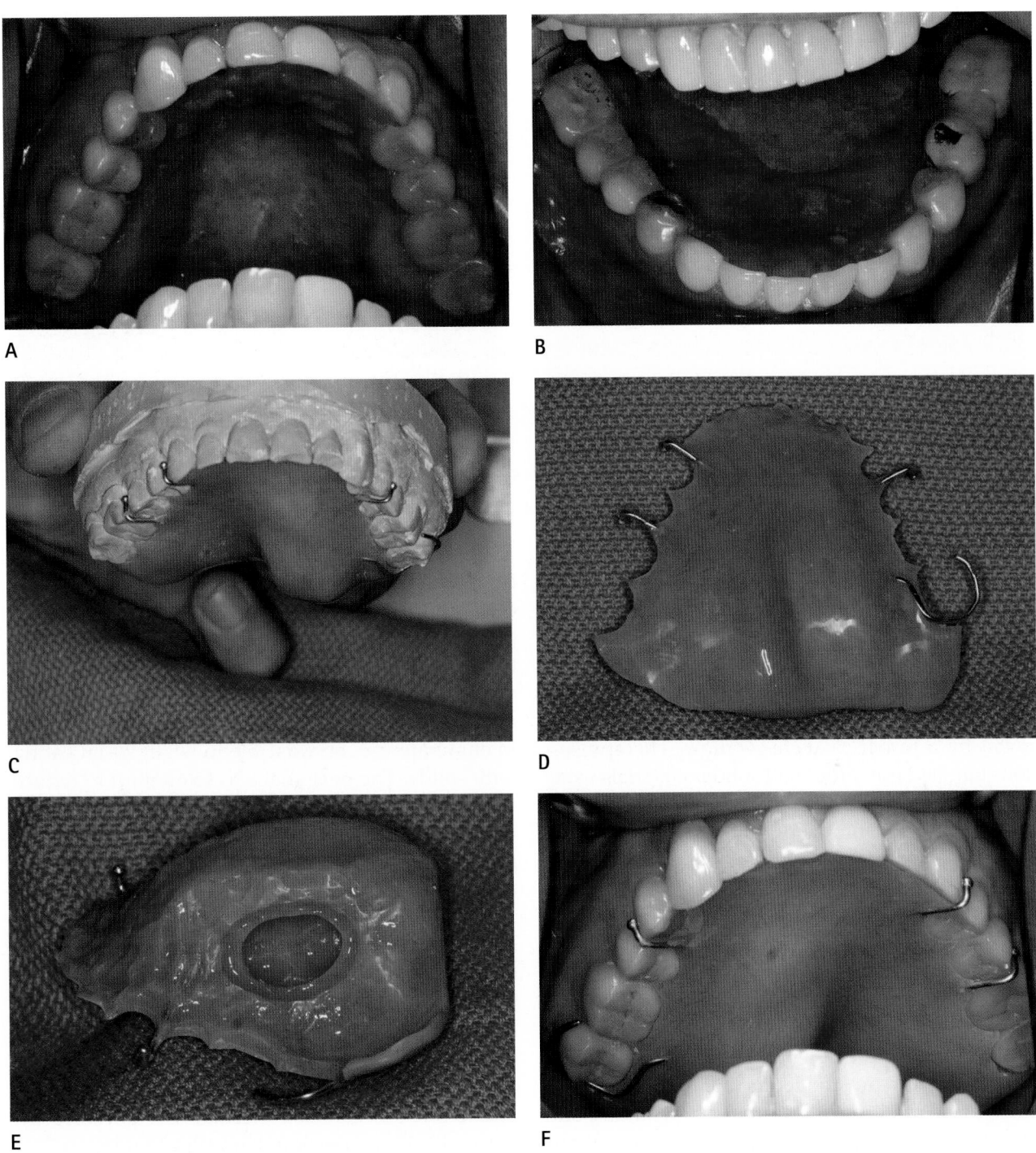

Figure 7–7. **A.** Mirror image of the maxillary arch. **B.** Mirror image of mandibular arch, flap reconstruction of the resected tongue. **C.** The original palatal augmentation prosthesis on the working cast model. **D.** Original palatal augmentation prosthesis. **E.** Hollowing of original palatal augmentation prosthesis to make it light. **F.** Mirror image of the original palatal augmentation prosthesis within the oral cavity. *continues*

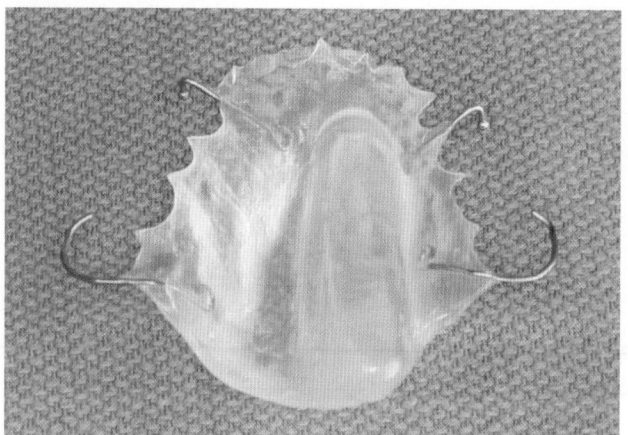

G

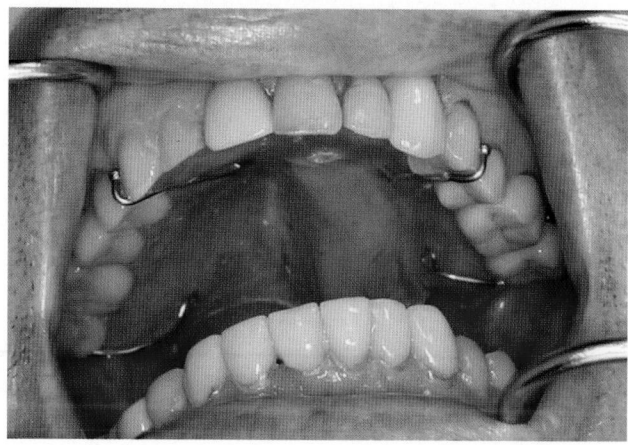

H

Figure 7–7. *continued* **G.** Current palatal augmentation prosthesis. **H.** Current palatal augmentation prosthesis within the oral cavity.

more room for the bolus transfer. This strategy was effective in eliminating his gag reflex on most solids. Once the patient was able to transfer solids to the right oral cavity, he was able to use a liquid wash, incorporating a breath hold, to transfer this to the pharynx, then swallowing multiple times followed by a throat clear/re-swallow. Therapy sessions targeted numerous soft solid bolus trials using this technique, initially starting with small bites of solid with large volume of liquid wash and using a mirror to monitor both placement and check for adequate mastication before moving the bolus posteriorly. Over time, the patient found it more comfortable and efficient to switch from using a plastic chopstick to a rubber-coated baby spoon for bolus manipulation. He was then able to learn to use the bulk of his palatal augmentation prosthesis to assist in "mashing" the food on the side where his flap was more bulky. The prosthodontist added more bulk to the left side of his prosthesis to assist with this, and this also improved his articulatory approximations for speech. The initial volume of liquid he required to clear a solid bolus was quite large (2–3 ounces per bite), resulting in early satiety. Additionally, mastication was inefficient (2 min for one small bolus). He therefore initially ate only small quantities of solids as he had to make sure he was taking enough cal-

ories from liquids/purees to continue to maintain oral nutrition. The patient developed a consistent pattern with this technique in 2 weeks and was able to discontinue use of the mirror to monitor as well as reduce mastication time to 20 to 30 s. As use of the mirror was limiting to social eating, once he was able to eliminate use, he was able to begin social eating with solids. The next goal was to attempt to reduce the amount of liquid required to follow a solid. This was accomplished by using a small amount of liquid prior to solid bolus placement to assist in lubrication of the oral cavity (the patient had postradiation xerostomia). The patient was then taught to use the rubber-coated baby spoon to assist in posterior bolus transfer. Once the bolus was in the posterior oral cavity, the patient required a smaller volume of liquid to transfer to and clear the pharynx. With 6 weeks of therapy targeting solid food intake using these strategies and his palatal augmentation, the patient was able to consume half of a "normal" portion soft solid meal with 16 ounces liquid assist in 15 min.

Soon, the patient began to experience greater difficulty placing/removing his palatal augmentation prosthesis. Vertical oral opening was remeasured and had declined to 28 mm (from 40 mm). The patient reported that he had reduced the frequency with which he completed his trismus home exercises in order to focus more on swallowing. With the realization that difficulty placing his prosthesis would have a direct impact on speech and swallowing, the patient resumed daily trismus exercises and was able to regain 5 mm of opening (to 33 mm) with 3 weeks of consistent practice.

Once the patient was more comfortable with his palatal augmentation, therapy sessions resumed with a target of successfully swallowing a greater range of foods, specifically more challenging solid foods, including sandwiches, tender steak, raw fruits and vegetables, and mixed consistencies (cereal, chunky soups). The patient demonstrated no overt indicators of aspiration during sessions as his diet was advanced. Larger bolus sizes were introduced as a means of assisting the maintenance of a more cohesive bolus for posterior transit. By this point, he was also able to eliminate any gag reflex with solids. He continued to have the most difficulty with posterior (velar) speech sounds. However, because his gag reflex had significantly diminished, he was then able to tolerate more bulk added to the posterior portion of his prosthesis. This additional bulk assisted the patient with achieving adequate articulatory approximation and intelligibility. Although the patient was discharged from regular speech therapy sessions, he continued to make some gains independently with speech and swallowing. By 8 months post treatment, he was maintaining oral nutrition on a mostly solid diet with liquid assist. He was communicating well, and with good intelligibility, in a variety of settings, including an online classroom where good intelligibility was reported by his students during live sessions.

The patient continues to follow intermittently with speech pathology and the prosthodontist for adjustments to his palatal augmentation prosthesis in order to maximize speech intelligibility. He is now 4 years post treatment, has been able to maintain his VO at 32 mm with a maintenance exercise program, continues to tolerate a solid diet, maintains his weight, eats out regularly with family and friends, has experienced no respiratory complications, continues to work full time, travels on a regular basis, and is gracious enough to assist in educating and motivating other patients who are facing this type of cancer treatment (Video 7–4, Video 7–5, Video 7–6).

Long-Term Dental Care and Follow-Up

The patient continues to see his general dentist on a regular basis for dental prophylaxis and monitoring of dental decay. It is vital that the patient continue to maintain teeth for the purpose of supporting the palatal augmentation prosthesis. The patient was prescribed fluoride therapy as lifelong therapy. He continues using the fluoride gel with his fluoride carriers on a daily basis for 10 min per day. The patient is seen yearly at the dental oncology clinic for evaluation of any oral and dental changes. The patient is monitored for trismus and any changes in vertical opening. Any decrease in vertical opening develops challenges in prosthetic rehabilitation in terms of making impressions and fitting the patient with the palatal augmentation prosthesis. The prosthesis needs bulk in order to contact with the flap. The bulk of prosthesis attached to the palatal portion can be increased for better contact and articulation. If the patient develops loss of vertical opening, the bulk would have to be reduced which may, in turn, affect articulation of speech. The palatal augmentation prosthesis has been remade yearly in the past 3 years due to post treatment changes both in the degree of maximum vertical opening as well postradiation therapy flap changes. The patient has done an excellent job with home care. He has only had minor dental restorative work and has not required any oral surgical interventions.

CONCLUSION AND CANCER SURVEILLANCE

The patient has been followed at regular intervals with physical exam by the head and neck surgeon as well as regular neck and chest imaging to follow the primary site, regional lymphatics, and previously noted indeterminate lung nodule. The patient has been without evidence of recurrent disease at the primary site or bilateral necks but was found to have progression of the lung nodule approximately 1 year post treatment which was suspicious for metastatic disease. This was biopsied and was positive for metastatic adenoid cystic carcinoma.

The patient was asymptomatic from this lesion and continued to undergo regular surveillance due to the typically slow growth of distant metastasis for adenoid cystic carcinoma. He has had some interval increase in size of nodules but no new masses, and he remains asymptomatic without immediate threat to the central airway or other structures. He has been offered treatment with radiation therapy but continues to opt for regular surveillance at this point.

REFLECTION AND ANALYSIS FOR FURTHER STUDY

1. This case demonstrated an important interplay between the patient's trismus and ability to progress with speech and swallow goals. As a clinician, what type of guidance would you offer your patient in order to maintain an optimal "balance" of therapeutic goals among trismus, speech, and swallow rehabilitation?
2. At one point this patient's hyperactive gag reflex seemed an insurmountable obstacle to resumption of significant amounts of semisolid and solid consistencies. How did the clinician's consistent use of progressive desensitization assist this patient in resuming oral intake?
3. This patient was able to achieve therapeutic gains even after leaving formal speech and swallow therapy. As a clinician, what strategies would you use to maximize the likelihood of your patient continuing to progress after discontinuing therapy?

REFERENCES

Buchbinder, D., Currivan, R. B., Kaplan, A. J., & Urken, M. L. (1993). Mobilization regimens for the prevention of jaw hypomobility in the radiated patient: A comparison of three techniques. *Journal of Oral Maxillofacial Surgery, 51,* 863–867.

Cohen, E. G., Deschler, D. G., Walsh, K., & Hayden, R. E. (2005). Early use of a mechanical stretching device to improve mandibular mobility after composite resection: A pilot study. *Archives of Physical Medicine and Rehabilitation, 86,* 1416–1419.

Dijkstra, P. U., Sterken, M. W., Pater, R., Spijkervet, F. K., & Roodenburg, J. L. (2007). Exercise therapy for trismus in head and neck cancer. *Oral Oncology, 43,* 389–394.

Duarte, V. M., Chhetri, D. K., Liu, Y. F., Erman, A. A., & Wang, M. B. (2013). Swallow preservation exercises during chemoradiation therapy maintains swallow function. *Otolaryngology-Head and Neck Surgery, 149,* 878–884.

Hoffman, M. R., Mielens, J. D., Ciucci, M. R., Jones, C. A., Jiang, J. J., & McCulloch, T. M. (2012). High-resolution manometry of pharyngeal swallow pressure events associated with effortful swallow and the Mendelsohn maneuver. *Dysphagia, 27*(3), 418–426.

Krisciunas, G. P., Sokoloff, W., Stepas, K., & Langmore, S. E. (2012). Survey of usual practice: Dysphagia therapy in head and neck cancer patients. *Dysphagia, 27*(4), 538–549.

Lazarus, C. L., Logemann, J. A., Song, C. W., Rademaker, A. W., & Kahrilas, P. J. (2002). Effects of voluntary maneuvers on tongue base function for swallowing. *Folia Phoniatrica et Logopaedica, 54,* 171–176.

Li, N., Xu, L., Zhao, H., El-Naggar, A. K., & Sturgis, E. M. (2012). A comparison of the demographics, clinical features, and survival of patients with adenoid cystic carcinoma of major and minor salivary glands versus less common sites within the SEER Registry. *Cancer, 118*(16), 3945–3953.

Marunick, M., & Tselios, N. (2004). The efficacy of palatal augmentation prostheses for speech and swallowing in patients undergoing glosectomy: A review of the literature. *Journal of Prosthetic Dentistry, 91*(1), 67–74.

Ohba, S., Yokoyama, J., Kojima, M., Fujimaki, M., Anzai, T., Komatsu, H., & Ikeda, K. (2014). Significant preservation of swallowing function in chemoradiotherapy for advanced head and neck cancer by prophylactic swallowing exercise. *Head & Neck.* doi:10.1002/hed.23913

Robbins, K. T., Bowman, J. B., & Jacob, R. F. (1987). Postglossectomy deglutitory and articulatory rehabilitation with palatal augmentation prostheses. *Archives of Otolaryngology-Head and Neck Surgery, 113*(11), 1214–1218.

Shaker, R., Kern, M., Bardan, E., Taylor, A., Stewart, E. T., Hoffmann, R. G., . . . Bonnevier, J. (1997). Augmentation of deglutitive upper esophageal sphincter opening in the elderly by exercise. *American Journal of Physiology, 272,* G1518–G1522.

Smith, B. G., Hutcheson, K. A., Little, L. G., Skoracki, R. J., Rosenthal, D. I., Lai, S. Y., & Lewin, J. S. (2015). Lymphedema outcomes in patients with head and neck cancer. *Otolaryngology-Head and Neck Surgery, 152*(2), 284–291.

Soares, E. C., Carreiro Filho, F. P., Costa, F. W., Vieira, A. C., & Alves, A. P. (2008). Adenoid cystic carcinoma of the tongue: Case report and literature review. *Medicina Oral, Patologia Oral y Cirugia Bucal, 13*(8), E475–E478.

Stubblefield, M. D. (2011). Radiation fibrosis syndrome: Neuromuscular and musculoskeletal complications in cancer survivors. *PM&R, 3,* 1041–1054.

Tacani, P. M., Franceschini, J. P., Tacani, R. E., Machado, A. P., Montezello, D., Góes, J. S., & Marx, A. (2014). Retrospective study of the physical therapy modalities applied in head and neck lymphedema treatment. *Head & Neck.* doi:10.1002/hed.23899

Toth, B. B., Chambers, M. S., & Fleming, T. C. (1996). Prevention and management of oral complications associated with cancer therapies: Radiotherapy/chemotherapy. *Texas Dental Journal, 113,* 23–29.

Yorkston, K., Beukelman, D., & Traynor, C. (1984). *Assessment of Intelligibility of Dysarthric Speech.* Austin, TX: Pro-Ed.

8

Minimally Invasive Approach to Treating Cancer of the Base of Tongue

Molly A. Knigge and Timothy M. McCulloch

HISTORY

Patient C is a 70-year-old female who first visited the clinic 4 years ago when she was diagnosed with a T1 N0 M0 squamous cell carcinoma of the left lateral tongue.

Medical History

At presentation, Patient C appeared to be in good health. Her medical history was significant for hypertension, anxiety, and gait abnormality, eczema, chronic obstructive pulmonary disorder (COPD), asthma, and heart murmur. She had a significant smoking history of 0.5 packs per day for 30 years (15 pack-year history). Examination of the neck revealed no palpable lymphadenopathy or masses. Tenderness of the left posterior tongue was reported by the patient on palpation. Direct examination of the tongue via flexible fiberoptic laryngoscope revealed a superficial ulceration of the left tongue base approximately 1.0 × 1.5 cm in size. Laryngoscopic examination of the larynx and pharynx was otherwise unremarkable.

Patient C underwent partial glossectomy to remove the left lateral tongue lesion, with a full-thickness skin graft from neck skin to tongue and left selective neck dissection of Levels I, II, and III. One year later, a new primary lesion was identified on the contralateral right palate, tonsil, and palatal-glossal sulcus. This lesion was treated surgically with a transoral robotic (TORS) technique. The resected T1 specimen was 2.3 × 1.4 cm in size, with clear margins. The resection site was allowed to heal without graft or flap repair. She did not undergo postoperative radiation treatment at that time. She attended regular clinic follow-up visits for 1.5 years showing no sign of recurrent or new primary disease. She did not require swallowing or speech services with a speech pathologist following either of the procedures, returning to a general diet without documented signs of dysphagia or aspiration.

The patient returned to the University of Wisconsin Otolaryngology clinic reporting a 2-week history of increasing pain in the left tonsil and tongue base region that worsened with coughing, swallowing, or sneezing. At the time of presentation, she rated this pain as 10 out of 10 on a subjective numeric pain rating scale. She self-administered ibuprofen or acetaminophen for pain control and had modified her diet to avoid solid foods in favor of softer textures to avoid pain. She denied the presence of any new neck masses or other symptoms.

Social History

Aside from the head and neck surgical history detailed above, Patient C was a well-educated, active, engaged woman with a busy social life, who lived independently.

DIAGNOSTIC WORKUP

Preoperative F-fluorodeoxyglucose (FDG)–positron emission tomography (PET)/computed tomography (CT) performed 3 weeks prior to surgery revealed an intensely hypermetabolic left base of tongue mass with extension inferiorly into the left pala-tine tonsillar region, highly suspicious for recurrent malignancy (Figures 8–1 and 8–2). There were two adjacent, mildly FDG avid subcentimeter left Level II cervical lymph nodes. There was no definitive evidence for distant FDG avid metastatic disease. An in-office transnasal flexible fiberoptic laryngoscopy was performed on the same day to obtain tongue base biopsies to confirm the presence of malignancy.

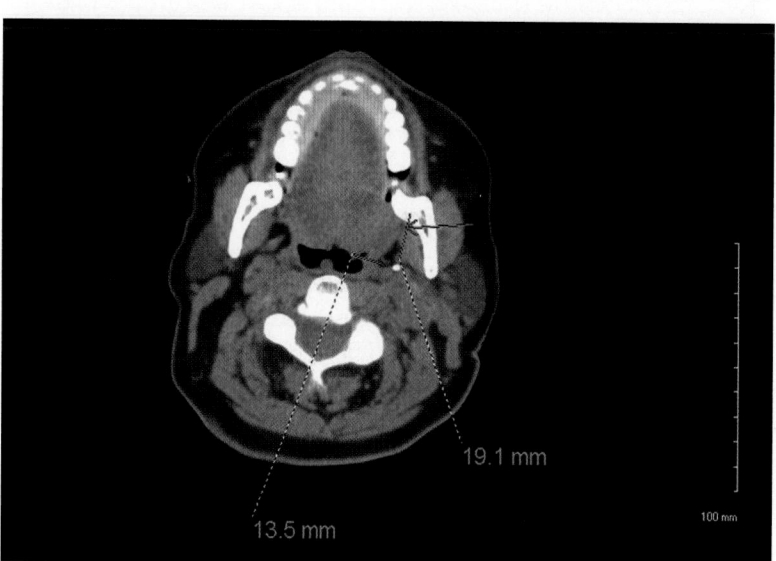

Figure 8–1. Preoperative CT imaging—Left base of tongue mass.

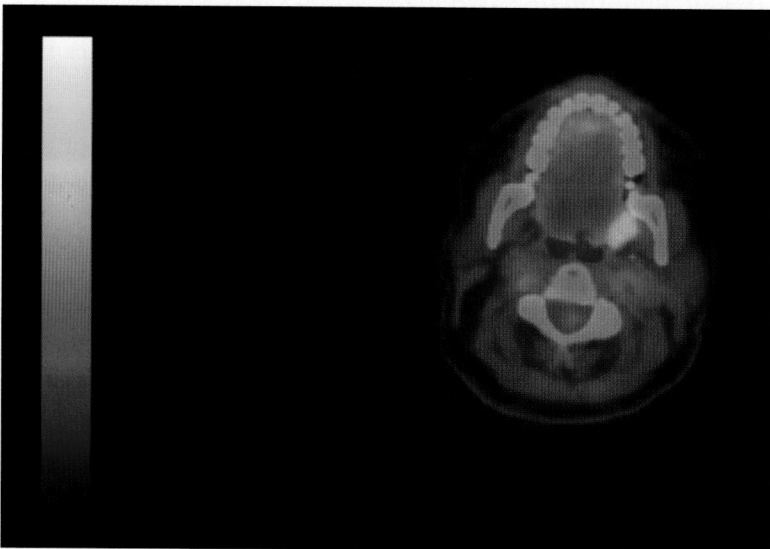

Figure 8–2. Preoperative PET imaging—Left base of tongue mass.

Pathology confirmed the presence of invasive, moderately differentiated squamous cell carcinoma within the specimen.

SURGICAL TREATMENT AND PATHOLOGY

Two weeks following diagnosis of recurrent disease, the patient underwent a robotic tongue base resection and left selective neck dissection of Levels II and III. The surgical resection was 4 × 1.7 × 1.5 cm, extending from the level of the glossotonsillar sulcus to the level of the epiglottis, with lateral margins extending from midline to the left peripharyngeal fat plane. Resection included the left tongue base lymphatic and superficial muscular tissues. The tumor stage was T1 N0 M0. The surgical area was left to heal without reconstruction of the defect undertaken. Pathology was reported as invasive, moderately differentiated squamous cell carcinoma, and tumor size measured as 2 × 1 × 0.9 cm. The tumor involved the tongue muscle, with separate margins set and all margins reported negative for tumor. Final pathology indicated no lymph-vascular invasion and no perineural invasion. Four regional lymph nodes sent were all negative for carcinoma.

POSTSURGICAL TREATMENT / SLP CONSULTATION

Three days following her surgical resection, while the patient was still hospitalized, orders for swallowing consultation were received by the University of Wisconsin Swallowing Service. Review of her medical chart revealed that she had progressed well after surgery, progressing rapidly from clear liquids to soft solids by postoperative Day 1. On postoperative Day 2, nursing documented coughing during meals, suggestive of possible aspiration.

Given these concerns, an instrumental swallowing assessment was recommended for Patient C on postoperative Day 3. She agreed to first complete a bedside clinical examination of swallowing in order to determine her readiness for a videofluoroscopic procedure. Medically, the patient appeared appropriate for evaluation. She was seated in a wheelchair in an upright position, and an IV line was noted to be in place. Cognitively, the patient was alert and oriented to self, place, time, and situation. All commands presented during the evaluation were observed to be followed without difficulty.

The patient denied any swallowing-related pain. Reduced range of lip movement was noted on the left side. The tongue was judged to be weak, with reduced speed of movement. Velar and mandibular movement appeared to be functional. Voice quality and loudness were judged to be within functional limits. She appeared to be managing her oral secretions well and was deemed ready for videofluoroscopic swallow study (VFSS).

The VFSS was completed with both lateral and anteroposterior views. The patient was presented graduated volumes of Varibar thin liquid barium contrast, Varibar nectar liquid, Varibar pudding, and a graham cracker solid coated with pudding contrast. A 13-mm barium tablet was also presented with nectar liquid as the medium for pill passage. The patient displayed mildly delayed oral transit during the oral phase for solid textures only. Complete nasopharyngeal closure was documented. Delayed pharyngeal swallowing response was noted, with boluses reaching the valleculae prior to pharyngeal swallow trigger. Incomplete retraction of the tongue base to the posterior pharyngeal wall was evident at the operative site. This appeared to contribute to bolus stasis and postswallow pharyngeal residue, which entered the laryngeal vestibule and was aspirated after the swallow. Reduced hyolaryngeal excursion was noted, resulting in aspiration of thin liquids and penetration of nectar thick liquids. Postural strategies were attempted, with chin tuck showing no benefit. Application of a head turn left with single sips prevented penetration with nectar liquid. Penetration-Aspiration Scale (Rosenbek et al., 1996) scores for all textures are listed in Table 8–1. Cues to the patient to cough following aspiration in order to clear the aspirated material from the trachea were ineffective, and her cough was noted to be weak. In the anteroposterior view, liquid bolus flows deviated toward the right side of the pharynx. Feeding strategies of alternated liquids and solids combined with reduced bolus size appeared beneficial.

Table 8–1. VFSS Penetration-Aspiration Scores (PASs) and Flexible Endoscopic Examination of Swallowing (FEES) Ratings by Texture

Bolus Type		VFSS Postop Day 3	VFSS Postop Day 10	FEES Postop Day 37
Thin	5 mL	2	–	–
	Cup	7	–	–
	Straw	–	–	Trace penetration
	Straw/HTL	–	8	–
Nectar	5 mL	2	2	–
	Cup	5	–	–
	Cup/HTL	1	–	–
	Straw	–	–	No P/A
	Straw/HTL	–	1	–
Pudding	5 mL	1	1	No P/A
Solid	¼ cracker	1	1	No P/A
13-mm tablet with nectar liquid		1	–	–

Note. HTL, head turn left; *P/A,* penetration/aspiration visualized endoscopically.

The patient was able to clear bolus material from the pharynx between presentations with cues to swallow repeatedly. She was successful in swallowing the 13-mm barium tablet with nectar liquid while turning her head to the left. Upper esophageal sphincter function appeared within normal limits (see Video 8–1).

Following VFSS the patient was diagnosed with mild-moderate oropharyngeal dysphagia characterized by mildly delayed oral transit of solid bolus volumes, impaired tongue base contact to posterior pharyngeal wall at the surgical site, asymmetry of pharyngeal constriction, and reduced closure of the laryngeal vestibule during swallows. Aspiration of thin liquids occurred both during and after the swallow, the latter being related to bolus residue spilling from the pharynx into the laryngeal vestibule after swallows.

The patient was counseled to adopt a modified diet of diced solids with nectar-thick liquids, and provided with education regarding the risks of uncompensated aspiration of thin liquids. She was advised to take medications with puree or nectar liquids. All textures required head turn to the left for safe and efficient bolus transit, and she was provided training in the requisite posture to simulate her performance during VFSS. A written checklist of recommended feeding strategies was also provided, including single sips, small volumes per bolus (1 tsp for puree and solid textures), decreased rate of feeding, and instructions for applying the head turn to the left. She was trained in nectar thick liquid preparation, provided starter packages of thickener for her discharge home, and given written instructions for acquiring thickener at the hospital or outside pharmacy. Due to her inpatient status, aspiration precaution orders were entered and recommendations communicated to her inpatient care team within the electronic medical record. This order entry resulted in a printed list that was posted at the patient's bedside for care providers who may not have access to the medical record, while recommendations for medication administration were electronically communicated to the handheld Medication Administration Record (MAR) device utilized by her registered nurse (RN). The patient was discharged later that day to her home with a plan established for postoperative ENT and swallow service follow-up on an outpatient basis in 1 week.

DISCHARGE COMPLICATION AND FURTHER ASSESSMENT

Five days following her hospital discharge, on postoperative Day 8, the patient presented back to the emergency department with a 1-day history of worsening shortness of breath. During her admission history-taking, she acknowledged "having trouble adhering to the thickened liquid diet." Chest imaging upon readmission showed mild pulmonary edema and suspected early stage aspiration pneumonia. She was treated with vancomycin, Zosyn, and ciproflaxin (later changed to Unasyn and Doxycycline). She was also assessed by a clinical dietician, who documented that the patient reported good appetite, exhibiting weight loss of only 2.5 lbs or 1.6% of her body weight since surgery. Repeat swallow service consult was requested to evaluate her swallow and inform the patient's ability to adhere to the previous recommendations. The patient was returned to NPO status awaiting swallowing evaluation and was placed on supplemental O_2 at a rate of 4 L/min, delivered via nasal cannula.

Clinical bedside swallowing examination was unable to be completed the day after readmission secondary to patient complaints of nausea but was successfully completed on Day 2. On questioning, the patient expressed a strong dislike of nectar-thick liquids and reported difficulty adhering to the recommendation for nectar thick liquids following her recent discharge from the hospital. She denied throat pain at rest or during swallowing. Oral mechanism examination revealed persistent left labial and facial weakness, lingual weakness, and incoordination. Vocal function and cough were judged to be within functional limits. The patient was then administered thin liquid, nectar liquid, and puree consistencies at bedside in order to compare her swallow function to that which was documented during her previous examination one week prior. She executed a head turn to the left with all textures given; however, throat clearing was noted

following one trial of thin liquids. A repeat VFSS was ordered for the following day to assess her current swallow status in the context of respiratory complications and difficulty adhering to thickened liquids. The patient remained NPO until her VFSS could guide her diet and swallowing strategy planning.

A repeat VFSS examination was performed in both lateral and anteroposterior views. Varibar Nectar thick liquid, Varibar Thin liquid, Varibar Pudding, and a graham cracker coated with pudding were administered during the study. Repeat Penetration-Aspiration scores are summarized in Table 8–1 where they can also be compared to those obtained during the prior VFSS. Prolonged chewing was noted on dry solids. Incomplete retraction of the tongue base to posterior pharyngeal wall was again noted at the surgical site. The pharyngeal swallowing response was delayed with the bolus reaching the valleculae prior to initiation. Impaired hyolaryngeal excursion was noted with reduced epiglottic inversion during swallows. Stasis of material was observed in the valleculae and pyriform sinuses after swallows, unilaterally on the left side. UES function appeared normal.

Analysis of VFSS findings revealed a persistent oropharyngeal swallowing delay combined with reduced pharyngeal constriction on the left side, leading to aspiration of thin liquids despite use of head turn to the left during swallow. Once again, a soft diet with nectar liquids was recommended and the patient was provided with further counseling regarding the importance of temporary use of thickened liquids. She was also advised to continue use of the head turn to the left to prevent aspiration of nectar liquids. She was trained in use of alternating liquids and solids to assist in vallecular clearance of semisolid and solid textures. She was capable of independent demonstration of all swallowing strategies upon discharge on postoperative Day #15.

PATIENT DISCHARGE

The patient was discharged to home with supplemental O_2 and home health services. Home health documentation revealed adequate intake; however, her home health nurse noted that the patient struggled to find foods to eat and frequently complained of persistent thirst resulting from intake of nectar thickened liquids. The patient reported moderate (4/10) pain only when swallowing or stretching.

POSTOPERATIVE RESULTS

On postoperative Day #37, the patient returned to the Otolaryngology clinic for examination and coordinated swallowing evaluation. The patient was administered the SF-12v2 Heath Survey Standard Version, with patient-rated health reported as "Very Good" postoperatively. Her regular daily activities were rated to be "limited a little" or affected "a little of the time" due to her baseline gait abnormality. She cited her physical and emotional health as interfering with social activities in the month prior to her outpatient follow-up "a little of the time." ENT examination revealed excellent healing at the tongue base surgical site.

POSTOPERATIVE SWALLOWING ASSESSMENT

Fiberoptic endoscopic evaluation of swallowing (FEES) performed by a speech pathologist, was recommended at follow-up to assess her swallow status and determine readiness for diet advancement. The patient reported improved adherence to the prescribed nectar liquids and head turn left postural strategy since her second hospital discharge. The Eating Assessment Tool, or EAT-10 (Belafsky et al., 2008), was used to gather patient-rated swallowing symptoms. Her perceived swallowing impairment ratings totaled 5, with 40 being the highest-rated difficulty on the instrument. She rated symptoms for swallowing difficulty resulting in weight loss and affecting the pleasure of eating, while the other eight questions on the instrument were rated as "No problem." She reported no pain in her throat at rest or during swallowing at this visit. She did note some changes in taste sensation as well as drooling from

the left side of her mouth that had been improving gradually. Oral mechanism examination revealed reduced range of labial movement on the left side. Facial, lingual, velar, and mandibular movements were noted to be within functional limits. Laryngeal function was judged to be within functional limits for voice quality and volitional cough. Salivary management during this visit was also judged to be functional (see Video 8–2).

On FEES, the patient demonstrated complete velopharyngeal closure during speech tasks. The pharynx and larynx were symmetrical with good vocal fold mobility noted bilaterally. Laryngeal and pharyngeal secretions appeared thin and clear without pooling. Nectar liquid via straw, thin liquid via straw, puree, and solid were presented. Oral phase appeared functional with adequate chewing and timely oral transit. Pharyngeal swallow trigger was timely with only trace penetration of thin liquids noted. When asked the swallow "normally" (i.e., without head turn or other compensatory strategy), the patient produced a timely and coordinated swallow without evidence of aspiration or postswallow pharyngeal residue.

Following FEES, the patient was determined to be safe to advance to a regular diet with thin liquids and discontinue use of postural swallow strategies. She was advised to take whole pills with water, though larger pills could be broken in half as needed for comfort. Given these minimal strategies required, no further swallowing therapy or management was recommended. Telephone follow-up at 3 months postop revealed no swallow complaints, and the patient reported that she felt she had returned to her baseline swallowing performance. Because of her history of recurrent disease, this patient continues to follow up with the Otolaryngology practice.

SUMMARY

This case highlights the importance of postoperative surveillance of swallow status in patients treated for head and neck cancer who are at elevated risk of aspiration. This patient's postoperative aspiration risk was amplified secondary to her underlying history of respiratory compromise (COPD). Patient values also play an important role in achieving optimal therapy and health outcomes. Upon repeat hospitalization, assessment of the barriers to adherence and enhanced counseling offered the patient further opportunity to comply with recommended diet modifications and swallow strategies during the acute postoperative period. This case also highlights the use of minimally invasive surgical techniques such as transoral robotic resection endeavors to reduce postsurgical complications and preserve long-term swallowing function. Although such techniques may not eliminate risk for aspiration consequences during acute recovery, the avoidance of treatment modalities such as radiotherapy may promise return to functional swallowing even in the context of multiple resections as demonstrated in this case.

REFLECTION AND ANALYSIS FOR FURTHER STUDY

1. What actions might have been taken during her initial postoperative stay to increase the likelihood of compliance with recommended dietary and swallow modifications?

2. Given the patient's complaint of persistent thirst with nectar thick liquids, could an alternative approach such as the Frazier Free Water Protocol have been considered without increasing this patient's risk of aspiration? Describe why or why not.

3. How can clinicians effectively monitor patient compliance or symptom exacerbation after discharge?

REFERENCES

Belafsky, P. C., Mouadeb, D. A., Rees, C. J., Pryor, J. C., Postma, G. N., Allen, J., & Leonard, R. J. (2008). Validity and reliability of the Eating Assessment Tool (EAT-10). *Annals of Otology, Rhinology, and Laryngology, 117*, 919–924.

Rosenbek, J. C., Robbins, J. A., Roecker, E. B., Coyle, J. L., & Wood, J. L. (1996). A Penetration-Aspiration Scale. *Dysphagia, 11*, 93–98.

SF-12® Health Survey © 1994, 2002 by Medical Outcomes Trust and QualityMetric Incorporated. All Rights Reserved. SF-12® is a registered trademark of Medical Outcomes Trust.

9

Management of SCCA of the Base of Tongue

Adam T. Lloyd, Henry Ho, Erin P. Silverman, and Bari Hoffman Ruddy

HISTORY

This case is a 75-year-old male referred to the Ear, Nose, Throat, and Plastic Surgery Associates in Orlando, Florida, by his primary care physician following a 1-month history of an enlarged lymph node localized to the left side of the neck, discovered during a routine physical examination. When he presented to our service, the patient reported a 6-month history of feeling as though he had "a lump" in his throat, along with a persistent need to clear his throat. Accompanying these symptoms was the perception of "fullness" in the right ear. The patient's past medical history was significant for hypertension, hyperlipidemia, cataracts, and nasal allergies. He underwent hernia repair several years prior and tonsillectomy as a child. The patient denied use of tobacco products and reported limited alcohol (approximately two glasses of wine per day) and caffeine (one caffeinated beverage per day) consumption. Family medical history was significant for laryngeal cancer, with the patient noting that his father ultimately succumbed to the disease.

DIAGNOSTIC WORKUP (WEEKS I TO 3)

Visual Examination

Initial physical evaluation revealed a firm prominence, approximately 3 cm in diameter, noted in the area of the left carotid bulb (Level II). Flexible fiberoptic endoscopy revealed a 1 × 1 cm mass on the left side of the vallecula. This was confirmed via neck computed tomography (CT) as an asymmetric left-sided supraglottic laryngeal/tongue base lesion measuring 2.5 × 1.6 × 1.7 cm, effacing the vallecula. There was also an irregular-appearing left Level II and left Level III adenopathy with necrosis. Additionally, a 6-mm right thyroid nodule was located and noted (Figure 9–1).

Direct Laryngoscopy With Biopsy

Direct laryngoscopy confirmed prior observations of a 2-cm mass in the left vallecula that was firm to palpation. Histopathological examination of this mass revealed an invasive, moderately differentiated, squamous cell carcinoma, p16 positive.

Imaging Studies. Chest CT revealed a reticulonodular opacity localized within the posterior upper lobe of the right lung, likely secondary to infectious or inflammatory changes. Dimensions of the dilated ascending aorta were stable when compared to a CT of the chest obtained 7 years prior. Additional observations included a small hepatic cyst and right renal cyst. A PET scan revealed a focal area of increased uptake in the left supraglottic region at the level of the left vallecula measuring 1.5 × 1.8 cm with a maximum SUV of 10.1. There was a Level III lymph node with a necrotic center with a maximum SUV of 5.6. Subcentimeter multifocal nodules were noted

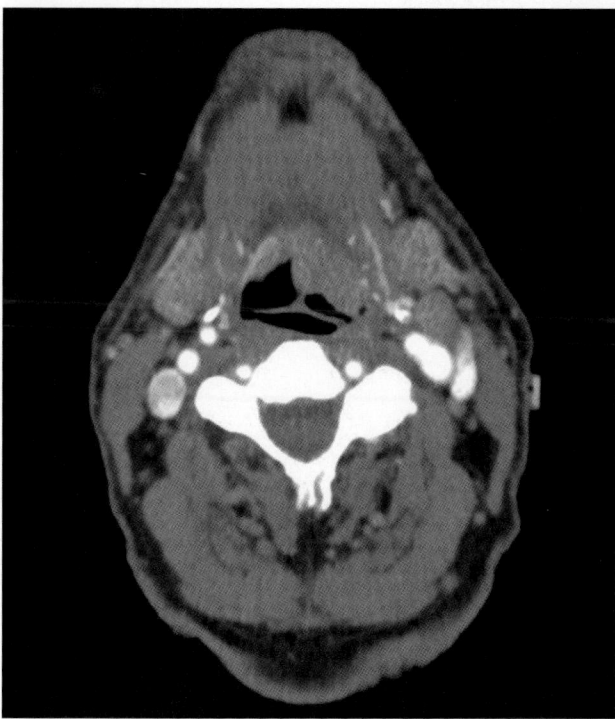

Figure 9–1. An initial CT scan of the neck.

in the lateral segment of the right middle lobe with a maximum SUV of 1.6. There was no evidence of metastatic disease (Figure 9–2).

Tumor Board Discussion

Over the course of diagnostic workup, the patient met with an otolaryngologist, radiation oncologist, and medical oncologist to discuss treatment options including transoral robotic surgery (TORS), radiation, and/or chemotherapy. After tumor board meeting, TORS with risk-adjusted adjuvant chemoradiation therapy (CRT) was recommended and the patient gave consent for the procedure.

TREATMENT (WEEKS 4 TO 13)

Surgical Management

One month after initial evaluation and biopsy the patient underwent transoral robotic partial tongue

base resection (TORS) utilizing the da Vinci surgical system. Mercante and colleagues (2013) found TORS to be a definitive treatment in selected T1–T2 cases of the base of tongue tumors without adverse features and allowed the possibility for deintensification of adjuvant treatments. A selective left neck dissection incorporating Levels II, III, IV was also performed. Surgical pathology revealed invasive, moderately differentiated squamous cell carcinoma within the tongue base specimen, involving the peripheral resection margin from 3 to 6 o'clock and a deep resection margin on the 6 o'clock half of the specimen. Intraoperative reexcision of margins were negative on frozen section. Evaluation of the neck dissection specimen revealed metastatic squamous cell carcinoma within two (of 27 total) lymph nodes at Level IIb. The initial plan was for deintensifying postoperative radiation and chemotherapy as frozen sections were negative. Unfortunately final pathology revealed positive margins, a more aggressive approach of combined modality radiation and chemotherapy was therefore indicated.

Staging

Staging of the primary tumor was based on the oropharyngeal and laryngeal exam, PET-CT scans and pathology. Histopathologic findings were IVA, T2N2bM0, grade 2 squamous cell carcinoma of the left base of tongue/vallecula (2 cm), P16 positive. P16-positive histopathologic findings suggest that the tumor was positive for human papillomavirus (HPV). Because HPV-positive tumors tend to respond well to postoperative radiation therapy (Bhayani, Holsinger, & Lai, 2010; Kaplan & Damrose, 2010), the decision was made to proceed accordingly.

Preradiation Swallowing Evaluation and FEES

One month following TORS, the patient began CRT. At this time the patient was referred to a speech pathologist for a clinical and fiberoptic endoscopic evaluation of swallowing (FEES) (see Video 9–1). As part of standard protocol in our otolaryngology practice, prior to starting radiation therapy, each patient completes a clinical swallowing assessment

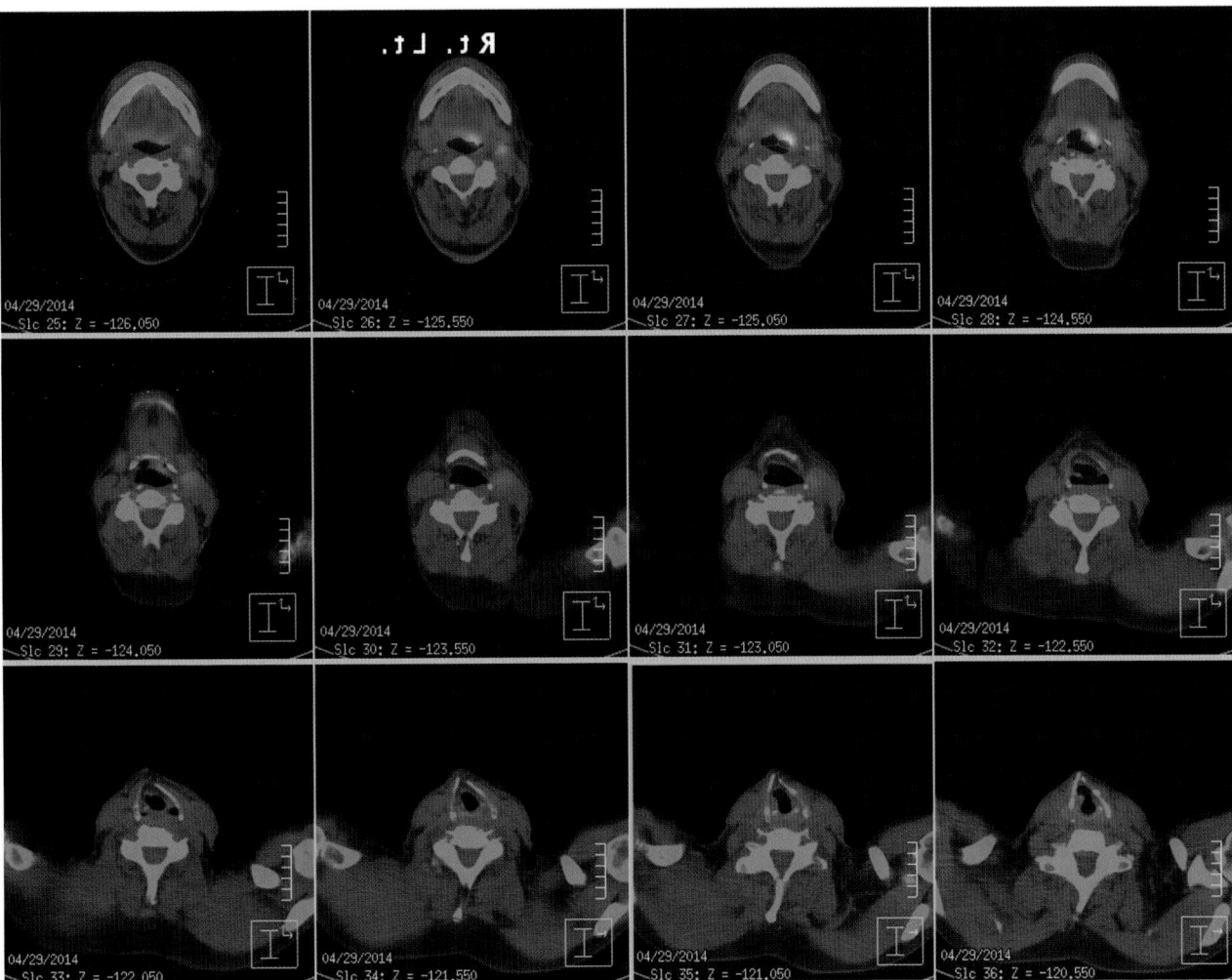

Figure 9–2. An initial PET scan.

and FEES study. This allows the speech pathologist to provide the patient with information regarding potential changes to swallow function resulting from radiation therapy. Following comprehensive assessment of swallow physiology, patients are provided with therapeutic strategies, including exercises to maximize swallow safety and function over the course of therapy (Denaro, Merlano, & Russi, 2013; Starmer, Gourin, Lua, & Burkhead, 2011). At the time of evaluation, the patient denied swallowing difficulties or xerostomia; however, he reported postnasal drainage and frequent throat clearing. FEES revealed mild pharyngeal-phase dysphagia characterized by reduced base of tongue propul-

sion and reduced pharyngeal constriction with mild postswallow residue noted within the valleculae, pyriform sinuses, and along the posterior pharyngeal wall.

A variety of compensatory strategies were attempted in order to assess the patient's ability to clear the residue remaining in the pharyngeal cavity post swallow. Chin tuck, liquid wash, and repeat swallow were successful at clearing this residue. Swallow compensatory strategies were discussed with the patient including multiple swallows per bolus, small bites and sips (reduced bolus volume), alternating liquids and solids, chin tuck before and during swallow, and use of an effortful swallow maneuver. The patient was encouraged to continue a fully oral diet and swallow often while receiving radiation therapy.

ADJUVANT TREATMENT

Prior to radiation therapy, a percutaneous endogastric (PEG) tube was placed due to the likelihood of significant odynophagia and dysphagia resulting from the location of the tumor and the field of radiation. Rutter and colleagues (2011) showed reduction in weight loss and hospitalization for nutrition deficits when a PEG-tube was placed prior to treatment. Dental fluoride trays were prescribed by his dentist in order to minimize the potential for radiation-related tooth decay. The patient underwent 10 weeks of radiation therapy, 5 days per week. He received 5040 cGy in 28 fractions to the primary tumor site, bilateral neck, and left supraclavicular fossa. Thereafter, the primary tumor site and involved left neck was boosted to an additional 900 cGy in five fractions to achieve a total tumor dose of 5940 cGy. Concurrently, a 6-week course of chemotherapy (Cisplatin) was initiated.

During the course of CRT, the patient developed significant mucositis, nausea, pain, and oral thrush for which he was prescribed a 14-day course of Diflucan 100 mg QD. He was given Neutra-Caine rinses, Neutra-Sal rinses, and Magic mouthwash, which were moderately successful in lessening this pain. The patient continued a full oral diet for the initial 2 weeks of chemoradiation therapy. However, by Week 3 the patient reported odynophagia, and consequently, elected to receive full nutritional support via his PEG tube.

POST RADIATION AND CHEMOTHERAPY TREATMENT (WEEKS 15 TO 26)

Post treatment Head and Neck Evaluation

Upon completion of 6 weeks of chemotherapy, the patient continued to receive radiation therapy for an additional 4 weeks. At the conclusion of radiation therapy, he returned to our service for a comprehensive posttherapy evaluation. The patient reported that he was followed weekly by his primary care physician throughout the entire course of his treatment. He continued to maintain a completely nonoral diet, meeting all nutritional and hydration needs via PEG tube. He voiced persistent complaints of odynophagia, dysphagia, dysphonia, and generalized fatigue and asthenia. An approximate 14-pound weight loss was noted since therapy initiation, and mucositis of tissues proximal to the treatment area was evident on examination. The patient was scheduled for a post treatment clinical swallowing evaluation with FEES in order to begin the process of swallow rehabilitation and resumption of oral intake (Leder & Murray, 2008; Logemann et al., 2008).

Post treatment Clinical Swallowing Evaluation and FEES

At the time of clinical swallow and FEES examination, the patient weighed approximately 141 pounds (down 15 pounds from his pretreatment weight of 156 pounds). He maintained a complete nonoral diet, taking eight cans (2400 calories) of Jevity and 54 ounces (351 calories) of Gatorade via PEG per day, in addition to frequent water flushes. Following completion of chemoradiation the patient reported experiencing increased xerostomia, a "burning sensation" in his throat (particularly while drinking water), and increased throat and oral secretions, necessitating frequent expectoration. He continued to use NeurtaSal and NeutraCaine daily for pain relief. Perceptual evaluation of speech revealed mildly reduced intelligibility and a mild "cul-de-sac" resonance compared to pretreatment status. Clinical swallowing evaluation and FEES were deferred for 2 weeks secondary to patient discomfort.

Two weeks later, the patient noted that the burning sensation in his throat had decreased and attributed some of this improvement to Biotene throat spray. He continued to experience some soreness in the mouth and throat, particularly on the left side for which he continued to use Prevention mouth rinse. Upon report of reduced pain, improved secretion management, and increased appetite, a repeat FEES examination was completed (see Video 9–2), revealing edema of the posterior pharyngeal wall as well as erythema of the vocal folds. Swallow was characterized by a mild to moderate pharyngeal phase dysphagia with reduced base of tongue propulsion and reduced pharyngeal constriction. As with the previous FEES, this contributed to postswallow residue in the valleculae and along the posterior pharyngeal wall. Residue was noted along the left side of the base of tongue near the site of the previous partial tongue base resection. This residue appeared to increase with increasing bolus viscosity. Slight penetration to the laryngeal surface of the epiglottis was evident; however, the patient was able to eliminate the penetrant with sips of thin liquid. The speech pathologist recommended reintroduction of regular solids and thin liquids PO. As the patient gradually increased his volume of PO intake, he was instructed to decrease the amount of Jevity 1.5 taken via the PEG tube from his present intake of eight cans per day, with the ultimate goal being complete elimination of PEG tube feeds. Strategies and exercises to enhance swallow safety were reviewed and practiced including small bites and sips, alternating liquids and solids, multiple dry swallows in between bites of solid foods, and chin tuck as necessary when liquid wash alone did not alleviate the feeling of residue in the mouth and throat.

Swallowing Therapy

Within 1 week of beginning swallow therapy, the patient began increasing his PO intake. However, beginning at swallow therapy Week 2 he began to experience significant discomfort and pain on the posterior left side of his tongue. He began using Magic Mouthwash before eating, and Prevention rinse after. This combination was reportedly effecting in reducing his pain. In spite of continued efforts to gradually advance PO, the patient continued to rely on the PEG tube for the majority of his nutrition, tolerating only small amounts of PO. The importance of meticulous dental care and head and neck stretches were stressed, and the patient was offered assurances that his discomfort and sensitivity would continue to improve. Tramadol (100 mg PRN) and viscous lidocaine (2% swish and spit) were pre-

scribed by the patient's radiation oncologist to be taken for pain, as needed.

The patient continued swallow therapy for several more weeks and reported that, over time, his pain level was significantly improved although he continued to experience some sensitivity and soreness of the posterior portion of the left side of his tongue and that he could not tolerate spicy foods. The patient kept a food-log, detailing the number of PO calories consumed per day. He indicated that he had been consuming approximately 2000 to 2800 PO calories per day for the preceding week and a half and had discontinued use of the PEG-tube entirely. During this time, his diet consisted of soft solids and thin liquids (including approximately 48 ounces of water per day) as well as two to three bottles of liquid high-calorie nutritional supplements such as Ensure Plus or Boost Plus. The PEG-tube was subsequently removed, and the patient was instructed to continue a diet of soft solids and thin liquids while meeting regularly with the speech pathologist to review the prescribed swallowing and exercises and monitor compliance with compensatory strategies. By this time his speech intelligibility and resonance were improved although not completely normalized.

During the patient's final session of swallowing therapy, he reported no difficulty swallowing and was consuming between 2100 and 2800 calories PO per day. His weight had stabilized around 145 pounds, just 10 pounds down from his pretreatment weight of 155 pounds. Persistent, yet improving soreness of the left mouth and tongue were reported along with minor perceived changes to his sense of taste. He reported persistent fatigue throughout the day; however, he continued to complete his daily swallowing exercises with frequent attempts to add regular solid consistencies to his soft diet and follow up with the speech-language pathologist as needed.

FOLLOW-UP FOR FURTHER CONCERNS

At 10 weeks following the conclusion of CRT, the patient returned to otolaryngology at the request of his dentist, who had observed some lesions on the left gum and left tongue. The patient noted continued pain in these areas, which he had been treating, with some limited success, with Magic Mouthwash. Aside from odynophagia, he continued to deny the presence of dysphagia symptoms.

PERCEPTUAL AND VISUAL EXAMINATION

Perceptual evaluation of voice status by the otolaryngologist revealed a mildly rough voice quality. Visual inspection of the oral cavity produced an area of subtle induration in the left posterolateral tongue measuring approximately 1.5 cm. There was also a small ulceration on the gingiva adjacent to teeth #18 and #19. There was generalized fullness of the left lateral tongue upon palpation. Differential diagnosis included radiation necrosis versus persistent cancer and a repeat PET scan was ordered and completed 3 days later.

Imaging Studies

The results of the PET scan included resolution of the hypermetabolic activity in the left palatine tonsillar region. There was FDG uptake in the region of the left base of the tongue and right vocal fold, which could represent postsurgical changes or metastatic disease. Resolution of the hypermetabolic left Level II cervical lymph node was noted and no new hypermetabolic lymph nodes were identified. There was a nonspecific interval decrease in size and FDG uptake within the right upper lobe pulmonary nodule (Figure 9–3). The combination of PET scan findings, which included increased activity within the left tongue base and right vocal fold, apparent lesions on physical examination, and patient reports of persistent pain suggested a need for diagnostic biopsy and frozen section

Repeat Direct Laryngoscopy With Biopsy

Direct laryngoscopy completed by the otolaryngologist who previously treated this patient revealed an essentially "normal" appearing larynx and tongue base, consistent with expected changes attributable to prior CRT and surgery, including significant fibrosis. No tumor was identified via visualization or palpation and histopathological examination of the left tongue base and right vocal fold was negative for malignancies.

CONTINUED FOLLOW-UP

Some weeks later, the patient reported marked improvement in pain, which he attributed to his use of Tramadol as needed. A follow-up with otolaryngology was recommended in 4 months. One month later, the patient was seen by oncology. Physical examination showed no evidence of pathologic adenopathy and the patient's weight had nearly returned to his pretreatment baseline of 155 pounds. Upon return visit to radiation oncology, the patient noted continued overall improvement and limited complaints including a persistent, minor cough and soreness around the left lower molars, which was being followed closely by his dentist. Hyperbaric oxygen therapy would be considered as a future treatment option if symptoms did not improve.

CONCLUSION

This case describes a multidisciplinary team approach for diagnosis, treatment, and rehabilitation of a patient with base of tongue cancer. The patient presented to his primary care physician with subtle symptoms that failed to improve with antibiotics. When subsequent workup revealed base of tongue cancer, the patient underwent an innovative, minimally invasive, organ-preserving transoral robotic surgery. Because of adverse features on final pathology, he received adjuvant CRT. The patient experienced swallowing difficulty and, by the end of CRT, was PEG-tube dependent for nutritional support. He required swallowing therapy and a repeat biopsy. Six months from initial diagnosis, following completion of CRT and swallowing therapy, the patient was able to resume a full oral diet. He continues to follow up regularly with otolaryngology, oncology, radiation oncology, primary care, and dentistry.

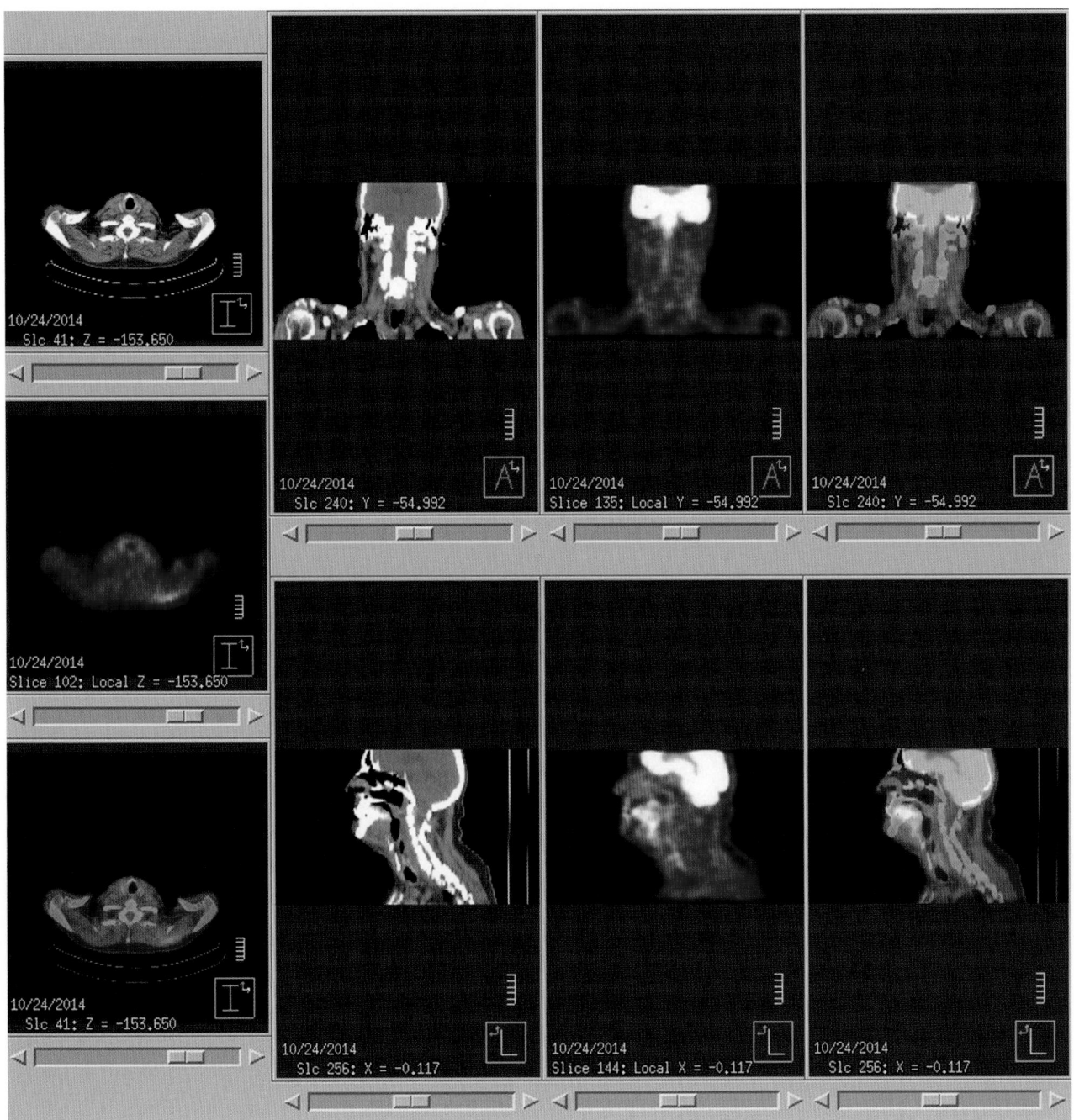

Figure 9–3. A post treatment PET scan.

REFLECTION AND ANALYSIS FOR FURTHER STUDY

1. As a clinician, how would you facilitate transdisciplinary communication among the members of your team?
2. What is the role of the PET scan in the diagnosis and staging of cancer?

REFERENCES

Bhayani, M. K., Holsinger, F. C., & Lai, S. Y. (2010). A shifting paradigm for patients with head and neck cancer: Transoral robotic surgery (TORS). *Oncology (Williston Park), 24*(11), 1010–1015.

Denaro, N., Merlano, M. C., & Russi, E. G. (2013). Dysphagia in head and neck cancer patients: Pretreatment evaluation, predictive factors, and assessment during radiochemotherapy, recommendations. *Clinical and Experimental Otorhinolaryngology, 6*(3), 117.

Kaplan, M. J., & Damrose, E. J. (2010). Transoral robotic surgery (TORS): The natural evolution of endoscopic head and neck surgery. *Oncology (Williston Park), 24*(11), 1022, 1025, 1030.

Leder, S. B., & Murray, J. T. (2008). Fiberoptic endoscopic evaluation of swallowing. *Physical Medicine and Rehabilitation Clinics of North America, 19*(4), 787.

Logemann, J. A., Pauloski, B. R., Rademaker, A. W., Lazarus, C. L., Gaziano, J., Stachowiak, L., & Mittal, B. (2008). Swallowing disorders in the first year after radiation and chemoradiation. *Head & Neck, 30*(2), 148–158.

Mercante, G., Ruscito, P., Pellini, R., Cristalli, G., & Spriano, G. (2013). Transoral robotic surgery (TORS) for tongue base tumours. *Acta Otorhinolaryngologica Italica: Organo Ufficiale Della Società Italiana Di Otorinolaringologia e Chirurgia Cervico-Facciale, 33*(4), 230.

Rutter, C. E., Yovino, S., Taylor, R., Wolf, J., Cullen, K. J., Ord, R., . . . Suntharalingam, M. (2011). Impact of early percutaneous endoscopic gastrostomy tube placement on nutritional status and hospitalization in patients with head and neck cancer receiving definitive chemoradiation therapy. *Head & Neck, 33*(10), 1441–1447.

Starmer, H., Gourin, C., Lua, L. L., & Burkhead, L. (2011). Pretreatment swallowing assessment in head and neck cancer patients. *Laryngoscope, 121*(6), 1208–1211.

10

An Interdisciplinary Approach to the Management of HPV-Positive Tonsil Cancer With Chemoradiation Therapy

Angela L. Campanelli, Jennifer R. Reitz, Wendy D. LeBorgne, and Matthew R. Garrett

HISTORY

This is a case of a 60-year-old male who we will refer to as "Patient X," a nondrinker, nonsmoker with HPV-positive squamous cell oropharyngeal carcinoma. This particular case was chosen for presentation because much of the history, diagnostic workup, therapeutic interventions, and clinical responses can be observed across patients with carcinoma specific to this region. Patient X is married with two daughters and is a college-educated safety officer. He is a lifelong nonsmoker and has a history of generally good physical health and maintained a regular exercise regime prior to his cancer diagnosis. His family history includes a mother who died at the age of 48 years from pancreatic cancer, father who survived testicular cancer, a sister with melanoma, and another sister with squamous cell carcinoma of the skin.

Past Medical History

Patient X was well-known to both the otolaryngology and voice and swallowing clinic for several years prior to his diagnosis of oropharyngeal carcinoma. His past medical history was significant for anxiety and depression. Additionally, he had a history of mandibular tori on the floor of mouth, contributing to a detectable lateral lisp, although his speech was 100% intelligible. He was diagnosed with oral herpes in his teenage years and continues to take an oral antiviral as needed for acute outbreaks. Prior to treatment, his medications included Wellbutrin, Lamictal, Protonix, MiraLAX, Valtrex, Ritalin, Skelaxin, and Tramadol HCl.

Patient X was first seen by otolaryngology in 1999 at the age of 43 and through 2001 was treated nonsurgically for environmental allergies and a deviated septum. In 2004, he returned with a complaint of epistaxis, for which he was treated. The following year, he presented with complaints of sour taste in the mouth and began treatment for laryngopharyngeal reflux (LPR). He was also referred to gastroenterology and found to have a stomach ulcer as well as esophageal narrowing for which he underwent esophagogastroduodenoscopy (EGD) with dilation. His initial visit to the voice and swallowing facility occurred in 2009, when he was referred with complaints of hoarseness, odynophagia, globus sensation, and left-sided throat pain. At that time, Patient X was found to have a left vocal process granuloma. Following his diagnosis, he was compliant with reflux diet and lifestyle precautions, medically managed with 40 mg of Protonix, and worked to eliminate phonotraumatic behaviors. The left vocal process granuloma was monitored at 3-month intervals with a final resolution documented in late 2010. After resolution of the granuloma, he enrolled in voice therapy focused on Vocal Function Exercises designed to strengthen and balance the laryngeal musculature (Stemple, Lee, D'Amico, & Pickup, 1994), as well as Resonant Voice Therapy (Verdolini, 2008) to promote a forward tonal resonance. He failed to fully follow through with a complete course of voice therapy entailing six to eight sessions over 3 to 4 months, instead attending three sessions, and remained mildly dysphonic after being lost to follow-up.

In 2001, prior to his diagnosis of cancer, he complained of dizziness that was determined to be idiopathic after physical examination, computed tomography (CT) scan, and magnetic resonance imaging (MRI). The dizziness reportedly resolved without treatment over the course of several months. The MRI completed as part of the diagnostic workup for the dizziness complaint did note the presence of a small disc bulge at C3-4 without evidence of focal disc herniation, as well as minimal disc bulge at C5-6 without evidence of herniation or stenosis. In 2007, he complained of headaches and underwent another MRI, which revealed incidental nonspecific white matter disease throughout the subcortical and periventricular white matter regions. These findings were consistent with patient reports of a several year history of back and neck problems causing both pain and range of motion restrictions. His back problems resulting from an injury that include thoracic and lumbar involvement of ruptured L4-5 disc L5-S1 discs. He underwent several rounds of physical therapy with variable success over the years.

After a several-year hiatus from otolaryngology care, the patient returned to the clinic in January 2014 with a complaint of palpable bilateral neck masses. Two weeks prior to this appointment, he had been placed on Ciproflaxin for a sinus infection diagnosed by his primary care physician.

Additional diagnostic tests were ordered and are as follows below.

Diagnostic Workup

- Fine-needle aspiration (FNA), left neck lymph node: Squamous cell carcinoma
- Positive emission tomography (PET)/ CT skull to thigh: 2-cm mass (SUV 12.2) in the right tonsillar region, suspicious for malignancy; small focus of moderate update (SUV 6.4) in the right lateral oral cavity, suspicious for malignancy; multiple bilateral neck adenopathy, right greater than left with the largest in the right in the jugulodigastric region measuring 2 cm (SUV 12.1); other lymph nodes in the right neck with SUV ranges from 6 to 10; on the left, the largest node measured 1.8 cm (SUV 6.2), and one in the lower neck measured 1.4 cm (SUV 7.3) (Figures 10–1 and 10–2)
- Direct laryngoscopy and right tonsil biopsy, rigid esophagoscopy: Firm lesion palpated in the right inferior-posterior tonsillar region, biopsied moderately differentiated invasive squamous cell carcinoma, p16 human papillomavirus (HPV) positive
- Rigid laryngeal stroboscopy (VLS): New finding of irregular, suspicious tissue in the right tonsillar area; persistent bilateral true vocal fold bowing, edema and erythema, and mild pachydermia in the interarytenoid area suggestive of laryngopharyngeal reflux consistent with comparative VLS in 2010 (see Video 10–1)

Tumor Board Discussion and Staging

This patient's diagnostic results were subsequently reviewed at an interdisciplinary care conference in which physician representation and input was gathered from hematology-oncology, radiation-oncology, and surgical otolaryngology. Also present for ancillary counsel were allied health professionals from speech-language pathology and radiation-oncology nursing. In accordance with the American Joint Committee on Cancer (AJCC) Cancer Staging Manual (2010), the patient was diagnosed with a clinical stage IVA T2 N2c M0 HPV-positive squamous cell carcinoma of the right tonsillar fossa.

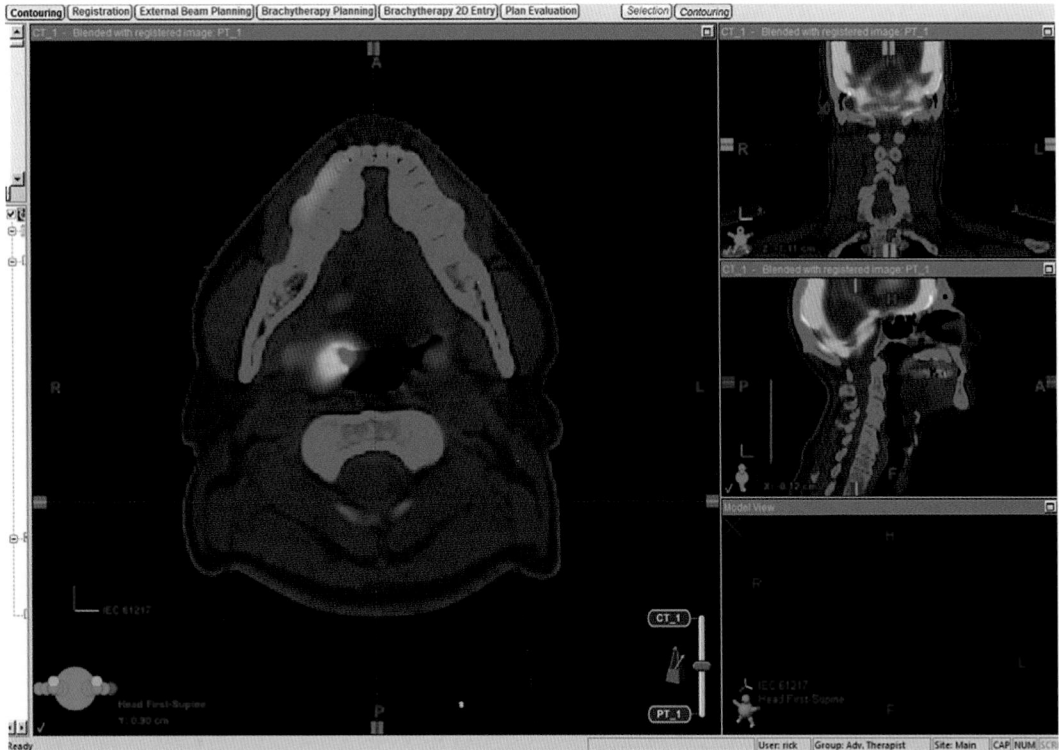

Figure 10–1. PET-CT Pre Treatment.

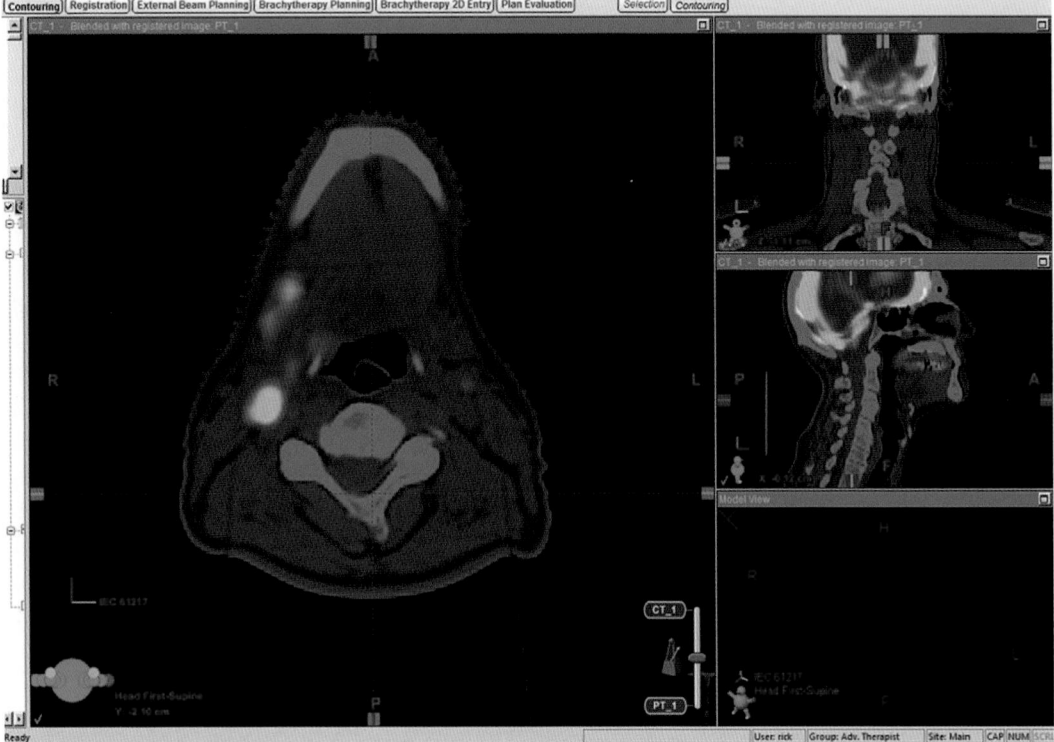

Figure 10–2. PET-CT Pre-TX.

In this integrative care setting, the medical team developed a plan of care that included medical treatment with multidisciplinary care and support from dietary, nursing, and speech-language pathology. The dietician's role included making recommendations for diet texture modification, food fortification, dietary counseling, and use of dietary supplements. The oncology nurse provided patient education, physical, psychological, social, and emotional support, acted as a link between interdisciplinary care professionals and medical facilities, and supported physicians in medical care procedures. The speech-language pathologist was consulted to perform assessment of swallow function and provide dysphagia therapy focused on maximizing swallow function during and after radiation therapy.

TREATMENT PLAN

Results of all tests and subsequent staging were reviewed with the patient, who agreed to the following medical treatment plan in accordance National Comprehensive Cancer Network (NCCN) Guidelines: Taxol at $40/m^2$ equals 80 mg and Carboplatin AUC of two for 8 weeks with radiotherapy beginning 6 days after the first systemic therapy using a 35 fraction intensity-modulated radiation therapy (IMRT) technique for tumor localization and sparing of normal tissue. The radiotherapy dose to the parotic glands was limited to less than 4000 centigray (cGy), and uninvolved lymph nodes as well as retropharyngeal nodes received 6000 cGy. Following 7000 cGy to the large fields, the patient had an additional two treatments delivering another 400 cGy over the area of the primary itself, resulting in a total dosage of 7400 cGy to the primary tumor. There was no disruption of treatment, with 50 elapsed days from first to last systemic therapy and 48 elapsed days from first to last radiotherapy treatment.

Speech-Language Pathology Assessment

Referral for a swallowing evaluation was done soon after a biopsy confirmed malignancy. The patient's pretreatment body weight was 183 pounds. The initial dysphagia evaluation was completed 4 days before the first radiation treatment and consisted of comprehensive assessment of swallow function, patient education, and introduction and practice of therapeutic swallowing exercises.

Neck rotation was functional at 70 degrees to the left and 80 degrees to the right. Vertical mandibular excursion was normal at 60 mm; this increased to 62 mm after verbal cues to stretch. Tongue strength for anterior press and lateral press was judged to be normal at 5/5, and range of motion on protrusion was within normal limits. Oral mucosa was intact and pink in color. Speech was mildly distorted due to the presence of tori filling the floor of mouth. Voice was judged to be mildly dysphonic characterized by a back-focused resonance and a gravelly quality (which had been his baseline norm) noted during stroboscopic exams. He had no complaints of dysphagia, and his swallow appeared grossly normal for liquids and solids with the exception of mildly reduced laryngeal elevation as determined by observation of the anterior neck during swallowing tasks. Here, the rise and anterior tilt of the thyroid cartilage/larynx are used as an estimate of hyolaryngeal elevation.

SPEECH-LANGUAGE PATHOLOGY INTERVENTION

Education provided by the speech-language pathologist complemented the instructions given by the radiation oncologist regarding oral hygiene and the changes that might be expected during chemoradiation therapy (CRT). The therapeutic process, including a detailed description of the potential benefits of therapy and compliance with swallowing exercises was explained. Among the strategies introduced and practiced was a tongue strengthening task that involved pressing the blade of the tongue to the alveolar ridge as an isometric approach to strengthening the body of the tongue. With practice, a patient is ideally able to generate a harder, stronger swallow with increased pharyngeal contraction and increased bolus clearance.

Patient X was also taught the Masako maneuver, which targets anterior excursion of the posterior pharyngeal wall above and below the second cervical vertebrae. The technique requires the tongue to be held between the teeth with lips parted then, using an anterior press, the patient swallow, while the tongue maintains its position between the teeth.

Carnaby-Mann, Crary, Schmalfuss, and Amdur (2012) demonstrated that muscle remodeling occurred when patients receiving radiation therapy were trained to execute effortful swallows. They reported less structural deterioration of the genioglossus, hyoglossus, and mylohyoid muscles occurred using measures from MRI T2 weighted images. This muscle remodeling was accompanied by superior functional gains among those in the effortful swallow group compared to sham. Other evidence exists to suggest that lingual and pharyngeal strengthening exercises while maintaining oral intake throughout radiation therapy results in 92% of those studied returning to a normal oral diet. In comparison, patients that did not undergo swallow strengthening therapy and discontinued oral intake during radiation therapy demonstrated a 65% return to normal oral diet status (Hutcheson et al., 2013).

Changes in taste, pain, and swallowing follow a generally predictable pattern and are expected complications of radiation therapy that affect oral intake. The severity of these changes is highly variable among patients, as well as unpredictable. Patient X was scheduled for 35 individual chemoradiation treatments (CRTs), to be administered over the course of several months. By CRT #7 Patient X had experienced only minimal changes, which were well tolerated. By CRT #14, accumulated radiation dosing had resulted in moderate to severe mucositis, neck skin burns, and painful swallowing (odynophagia). By CRT #25 gastric feeding tube placement was necessary secondary to systemic dehydration, physical weakness, and pain. By the time his feeding tube was placed, Patient X had lost a total of 12 pounds.

Patient X's speech therapy attendance was poor throughout the course of CRT, amounting to one session of swallow therapy during the fifth week of treatment. Lingual strength was judged to be moderately to severely reduced at that point, and the patient was 100% dependent on tube feedings for nutritional support. Neck rotation was measured in order to determine the effects of radiation on the upper trapezius and all neck muscles including the highly targeted sternocleidomastoid, and the pharynx. He was unable to perform any of the neck rotation tasks due to documented third-degree burns.

Poor compliance with adjuvant therapies during radiation treatment is a common phenomenon. Adherence to a dysphagia exercise program consisting of only two sessions during radiation therapy was poor in the 109 patients interviewed by Shinn et al. (2013). They found 13% reported full adherence and 32% were partially adherent. To counter this tendency, the speech-language pathologist should consider the first session as a "sales negotiation." The patient must buy into the recommended treatment and perceive a tangible benefit in the initial visit in order to begin to realized the benefits of repeat visits. This can be a challenging proposition, as many patients do not develop dysphagia symptoms until later on during radiation treatment as radiation doses accumulate. Physician support and direct discussion with the patient have anecdotally been shown to be effective at improving patient compliance.

POSTRADIATION SWALLOWING ASSESSMENT

A laryngostroboscopy was completed at 10 weeks post completion of CRT. Patient X displayed coughing and choking following water intake on examination, positive signs of aspiration, and swallow compromise. The entire laryngopharyngeal complex appeared edematous and erythematous with slight narrowing of the pharynx (see Video 10–2).

A videofluoroscopic exam of swallow status (VFSS) was conducted 3 months post CRT in order to characterize the extent and nature of Patient X's swallow impairment. The VFSS report noted concern over the adequacy of the upper esophageal sphincter (UES) lumen with an attempted pill swallow. Additionally, solid food stasis was noted at the esophageal inlet post swallow. Cervical osteophytes and anterior webbing in the pharynx contributed to observations of pharyngeal narrowing. Moderate stasis was noted in the valleculae suggestive of base of tongue weakness/reduced retraction. Transient, trace airway penetration occurred with thin, nectar, and solid consistencies. The patient coughed every time contrast passed the arytenoid cartilages suggestive of irritable larynx/hypersensitivity. Recommendations resulting from this examination included breath hold with effortful swallow, and to continuation of the Masako and Shaker maneuvers. Patient X was on Famotidine, and re-evaluation of reflux medication was suggested for reducing laryngeal hypersensitivity.

Subsequent swallow therapy sessions involved active neck rotation, vertical mandibular excursion (jaw opening), and pharyngeal and base of tongue strengthening exercises. At 3 months post CRT, he had attended only four therapy sessions, and his oral intake was limited to small sips of water.

At this time he began attending twice weekly lymphedema therapy. This common side effect may manifest both internally and externally. Therapy was carried out by an occupational therapist certified in lymphedema therapy, and involved soft tissue manipulation and fitting of a compression garment to reduce submandibular fibrosis and fullness from lymphedema.

CONTINUED SWALLOW THERAPY OUTCOMES

At 4 months post completion of CRT, additional exercises were able to be added. These included the Mendelsohn maneuver (actively sustaining laryngeal elevation during the swallow), a modified Shaker maneuver, and the super-supraglottic swallow. The Shaker maneuver was designed by the gastroenterologist Reza Shaker to increase upper esophageal sphincter opening by strengthening the mylohyoid, thyrohyoid, geniohyoid, and anterior belly of the digastric muscles, responsible for the upward and forward motion of the hyolaryngeal complex during swallow to facilitate pharyngeal clearance and reduce aspiration risk. The super-supraglottic swallow consists of the sequence of effortful breath hold (Valsalva with bearing down), effortful swallow, volitional cough/expulsion of air prior to inhalation, and repeat (dry) swallow.

A sensory stimulation therapy called thermal-tactile stimulation was also added to Patient X's treatment plan. This involved applying an ice-cold #00 laryngeal mirror to the anterior faucial pillars to enhance sensory input (onset time of the swallow reflex) for increased motor output. Ideally, the patient is able to demonstrate a timelier swallow with strong laryngeal elevation. This patient's gag reflex was diminished suggesting reduced sensory perception/motor integration. Our patient reported immediate sense of ease of swallowing when a bolus of 3 cc pudding was preceded by this sensory stimulation. Ice-cold stimulation to the velum did not trigger any elevation, suggestive of a sensory-motor deficit. The physical therapy literature supports that motor output is dependent on appropriate sensory input. Because radiation therapy affects neural and muscle fibers, and chemotherapy may affect both, sensory-motor deficits are common side effects of CRT.

Jaw opening was targeted through guided stretching tasks wherein the patient was given moderate cues to gently open, exhaling for optimal stretch, and 40 mm was achieved. This degree of jaw opening is not optimal; at this 35- to 40-mm range, there are limitations to the ability to take food from a utensil or even take a bite of a sandwich. Normal vertical excursion is relative to an individual's body structure. This is generally accepted to be three stacked fingers inserted between the lower and upper incisors. Patient X's vertical mandibular excursion was measured at 35 mm, suggesting that he was not compliant with completing the stretching exercises at home.

Pain decreased significantly between 4 and 5 months post CRT with patient self-rating reduced to 2/10 (from 6/10) with successful wean from morphine.

FIVE-MONTH FOLLOW-UP

At 5 months post completion of CRT, the patient had effectively weaned from morphine and was reporting mild (2/10) pain in the affected regions. His weight was at an all-time low of 154 pounds, and gastric feeds were decreased in order to stimulate greater appetite. When asked about his weight loss post CRT, he cited poor appetite and lack of desire to eat, along with difficulty swallowing foods. Specifically, he felt as if foods stuck in his throat, frequently eliciting a gag response. Stricture or narrowing of the upper esophageal lumen was suspected; and referral to a gastroenterologist was made. He had multiple risk factors for stricture formation including past administration of Cisplatin, and a known history of LPR. Though prescribed appropriate therapy, he had been crushing the Pantoprazole (because of his swallowing impairment) which reduces bioavailability. On presentation to gastroenterology, his esophageal lumen size was documented as starting at 12 mm (36 Fr) by the gastroenterologist, comparable to the size of an aspirin. The upper esophageal sphincter is pliable and resilient when healthy; however, this is greatly diminished in the presence of stricture. In the case of Patient X, even small (20 cc) thin-liquid swallows were laborious and required the patient to employ two to three swallows to clear. Though normative data are not available on the average maximum UES lumen distention, weighted bougie dilators will dilate to 20 mm (60 Fr). At this visit the patient underwent UES dilation.

At 7 months after completion of CRT, a second UES dilatation was performed in the typical 4-week interval. His esophagus was dilated from 36 to 45 Fr, and his feeding tube was removed, necessitating that the patient make more frequent attempts at swallowing. He reported drinking two to three cans of Two Cal, a liquid nutritional supplement which has 475 calories per 8 ounces. His weight remained at 153 pounds.

At 11 months post CRT, he began seeing a licensed massage therapist trained in Cranial Sacral Therapy. The goal of massage therapy was to address pain, improve his sense of well-being, and treat trismus via soft tissue manipulation. He continued to attend outpatient dysphagia therapy which, by this time, involved myofascial release for treatment of trismus, review of previously introduced swallowing exercises, and ongoing encouragement of compliance for follow-up gastroenterology for serial esophageal dilatations.

ONE-YEAR FOLLOW UP

Approximately 1-year post diagnosis and 9 months post completion of CRT, Patient X remained in

therapy and was dependent solely on nutritional supplements. He was able to tolerate a National Dysphagia Diet Level 2 to 3, consisting of approximately one cup of soft moist foods per day. Eating was laborious and painful due to the presence of a persistent 3-mm ulceration along the inferior mandible/base of tongue area as well as areas of highly sensitized mucosal erythema. He was prescribed an intensive oral hygiene program by the radiation oncologist. This included alternating Neutrasal and use of diluted baking soda and saltwater rinse. (The formula was 32 ounces of water, 1 teaspoon of baking soda, and 1 teaspoon of salt.) He underwent his third esophageal dilatation achieving the previous 45 Fr. Per the patient's report, the gastroenterologist was not hopeful for further lumen expansion. At that time, he had been back to work for 2 months, appeared and reported being in good spirits, and seemingly adjusting to his new normal. Weight remained at 154 pounds.

A final objective measure was obtained via fiberoptic endoscopic exam of the swallow (FEES) 14 months post completion of CRT. Five weeks prior to this exam, the upper esophagus was dilated to 48 Fr (16 mm). He reported tolerating a soft diet, with poor tolerance of white meat chicken. This was an interval improvement as he was reliant on liquid supplements 9 months post completion of CRT. Results of the exam are as follows. With meat, premature spillage occurred with high risk of aspiration. Reduced anterior excursion of the posterior pharyngeal wall was noted. He did not employ effortful swallows resulting in residual particles of food on the base of tongue, stasis on the posterior pharyngeal wall, as well as moderate to severe stasis in the vallecular space. He was cued for an effortful swallow and liquid rinse using Ensure, resulted in trace coating of the hypopharynx and clearance of most solid residual. After water swallows, the pharynx was clear of all residual. No evidence of gross aspiration was noted though one limitation of this exam is that the view is obstructed during the swallow. After the swallow, small particles of food were seen on the superior portion of the laryngeal surface of the epiglottis. This is a risk factor for aspiration. There were small particles noted in the upper airway confirming silent aspiration. Findings were used to educate the patient on the need for ongoing home program and compliance with compensatory strategies. Compensatory strategies for dysphagia included liquid push/assist while preparing solid food bolus, and an immediate liquid rinse with an effortful breath-hold and effortful swallow. A prophylactic strong cough after every session of eating was recommended. Interval functional improvement may have been largely attributable to esophageal dilation, as he reported decreased compliance in home exercises. A 6-month follow-up exam was agreed upon. He agreed to continued compliance with medical therapy for acid reflux (see Video 10–3).

CONCLUSION AND SUMMARY

Patient X was medically followed post treatment by his physicians from otolaryngology, radiation oncology, and medical oncology. He underwent a follow-up PET/CT scan 3.5 months post treatment that revealed no residual disease within the oropharynx. There was a 1.9-cm mass with an SUV of 1.9 in the right middle lung lobe. The patient was given the option of close monitoring with repeat imaging in 3 months versus biopsy, and chose to undergo a CT scan-guided biopsy that revealed "inflammation." In accordance with NCCN guidelines, he saw each of his three cancer care physicians at least once per month for 3 months post treatment, and then at least once every 3 months for the first year post treatment. At this time, Patient X is just over 1-year post treatment and will continue to be followed by otolaryngology for physical examination every 2 to 4 months in post treatment Year 2, every 4 to 6 months in post treatment Years 3 to 5, and every 6 to 12 months in post treatment Years 5 and beyond (Figures 10–3, 10–4, and 10–5).

This case is representative of the growing population of patients with HPV-positive oropharyngeal

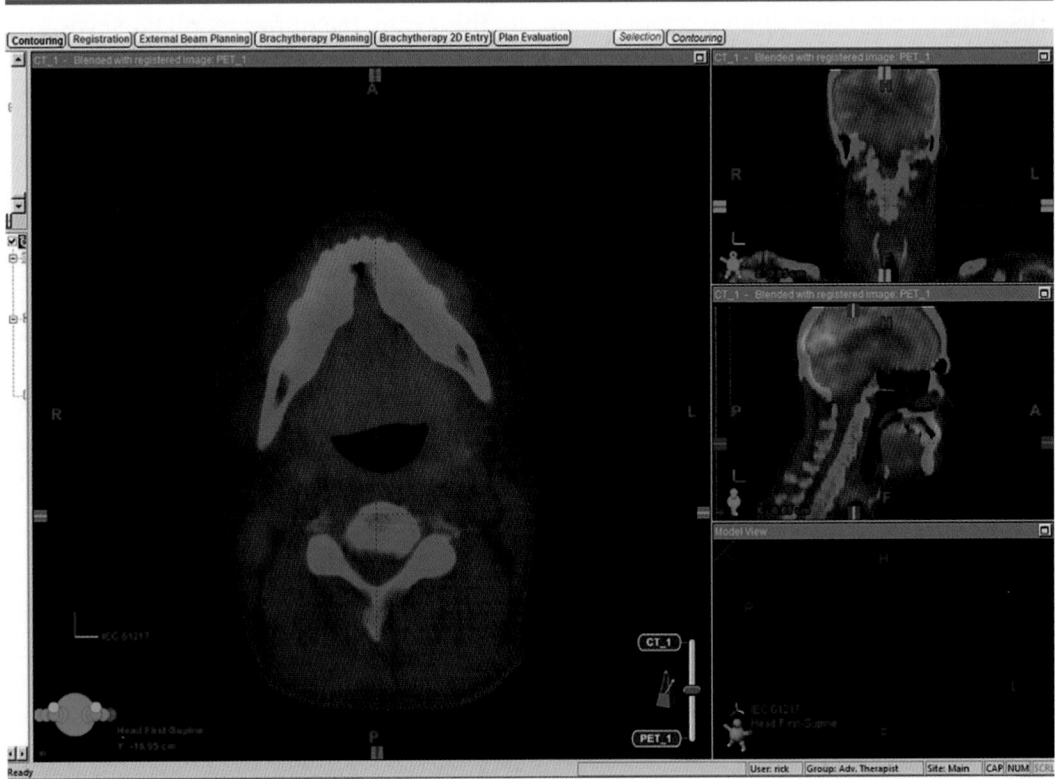

Figure 10–3. PET-CT Post Treatment.

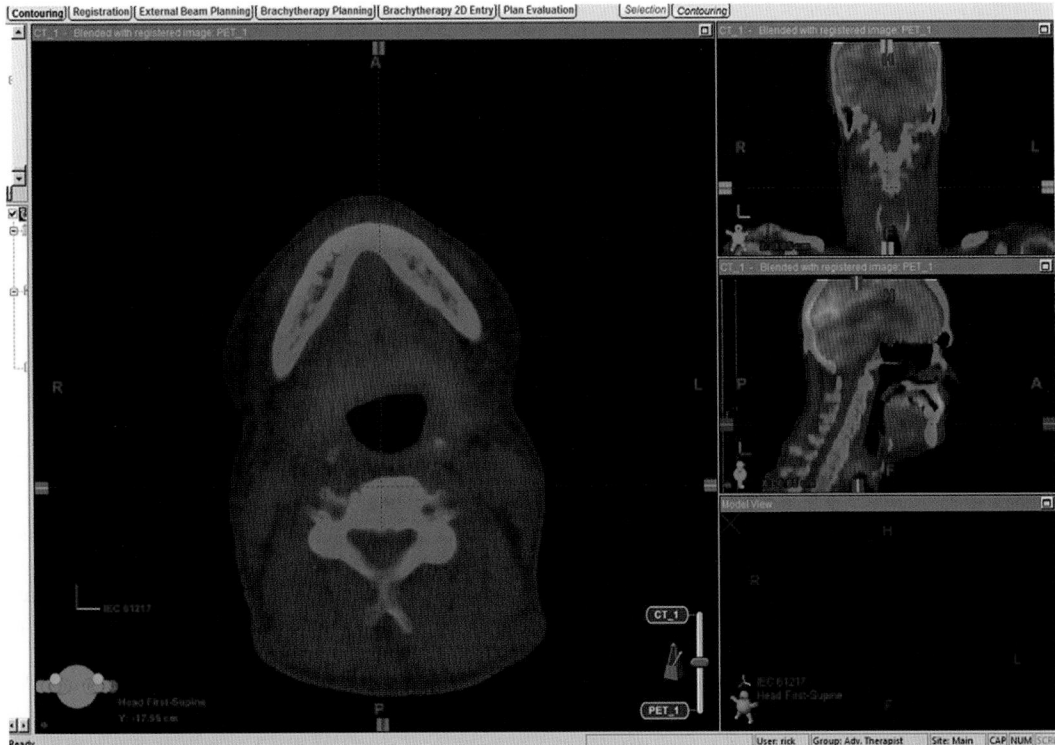

Figure 10–4. PET-CT Post-Treatment.

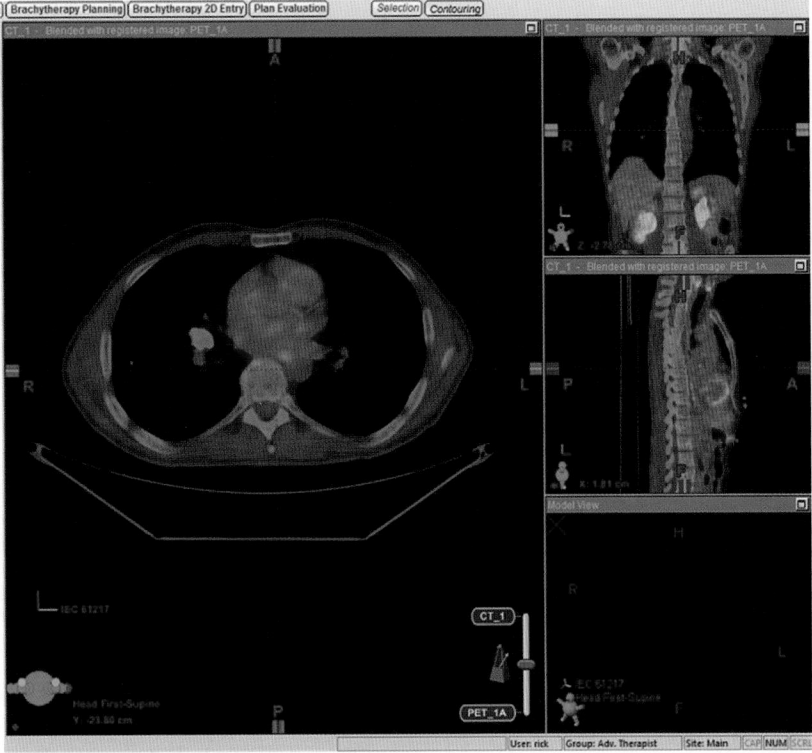

Figure 10–5. PET-CT Post-Treatment.

cancer, and the typical complications that may occur with CRT. He was unique in that he became more motivated and compliant several months after completion of radiation therapy. This underscores the importance of perseverance on the part of the clinician, as his gratitude and recovery were well worth the wait.

REFLECTION AND ANALYSIS FOR FURTHER STUDY

1. Many patients with head and neck cancer who receive radiation treatment develop swallowing issues later on as the radiation doses accumulate. Do you believe that the introduction to speech pathology services should be deferred? Why or why not?
2. What are the potential advantages and disadvantages to early introduction of speech-language pathology services?
3. When working with patients with a multitude of speech, voice, and swallow issues, what can the speech-language pathologist do to minimize "patient overload" and increase the likelihood of patient compliance with treatment recommendations?

REFERENCES

Carnaby-Mann, G., Crary, M. A., Schmalfuss, I., & Amdur, R. (2012). Pharyngocise: Randomized controlled trial of preventative exercises to maintain muscle structure and swallowing function during head-and-neck chemoradiotherapy. *International Journal of Radiation Oncology, Biology, Physics, 83*(1), 210–219.

Centers for Disease Control and Prevention. (2012). Human papillomavirus-associated cancers—United States, 2004–2008. *Morbidity and Mortality Weekly Report, 61*(15), 258–261. Retrieved from http://www.cdc.gov/mmwr/preview/mmwrhtml/mm6115a2.htm

Chaturvedi, A. K., Engels, E. A., Pfeiffer, R. M., Hernandez, B. Y., Xiao, W., Kim, E., & ... Gillison, M. L. (2011). Human papillomavirus and rising oropharyngeal cancer incidence in the United States. *Journal of Clinical Oncology, 29*(32), 4294–4301.

Hutcheson, K. A., Bhayani, M. K., Beadle, B. M., Gold, K. A., Shinn, E. H., Lai, S. Y., & Lewin, J. (2013). Eat and exercise during radiotherapy or chemoradiotherapy for pharyngeal cancers: Use it or lose it. *Otolaryngology-Head and Neck Surgery, 139*(11), 1127–1134.

National Comprehensive Cancer Network. (2013). *NCCN clinical practice guidelines in oncology* (v.2.2013), 20–25. Retrieved from http://oralcancerfoundation.org/treatment/pdf/head-and-neck.pdf

Stemple, J., Lee, L., D'Amico, B., & Pickup, B. (1994). Efficacy of vocal function exercises as a method of improving voice production. *Journal of Voice, 8*(3), 271–278.

Verdolini, K. (2008). *Lessac-Madsen Resonant Voice Therapy.* San Diego, CA: Plural.

PART IV

Hypopharyngeal and Supraglottic Cases

II

Overview of Multidisciplinary Management for Hypopharyngeal Cancer

Paula A. Sullivan, Ilona Schmalfuss, Charles E. Riggs, Jr., William M. Mendenhall, Elizabeth Leon, and Annette N. Askren; Illustrations by Carl C. Askren

INTRODUCTION

Squamous cell carcinoma (SCC) of the hypopharynx is relatively rare and comprises only 3% to 5% of all head and neck cancers (Cooper et al., 2009). The hypopharynx, or laryngopharynx, is a hollow tube about 5 inches long that connects superiorly with the oropharynx and inferiorly with the esophagus. The hypopharynx lies behind the larynx in front of cervical vertebrae 3–6 and projects laterally onto each side of the larynx. The hypopharynx is composed of three anatomic subsites: the piriform sinus, the posterior pharyngeal wall, and the posterior cricoid area (pharyngeal-esophageal junction). Approximately 65% to 85% of hypopharyngeal cancers involve the piriform sinuses. Tumors in this region are difficult to detect in the earliest stages, as they are hard to visualize by mirror and/or endoscopic examination. In addition to the disadvantage of poor visualization, hypopharyngeal cancer symptoms are commonly vague, nonspecific, and late in presentation. Sixty to 80% of patients with late-presenting disease have ipsilateral nodal metastasis (Gourin & Terris, 2004), and up to 40% have contralateral occult nodal tumors (Buckley & MacLennan, 2000). Accompanying swallowing dysfunction and advanced local and regional spread result in limited treatment options, poor outcomes, and poor survival.

Organ-preservation therapy (combined chemotherapy and radiotherapy) has become the treatment of choice for advanced hypopharyngeal cancer over the past decade or so. It avoids surgical resection and reconstruction, which may involve high risks of morbidity and mortality, and can also spare anatomy, including the neighboring larynx. However, patients with high-volume T3-T4 tumors greater than 6 to 8 cc have a low probability of cure with a functional larynx; in such cases, surgery followed by postoperative irradiation is preferred. A meta-analysis by Pignon, le Maître, Maillard, and Bourhis (2009) demonstrated a survival benefit for concurrent chemoradiotherapy (CRT) compared with radiotherapy alone in the treatment of advanced head and neck cancer. Although CRT may improve disease control, it commonly results in significant acute and chronic treatment-related toxicities, most notably xerostomia, mucositis, and dysphagia, sometimes necessitating gastrostomy feeding tube placement. In a retrospective review of 73 patients treated with CRT for advanced hypopharyngeal cancer, Keereweer and colleagues (2011) reported survival rates of 41%, local disease control rates of 71%, and regional disease control rates of 97%. However, dysphagia and xerostomia persisted during long-term follow-up, resulting in the conclusion that despite organ preservation, the significant acute and long-term treatment toxicities do not necessarily result in preservation of function and better quality of life.

Due to the complex management of patients with head and neck cancer, the National Comprehensive Cancer Network (NCCN) published evidence and consensus-based guidelines (NCCN, 2013) for optimal treatment and outcomes, including work-up and staging, treatment, and follow-up/ surveillance of hypopharyngeal cancers. Emphasis is placed on the necessity of a multidisciplinary team to manage and prevent common treatment sequelae, most notably dysphagia, significant weight loss, and accompanying deterioration in quality of life. Additionally, the NCCN Guidelines state that for patients with chronic dysphagia, follow-up may need to be indefinite given the late-occurring effects of complications, including cranial neuropathy, trismus, radionecrosis, stricture, pneumonia, and gastrostomy dependence (Hutcheson et al., 2012).

This chapter discusses the complex and ongoing management of a patient presenting with advanced-stage hypopharyngeal cancer of the right piriform sinus. Additionally, the chapter highlights the importance of an integrated, comprehensive multidisciplinary team throughout the continuum of care to date, further optimized by the use of Telehealth/ Skype technology to improve intensity of rehabilitation and subsequent outcomes.

A CASE OF ADVANCED HYPOPHARYNGEAL CANCER (RIGHT PIRIFORM SINUS)

History

Medical History

Patient T, a 56-year-old Caucasian male, presented to the Department of Veterans Affairs Ear, Nose, and Throat (VA ENT) clinic with a 4-month history of progressive, persistent right ear pain (otalgia), worsened with chewing, coughing, and swallowing. The patient denied any change to hearing but endorsed chronic right tinnitus that was continuous and non-pulsatile. He was treated with neomycin eardrops for approximately 1 month prior without relief. Recent mandibular x-ray showed no evidence for temporomandibular joint arthritis or other pathology.

The past medical history revealed an allergy to latex products. Patient T had a 20-year history of cutaneous psoriasis, treated for the past 10 years with etanercept (Enbrel). He had undergone left ethmoidectomy for ethmoiditis 10 years before presentation, and left low cervical foraminotomy for left arm numbness and weakness 8 years earlier. Smoking history (cigarettes) was quantified at 25 pack-years. He quit smoking and was diagnosed with chronic obstructive pulmonary disease 6 years prior to presentation. There was no history of current alcohol use. Review of systems confirmed bilateral sensorineural hearing loss, quantified as moderately severe by audiometry; stable weight; major depressive disorder with chronic anxiety; and no diabetes or thyroid disease.

Social History

Patient T is a retired, service-connected Gulf War veteran with 20 years of military service in both the U.S. Navy and U.S. Marine Corps Infantry. His military occupational specialty included lengthy and intense exposure to chemicals, including petroleum and asbestos. Patient T is divorced and resides with his adult daughter who is enrolled in nursing school. The patient is the second youngest of five siblings and remains in close contact with a brother and sister who live nearby. His younger brother has Prader-Willi syndrome and lives in a group home, and his mother resides in a nursing home.

Diagnostic Work-Up

On the day of presentation to the VA ENT clinic, flexible fiberoptic laryngoscopy revealed a large verrucous lesion involving the medial and lateral walls of the right piriform sinus that extended to the piriform sinus apex, limiting vocal fold mobility on the right. The mass was seen to track along the lateral wall of the aryepiglottic fold, with right lateral pharyngeal wall involvement. Physical examination of the neck and supraclavicular areas revealed no palpable cervical lymphadenopathy. Ear examination was normal. Simultaneous working channel biopsy of the mass was performed.

The patient underwent computed tomography (CT) of the neck and chest with IV contrast, following biopsy. A positron emission tomography/computed tomography (PET/CT) imaging study was performed 1 week later for staging purposes.

Biopsy results yielded moderately differentiated, invasive squamous cell carcinoma, nonkeratinizing, with positive staining for the p16 marker, but negative in situ hybridization for human papillomavirus (HPV−).

A growing body of evidence suggests that patients undergoing organ preservation treatment, followed regularly in a swallow preservation program during their course of radiation therapy, demonstrate improved functional outcomes, including improved quality of life (Kulbersch et al., 2006), improved swallowing function (Carroll et al., 2008), and maintenance of muscle structure (Carnaby-Mann, Crary, Schmalfuss, & Amdur, 2012). Thus, it was recommended that Patient T be followed per the speech pathology department's organ preservation practice guideline, including pretreatment assessment, weekly visits to review swallowing exercises and provide dysphagia intervention throughout course of treatment, initial post treatment evaluation (approximately 4–8 weeks after completion, per tolerance to treatment), 3 months following initial post treatment visit, 6 months thereafter, 12 months thereafter, and ongoing intervention, as necessary. Multiple baseline clinical swallowing examination measures of health status, function, performance, and quality of life were obtained, including the Montreal Cognitive Assessment Screening (MoCA), Karnofsky Performance Scale, EAT-10, MD Anderson Dysphagia Inventory (MDADI), Functional Oral Intake Scale (FOIS), and the Performance Status Scale-Head and Neck Cancer (PSS-HNC) Normalcy of Diet Subscale.

Speech Pathology Assessment Outcomes

Patient T's presenting complaints to speech pathology included right otalgia, rated 8 to 9 out of 10

in severity, progressive dysphagia to solids, and extreme sensitivity to cold and carbonated beverages. Weight loss was denied. The patient denied any vocal changes, although mild dysphonia characterized by hoarseness was noted. Flexible endoscopic examination of swallowing (FEES) was performed at this initial evaluation and confirmed reduced mobility of the right true vocal fold, pharyngeal asymmetry, laryngeal penetration of both liquids and solids, and vallecular residue (Figure 11–1). In light of baseline dysphagia, tumor location, and staging, the recommendation for a prophylactic percutaneous endoscopic gastrostomy (PEG) tube placement was discussed with Patient T, who adamantly declined this recommendation.

A daily program of prophylactic swallowing exercises was provided. The active exercise regimen adhered to general principles of neuromuscular exercise science to target strengthening and range of motion (Clark, 2003). Force (an index of strength) and endurance served as primary goals of strengthening—force being targeted via an increased level of resistance during a maneuver, and endurance being targeted with increased number of repetitions of a low-resistance maneuver. Active range-of-motion

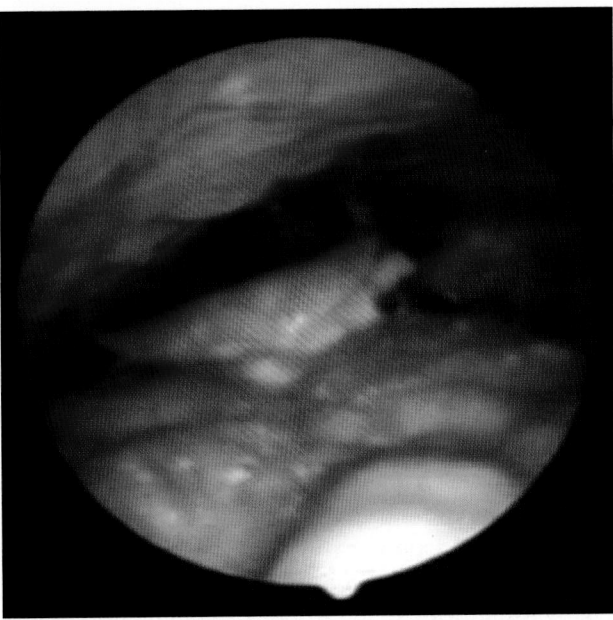

Figure 11–1. Pretreatment fiberoptic endoscopic evaluation of swallow (FEES) exam, performed by Speech Pathology.

techniques were included to target inhibition of stretch reflexes and support strength training. For example, the Mendelsohn maneuver enlists both active range of motion (or patient-regulated stretching) and strengthening techniques by requiring increased range coupled with maintenance of a laryngeal posture against resistance (Clark, 2003). Frequency of engagement in the prescribed regimen of active exercises promoted adequate overload and specificity of training. Patient T was encouraged to begin this exercise regimen prior to the initiation of conformal radiation treatment (CRT).

Dental Consultation

Following his speech pathology consultation, a dental evaluation noted that the patient was partially edentulous with a lower partial dental plate. Although dental caries were noted in one tooth, extraction was not recommended, as the radiotherapeutic field did not involve the tooth-bearing areas of the jaw. Additionally, Patient T was seen by the Head and Neck Dietitian for pretreatment evaluation with subsequent close follow-up throughout the continuum of care.

Multidisciplinary Tumor Board

Following completion of diagnostic work-up, findings were presented at the VA Medical Center's multidisciplinary Head and Neck Tumor Board conference. Representatives from Otolaryngology, Medical Oncology, Radiation Oncology, Radiology, and Speech Pathology were present. The neck CT (Figure 11–2) was reviewed showing an infiltrating lesion in the right piriform sinus that primarily affected the anterior and lateral walls of the right piriform sinus, as seen on clinical examination. In addition, a small area of involvement was noted along the posterior wall. The CT examination also demonstrated early involvement of the right posterior false and true vocal cords along the paraglottic fat planes. Often, this cannot be detected on clinical examination, as the tumor grows in submucosal fashion; however, it may be suggested by abnormal

vocal cord movement. No abnormal cervical lymph nodes were noted. There were no erosions of the laryngeal cartilages or extension to the piriform sinus apex. Chest CT showed no metastatic disease.

The PET/CT imaging (Figure 11–3) revealed intense FDG uptake in the right pyriform sinus mass, with a SUV equal to 31. PET/CT also showed bilateral hypermetabolic cervical lymph adenopathy in Level IIA concerning for metastatic disease. Based on imaging and clinical findings, the patient's tumor was thus staged as Stage IVA (T2N2cM0) invasive SCC of the right piriform sinus.

Discussion included surgery (partial laryngopharyngectomy, probable flap reconstruction, neck dissection) coupled with possible postoperative radiation versus CRT. In the face of the high-volume, node-positive disease, the Tumor Board ultimately recommended definitive treatment with curative intent with larynx-preserving, concomitant CRT therapy, to which the patient consented.

As Patient T resided approximately 150 miles north of the treating facility, housing during the planned course of organ preservation treatment was arranged in the local American Cancer Society Hope Lodge, a hotel at no cost to veterans and other patients who require frequent medical center treatments over a lengthy period of time.

Treatment

The CRT treatment plan included delivery of 74.4 gray (Gy) at 1.2 Gy per twice-daily fractions, 5 days per week, with intensity-modulated radiotherapy (IMRT) with six MV x-rays over 31 treatment days in a continuous course. The IMRT target volume included the primary tumor, the retropharyngeal nodes, and both sides of the neck. Because of the patient's hearing loss, the preferred chemotherapy regimen was planned to consist of concomitant weekly carboplatin AUC = 2, plus paclitaxel at 45 mg/m^2. Patient T initially elected against placement of a subcutaneous venous access port and PEG tube. However, by Week 3 of therapy, the patient was suffering progressively painful stomatitis, oral candidiasis, anorexia, dysgeusia, dysphagia, odynophagia, and prostration. He required admission to the VA hospi-

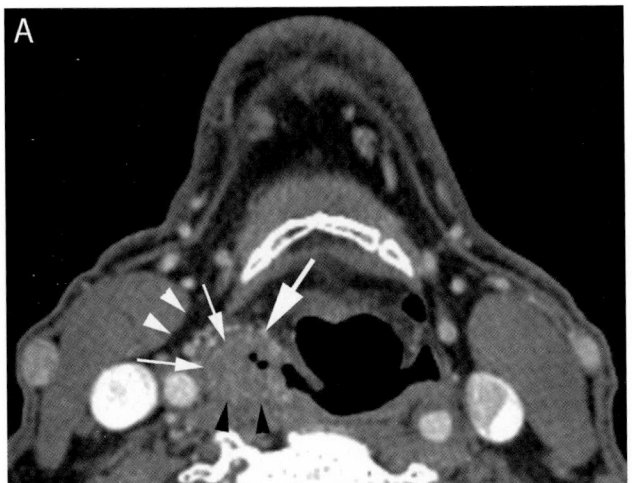

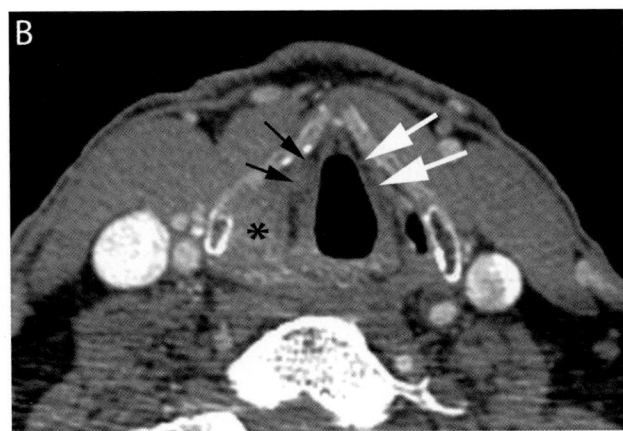

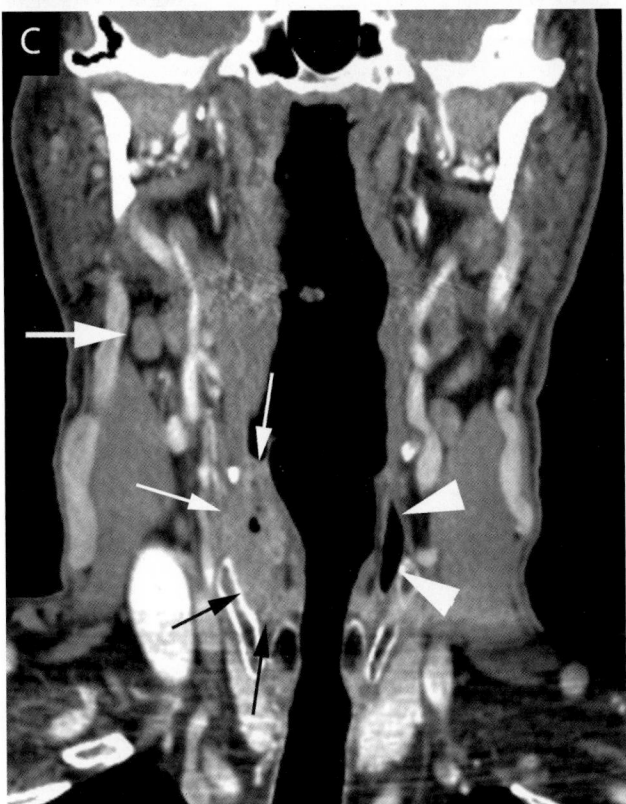

Figure 11–2. Pretreatment computed tomography (CT) imaging presented to Head and Neck Tumor Board for staging. **A–B.** Contrast-enhanced CT images of the neck in axial plane reveal a mass that is affecting the anterior (*large white arrow in A*), lateral (*small white arrows in A*), and posterior (*black arrowheads in A*) walls of the right piriform sinus. The mass displaces the superior laryngeal neurovascular bundle laterally with preservation of the adjacent fat planes (*white arrowheads in A*), indicating that the tumor is limited to the visceral compartment. The mass extends inferiorly to fill up and enlarge the right piriform sinus (*star in B*). In addition, it shows anterior extension into the right false vocal cord with subtle obliteration of the paraglottic fat plane (*small black arrows in B*) when compared to its normal appearance on the left (*large black arrows in B*). **C.** The coronal reformation image of the volumetric CT data set better illustrates the full extent of the piriform sinus mass on the right (*small arrows in C*) when compared to its normal air filled appearance on the left (*arrowheads in C*). A normal-sized Group IIA lymph nodes with unremarkable internal architechture is seen on the right (*large arrow in C*).

tal for fluid resuscitation, analgesia, and antibiotics. During this admission, a port device and PEG tube were placed, and paclitaxel was permanently discontinued from the chemotherapy regimen because of its greater potential to cause mucositis. The patient experienced considerable difficulties adapting to enteral tube feeding. He suffered early satiety, abdominal bloating, nausea, and intermittent vomiting. CRT was continued, with weekly carboplatin, and concluded in the seventh week after initiation.

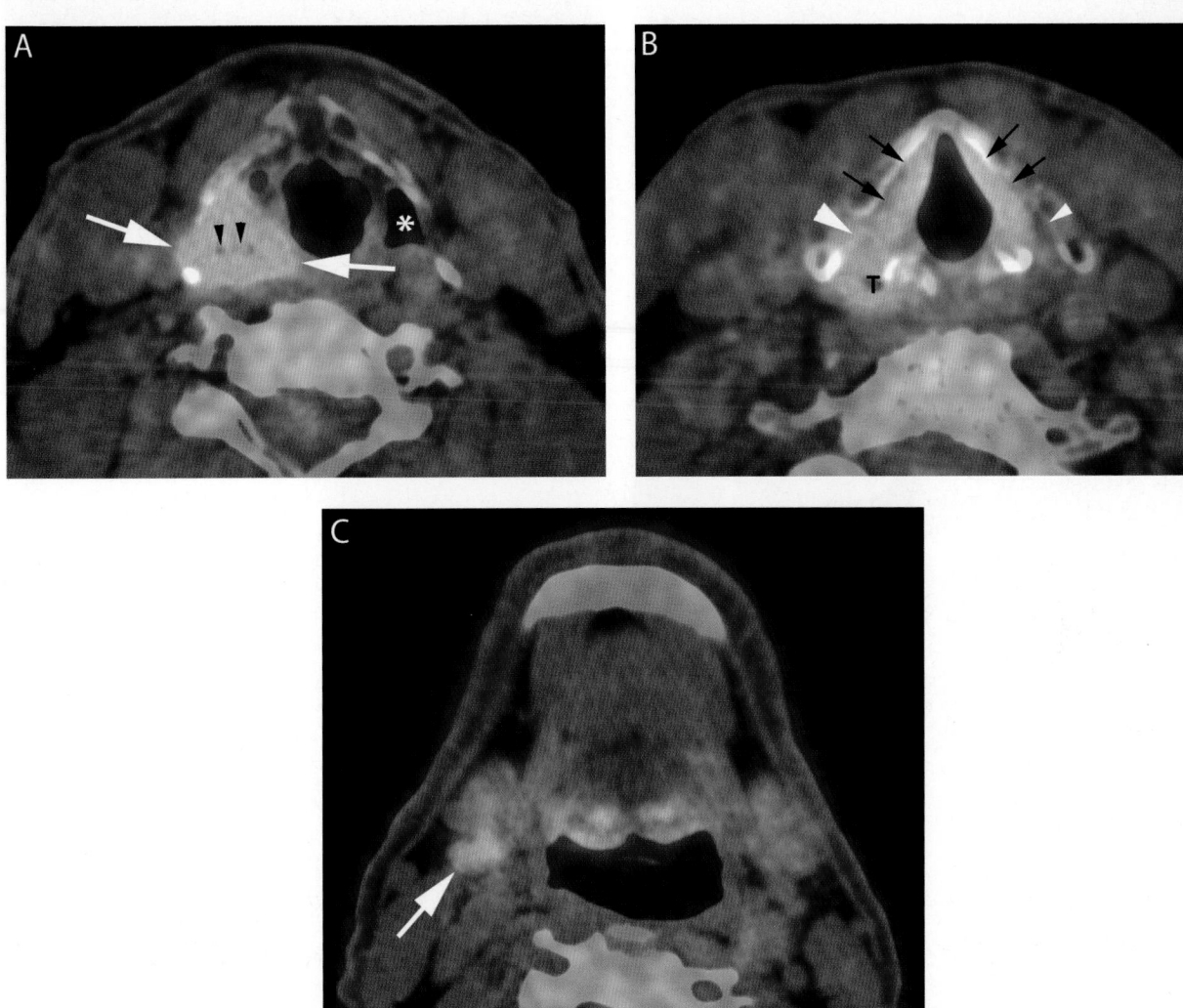

Figure 11–3. Pretreatment positron emission tomography/computed tomography (PET/CT) imaging presented to Head and Neck Tumor Board for staging. **A–C.** Axial fused FDG PET/CT images confirm the large mass that is circumferentially affecting the right piriform sinus (*between arrows in A*). The mass significantly narrows the right piriform sinus with only a small air-filled lumen visualized (*arrowheads in A*). Notice the normal, air-distended piriform sinus on the left (*asterisk in A*). The tumor (*T in B*) extends inferiorly to the level of the true vocal folds. The true vocal folds show marked FDG uptake (*arrows in B*), which is physiologic in nature when the patient talks during the FDG radiotracer uptake phase. Notice, however, the subtle difference in the FDG uptake within the posterior true vocal folds with no FDG uptake on the left (*small arrowhead in B*) when compared to marked FDG uptake on the right (*larger arrowhead in B*). This FDG uptake is confluent with the tumor (*T in B*) in the inferior piriform sinus and indicative of early posterior true vocal cord involvement. This explains the patient's slightly abnormal vocal cord motion on clinical examination and is not visible on endoscopic examination due to its submucosal location. In addition, there is marked FDG uptake in the previously noted normal-sized Group IIA lymph node (*arrow in C*) that is concerning for metastatic disease. No metastatic disease was detected in the body (*not shown*).

A total of 73.2 Gy was delivered to the primary site and positive nodes, 58.8 Gy to bilateral neck fields, and 49.2 Gy to bilateral supraclavicular fields. A total of five doses of carboplatin were delivered, in addition to two weekly paclitaxel doses.

At the time of this hospitalization during Week 3 of therapy, Stage IV mucositis precluded any oral intake. Following PEG and port placement, the patient required continued hospitalization during the remainder of his CRT due to poor tolerance of tube feedings, development of a purulent cellulitis around the PEG tube, and his significantly deconditioned status. Speech pathology continued to follow the patient during his extended hospitalization for ongoing support, education, and intervention as feasible. However, the patient's protracted recovery prevented his active participation in the previously prescribed swallow preservation program, and he remained NPO with all nutrition and hydration obtained via PEG tube.

Post Treatment

At the conclusion of the CRT, Patient T was discharged to a skilled nursing facility in his community and recovered essentially no swallowing function during that time. Three weeks later, he was readmitted to the VA medical center and was felt to have recalcitrant mucositis, oral candidiasis, generalized weakness and fatigue, and continued poor tolerance of enteral nutrition, despite recent conversion to a gastrostomy-jejunostomy (G-J) feeding tube. Nausea and early satiety were felt to be due to chronic narcotic use and reduced mobility, causing gastroparesis. He received some relief with a trial of azithromycin suspension.

Speech pathology assessment and intervention were resumed. In light of the patient's G-J tube dependency, severe oropharyngeal dysphagia, recent onset of patient-reported hypersensitive gag reflex, and limited home support, speech pathology, supported by the multidisciplinary team, advocated for Patient T's subsequent discharge to the VA hospital's Community Living Center (CLC) for a short period of skilled, intensive swallowing rehabilitation not available in his local community. Although the patient did not meet admission criteria, advocacy efforts were successful in facilitating admission to the CLC for a 3-week stay.

During this subacute period, some slow improvement in well-being was established. Although limited in scope due to poor patient tolerance, a videofluoroscopic swallow study (VFSS) was performed by Speech Pathology to guide rehabilitation. The VFSS revealed moderate-severe oropharyngeal dysphagia characterized by aspiration of thin liquids and significant pharyngeal residue (Figure 11–4). Airway compromise during the swallow was successfully mitigated with a head-turn-right compensatory posture coupled with a super-supraglottic swallow maneuver, a technique during which the patient is instructed to hold his breath and bear down promoting anterior tilt of the arytenoid cartilages and

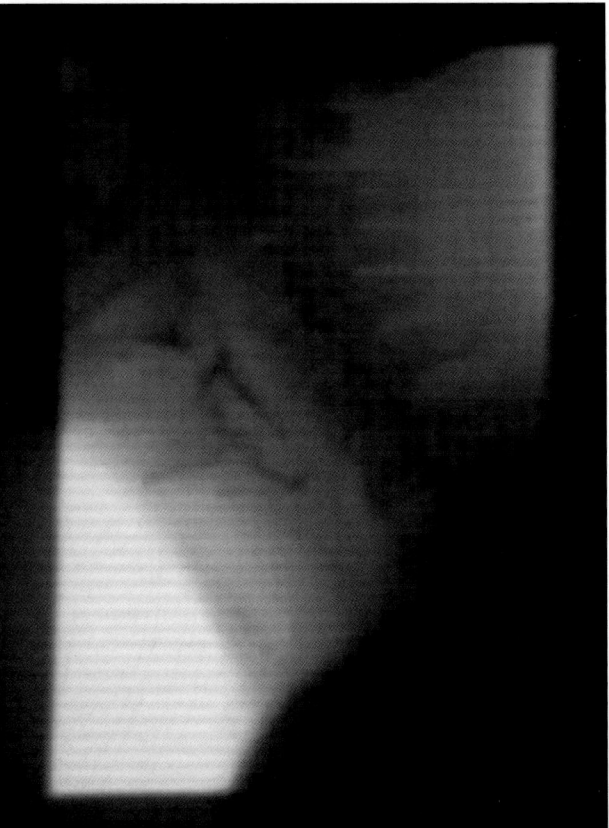

Figure 11–4. Still image of initial post treatment videofluoroscopic swallow study (VFSS).

adduction of the vocal cords, swallow while holding his breath, and complete the maneuver with a volitional cough to clear the laryngeal vestibule of material (Logemann, 1998). Postswallow aspiration risk from piriform sinus residue was considered to be high. The patient was followed for daily, intensive swallowing intervention.

Dysphagia intervention was continued by progressively desensitizing the patient's reported hypersensitive gag reflex. Toothette oral swabs, coated in various beverages, were introduced multiple times throughout the day by Speech Pathology and proved to effectively desensitize reported gag reflex to tolerate therapeutic liquid trials via teaspoon. Additionally, therapeutic swallowing exercises, including those to target the lingual and pharyngeal musculature of critical oropharyngeal areas (Figure 11–5) were drilled, twice daily, to include approximately 10 repetitions of each exercise. Exercise regimen (Figure 11–6) included tongue base retraction repetitions, the Masako maneuver, the Mendelsohn maneuver, and the Shaker exercise sequence.

Following Patient T's discharge home from the VA hospital's CLC, bimonthly swallowing rehabilitation via Telehealth/Skype technology was initiated to continue high-frequency swallowing exercises established in-house during CLC admission. How-

ever, the patient was admitted yet again to acute care for nausea, hypotension, and generalized malaise. Blood cultures yielded *Klebsiella pneumoniae*, subsequently proven to be related to contaminated subcutaneous venous access port catheter. This device was removed, and he recovered well. Once again, bimonthly swallowing rehabilitation via Telehealth/Skype technology was resumed after the patient returned home.

One month after completion of treatment, Patient T underwent a restaging CT of the neck and chest with IV contrast, and images were reviewed at the Head and Neck Tumor Board conference (Figure 11–7). The neck CT showed marked decrease in size of the right piriform sinus mass and persistent obliteration of the right posterior paraglottic fat planes. Residual fullness at the primary site is a common finding on neck CT examination performed only 1 month after completion of CRT. In general, diffuse fullness without a discrete mass or a mass less than 1 cm in diameter usually resolves on subsequent imaging while a residual lesion of more than 1 cm in size has a 50% chance of persistent disease. The CT of the chest continued to be negative for metastatic disease. The Tumor Board therefore recommended a PET/CT with a contrasted neck CT to be performed at 12 weeks after completion of his CRT.

At 12 weeks post treatment, the patient was examined in the VA ENT clinic. He reported that he was unable to swallow and was taking all nutrition via G-J tube. Fiberoptic laryngoscopy revealed diffuse postradiation edema of the supraglottis and glottis, with subtle submucosal fullness in the right piriform sinus. There was no obvious mucosal lesion. There was also no palpable cervical lymphadenopathy. The patient's PET/CT done at 12 weeks after treatment revealed complete response at the primary site with associated, expected postradiation edema (not shown) and no signs of metastatic disease. The Tumor Board recommended a repeat PET/CT with diagnostic neck CT to be performed at 6 months after treatment.

Six months after completing therapy, the patient was seen by ENT and speech pathology. Patient T reported that he was only able to take small amounts of thin liquids by mouth with subsequent hang-up in his throat, resulting in coughing and choking.

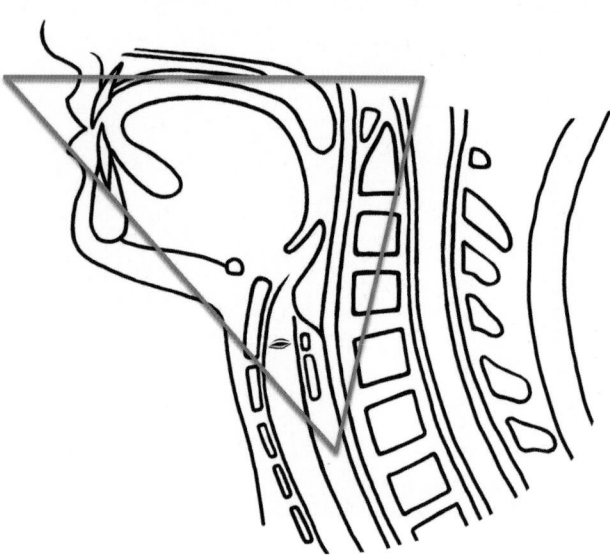

Figure 11–5. Critical areas targeted in the patient's dysphagia rehabilitation.

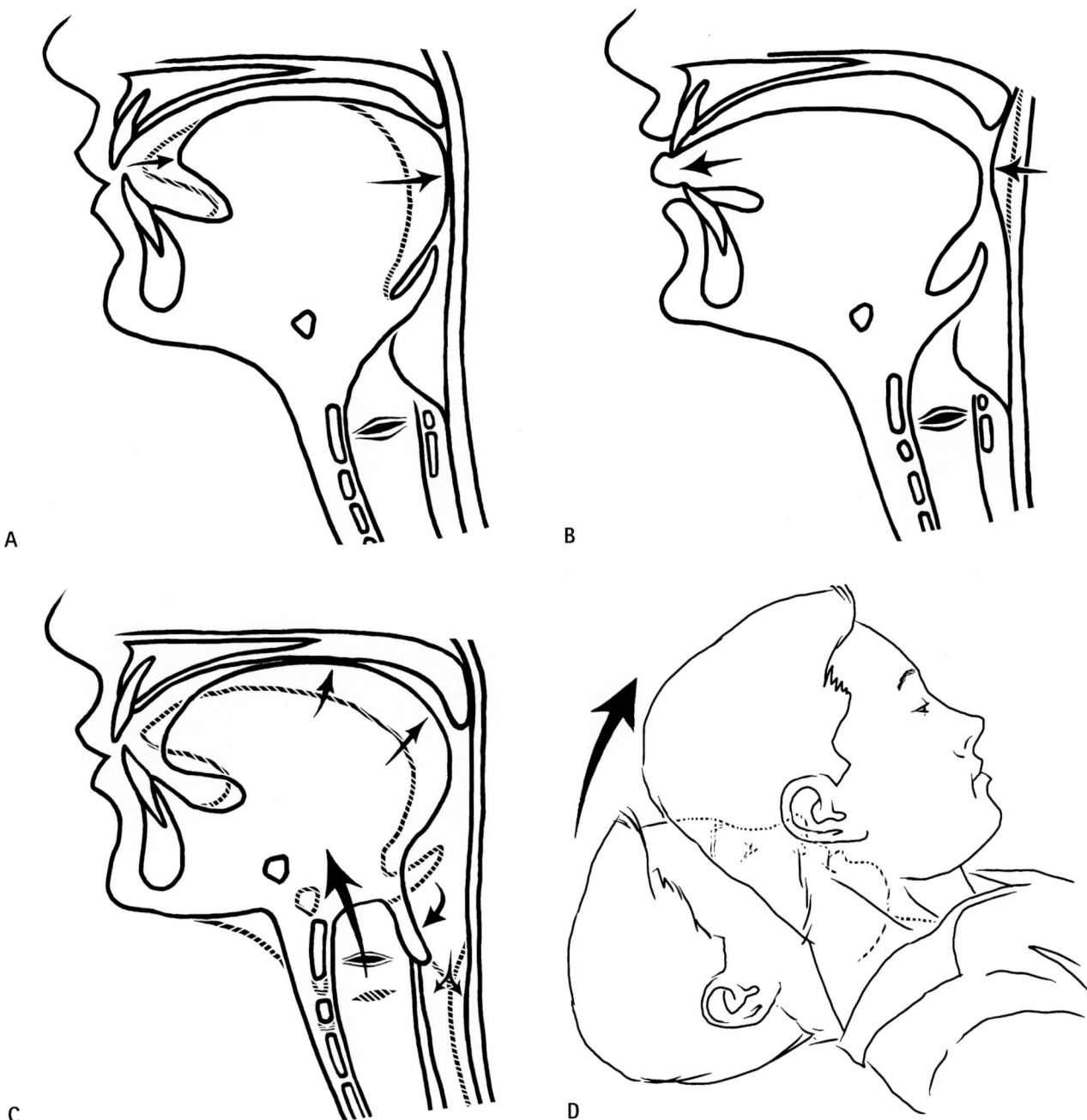

Figure 11–6. Various swallow exercises introduced prior to CRT and during therapeutic rehabilitation. **A.** Tongue-base retraction exercise includes extreme retraction of the lingual body toward the posterior pharyngeal wall and holding for 10 s, targeting base of tongue strength and range of motion. **B.** Masako/tongue-hold maneuver anchors the lingual apex while swallowing, promoting increased resistance at the tongue base and thus improving strength and range-of-motion of the tongue base, bulging of the posterior pharyngeal wall during swallowing, and increased pharyngeal squeeze during swallowing. **C.** Mendelsohn maneuver requires voluntary prolongation of hyolaryngeal excursion at the midpoint of the swallow to target increased range of motion of the hyolaryngeal complex and augment UES relaxation. **D.** Shaker sequence, during which the patient is instructed to lift the head and hold for 1 min then continue with 30 head-lift repetitions, targets anterior excursion of the larynx with subsequent UES opening.

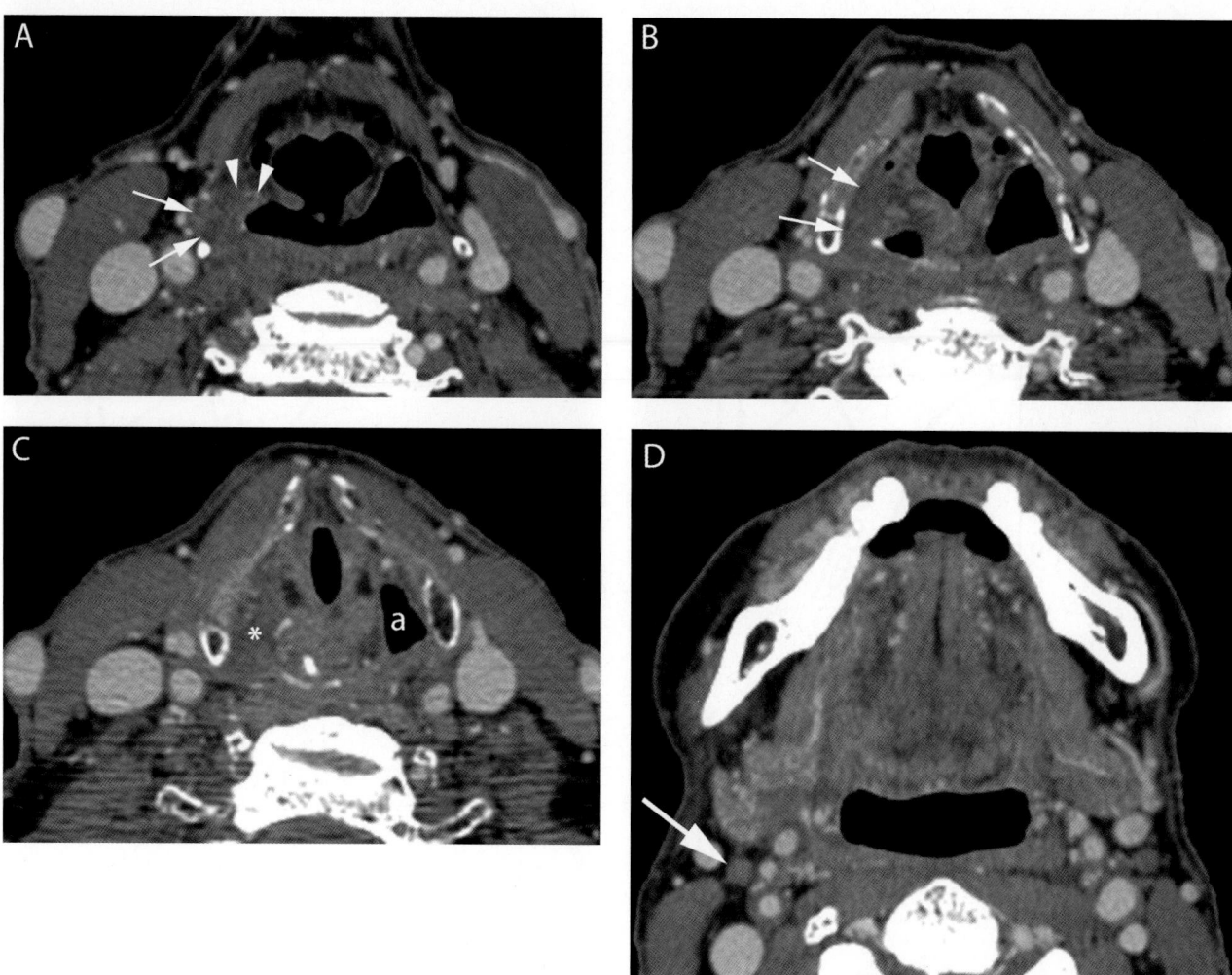

Figure 11–7. Contrast-enhanced follow-up CT images of the neck in axial plane (**A–C**) demonstrates marked decrease in size of the right piriform sinus mass when compared to the pretreatment CT study (see Figure 11–3). Nevertheless, there remains marked fullness along the anterior (*arrowheads in A*) and lateral (*small arrows in A and B*) walls of the piriform sinus entrance site which progresses in craniocaudal direction and results in complete obliteration of the right inferior piriform sinus (*star in C*) when compared to the normal, air-distended left piriform sinus (*a in C*). Notice that the areas of fullness are lower in density than the original tumor (see Figure 11–3) indicating significant response to CRT. **D.** The previously seen Group IIA lymph node (*large arrow in D*) also markedly decreased in size and maintains normal imaging characteristics.

He remained dependent on G-J tube feedings for primary means of nutrition. A videofluorographic swallowing study (VFSS) conducted by speech pathology at this time revealed improved retraction of the tongue base and elevation and excursion of the hyolaryngeal complex with essentially no relaxation of the upper esophageal segment (UES) with subsequent postswallow aspiration of contrast stasis (Figure 11–8). Use of various swallowing compensations did not facilitate upper esophageal sphincter UES opening. Repeat PET/CT 6 months after treatment showed continued locoregional control of disease without signs of metastatic disease (Figure 11–9).

Seven months after completion of CRT, at the recommendation of speech pathology, ENT performed a direct laryngoscopy, esophagoscopy, and esophageal dilation under general anesthesia. At that time, close inspection showed no mucosal lesion

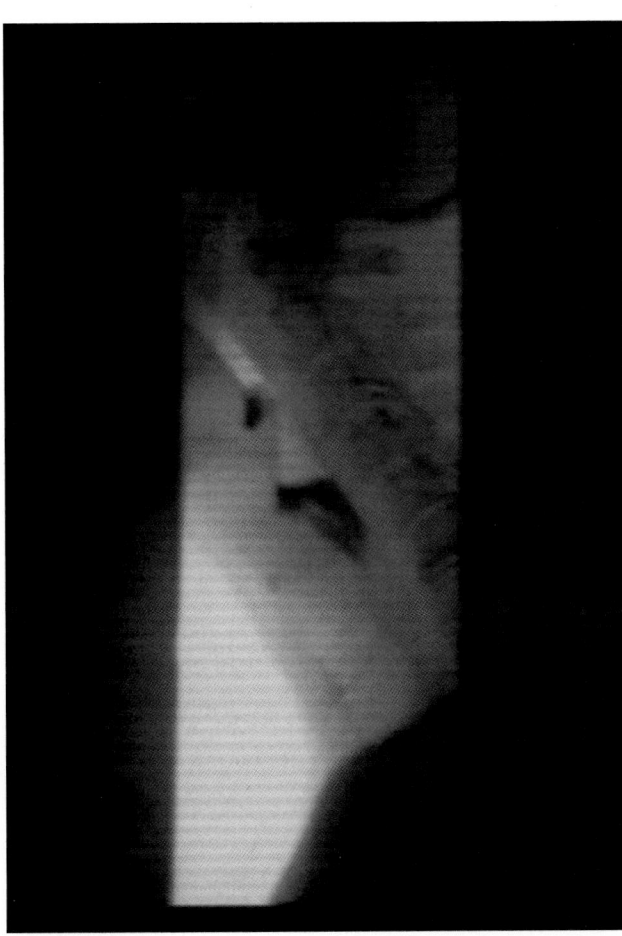

Figure 11–8. VFSS demonstrates essentially absent relaxation of the UES.

of the right piriform sinus. A proximal cervical esophageal stricture was found and serially dilated without difficulty or complication. Tapered rubber esophageal bougies were used. The day following the procedure, the patient was seen in speech pathology for intensive postdilation swallow therapy. Guided by two subsequent VFSSs, speech pathology recommended repeated dilations. ENT repeated the dilations with similar technique and findings 3 and 5 months later, for a total of three dilations. After each dilation, the patient was seen the subsequent day by speech pathology for intensive swallow therapy. The patient reported and demonstrated under videofluoroscopy progressive functional improvement in swallowing after each dilation.

During this time, Patient T continued to have bimonthly head and neck cancer surveillance in the ENT clinic, with complete head and neck exams including fiberoptic laryngoscopy. A contrasted neck CT examination at 1 year post treatment showed persistent control at the primary site without evidence of metastatic disease. VFSS conducted 1 year after treatment completion revealed significant improvement in all oropharyngeal parameters, including tongue-base retraction, hyolaryngeal elevation and excursion, and UES relaxation with moderate, persistent dysphagia. Intermittent, mild thin liquid aspiration per videofluoroscopy was effectively cleared from the airway by patient's spontaneous use of

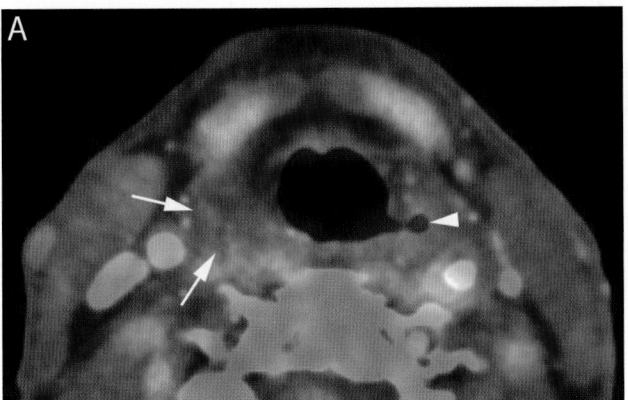
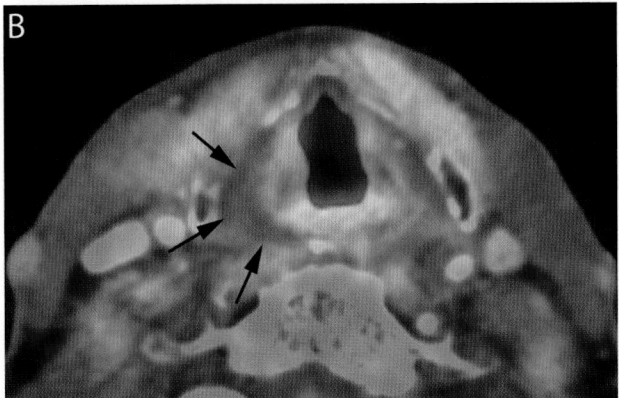

Figure 11–9. Fused FDG PET/CT images of the neck in axial plane performed 6 months after completion of radiation therapy confirm the persistent fullness in the right piriform sinus (*arrows in A and B*) but without any abnormal FDG activity indicating expected postradiation edema. Notice that the left piriform sinus is now partially obliterated (*arrowhead in A*) as it is also affected by postradiation edema. No metastatic disease was visualized in the neck or body (*not shown*).

the super-supraglottic swallow maneuver. Use of a second swallow combined with a head-turn-right posture moderately reduced pharyngeal residue (Figure 11–10). The G-J tube was removed 3 months later, as the patient was maintaining his weight with an essentially soft solid diet. Readministration of baseline clinical swallowing examination measures of health status, function, performance, and quality of life revealed global improvement.

Plans include continued head and neck cancer surveillance every 3 months. Additionally, Patient T will continue ongoing swallowing monitoring and intervention by speech pathology to further improve, and hopefully stabilize, swallowing function and subsequent quality of life.

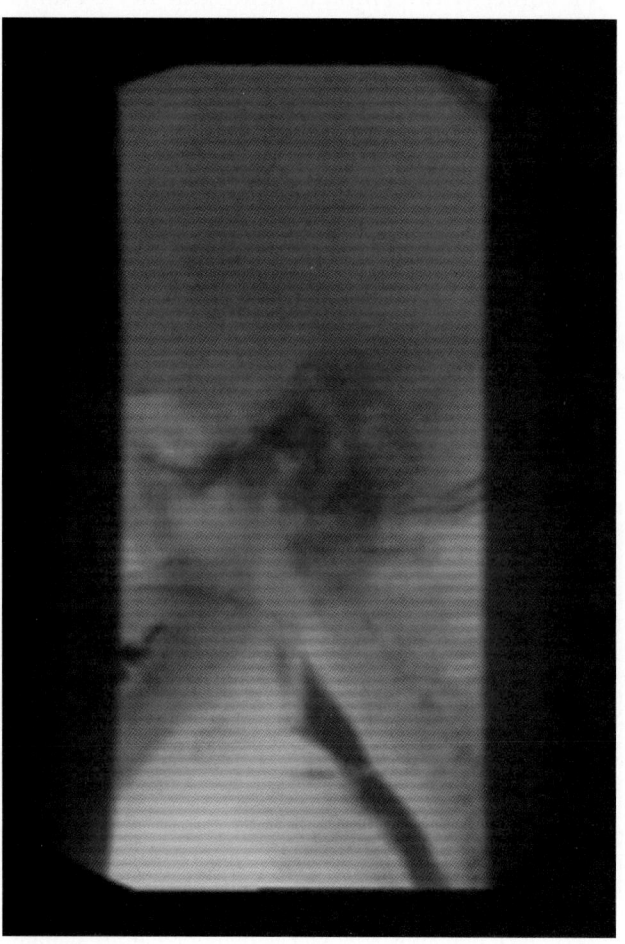

Figure 11–10. VFSS after repeated dilations of the proximal esophagus.

REFLECTION AND ANALYSIS FOR FURTHER STUDY

1. In what ways is the patient with head and neck cancer different than other patients treated for voice and swallow difficulties?
2. Radiation treatment is an option for many patients with head and neck cancer. Critically examine the role of the speech pathologist in patient counseling, and construct a readily understandable explanation of side effects of radiation treatment for head and neck cancer with regard to the voice and swallow functions of head and neck structures.
3. Analysis of this case illustrates the major role of the speech-language pathologist in ensuring that swallowing function was safe for this patient following the surgical procedure. Did you agree with the choices made by the speech-language pathologist on the timeline in which the therapy selections were completed? Provide two examples of what you agreed with and provide one example of what you might have changed and give the rationale and justification for your opinion.

REFERENCES

Buckley, J. G., & MacLennan, K. (2000). Cervical node metastasis in laryngeal and hypopharyngeal cancer: A prospective analysis of prevalence and distribution. *Head & Neck, 22*(4), 380–385.

Carnaby-Mann, G., Crary, M. A., Schmalfuss, I., & Amdur, R. (2012). "Pharyngocise": Randomized control trial of preventive exercises to maintain muscle structure and swallowing function during head and neck chemoradiotherapy. *International Journal of Radiation Oncology, Biology, Physics, 83*(1), 201–219.

Carroll, W. R., Locher, J. L., Canon, C. L., Bohannon, I. A., McColloch, N. L., & Magnuson, J. S. (2008). Pretreatment swallowing exercises improve swallow function after chemoradiation. *Laryngoscope, 118*(1), 39–43.

Clark, H. (2003). Neuromuscular treatments for speech and swallowing: A tutorial. *American Journal of Speech-Language Pathology, 12*, 400–415.

Cooper, J. S., Porter, K., Mallin, K., Hoffman, H. T., Weber, R. S., Ang, K. K., . . . Langer, C. J. (2009). National Cancer

Center Database report on cancer of the head and neck: 10-year update. *Head & Neck, 31*(6), 748–758.

Gourin, C. G., & Terris, D. J. (2004). Carcinoma of the hypopharynx. *Surgical Oncology Clinics of North America, 13*(1), 81–98.

Hutcheson, K. A., Lewin, J. S., Barringer, D. A., Lisec, A., Gunn, G. B., Moore, M. W. S., & Holsinger, F. C. (2012). Late dysphagia after radiotherapy-based treatment of head and neck cancer. *Cancer, 118*(23), 5793–5799.

Keereweer, S., Kerrebijn, J. D., Al-Mamgani, A., Sewnaik, A., Baatenburg de Jong, R. J., & van Meerten, E. (2012). Chemoradiation of advanced hypopharyngeal carcinoma: A retrospective study on efficacy, morbidity and quality of life. *European Archives of Otorhinolaryngology, 269*(3), 939–946.

Kulbersh, B. D., Rosenthal, E. L., McGrew, B. M., Duncan, R. D., McColloch, N. L., Carroll, W. R., & Magnuson, J. S. (2006). Pretreatment, preoperative swallowing exercises may improve dysphagia quality of life. *Laryngoscope, 116*(6), 883–886.

Logemann, J. A. (1998). *Evaluation and treatment of swallowing disorders* (2nd ed.). Austin, TX: Pro-Ed.

National Comprehensive Cancer Network. (2013). *Clinical practice guidelines in head and neck cancers* (2nd ed.). Retrieved from http://www.nccn.org

Pignon, J. P., le Maître, A., Maillard, E., & Bourhis, J. (2009). Meta-analysis of chemotherapy in head and neck cancer (MACH-NC): An update on 93 randomised trials and 17,346 patients. *Radiotherapy and Oncology, 92*(1), 4–14.

12

Rare Chondrosarcoma of the Supraglottis

Jonathon O. Russell, Joseph Scharpf, and Claudio F. Milstein

HISTORY

Mr. K is a 47-year-old gentleman with an unremarkable past medical history who presented to the Head and Neck Institute at the Cleveland Clinic for evaluation of a large submucosal mass. The mass was attached to the left laryngeal aspect of the epiglottis and obstructed visualization of the glottis. The true vocal folds were mobile bilaterally as previously examined by the referring community otolaryngologist. Mr. K had a 4-month history of globus sensation, left otalgia, and postnasal drainage that was refractory to a course of antibiotics. At the time of presentation to the Head and Neck Institute, he also complained of some dysphagia as well as an intermittent cough with perioral (PO) intake. His wife noted some dysphonia that she described as having an "echoic" quality, with the dysphonia having progressed over the preceding 2 to 3 months. There was no reported weight loss, and no symptoms suggestive of reflux. Additionally, his wife noted an increase in snoring.

Social History

Social history was relevant for moderate alcohol consumption, and no history of tobacco use. He had no additional medical comorbidities or known risk factors, environmental exposures, or genetic/familial history of cancer.

Medical History

No other significant medical history was reported.

DIAGNOSTIC WORKUP

At presentation to our clinic, a flexible nasopharyngoscopy was repeated with the above findings confirmed. A thorough discussion was had with the patient regarding the need for further diagnostic workup including further imaging studies and evaluation under anesthesia with direct operative laryngoscopy and biopsy. The discussion did consider the possible need for tracheostomy as well as possible tumor debulking pending frozen intraoperative pathology. In addition, computerized tomography (CT) scan images (with and without contrast) of the neck and (with contrast) of the chest were ordered by the Head and Neck surgeon as part of the preoperative workup.

Imaging

The CT scan images demonstrated a 3.0 × 2.3 × 2.4 cm heterogenously enhancing lesion attached to the left anterior surface of the epiglottis that was abutting the tongue base and appeared to obliterate the normal preepiglottic fat along the left lateral pharyngeal wall. Asymmetric soft tissue was noted to extend inferiorly along the left aryepiglottic fold and abut the ipsilateral thyroid cartilage. The cricoid cartilage and pyriform sinuses were symmetric, and the lesion did not extend laterally from the aryepiglottic fold. There was no pathologic lymphadenopathy in the neck or chest. These findings are illustrated in Figure 12–1.

Direct Laryngoscopy Procedure and Results

The patient was taken to the operating room, where he underwent a successful direct laryngoscopy with biopsies. Intraoperatively, the oral cavity and tonsillar fossae were unremarkable. The base of tongue was full and indurated on the left to palpation, and the large supraglottic mass appeared to have eroded through the both the laryngeal and lingual aspects of the epiglottis and involve the base of tongue and vallecula, with no obvious cleavage plane between the mass and the base of tongue. The residual epiglottis was displaced to the right. The tumor was biopsied and sent for both frozen and permanent histopathologic review. Intraoperative findings were consistent with a probable cartilage malignancy or an unspecified chondroid tumor with deferment to

final pathology. Hemostasis of the supraglottis was readily obtained with a pledget soaked in 1:10,000 epinephrine. At the conclusion of the case, the glottis was readily visualized and normal, and so the decision was made to not complete tracheotomy at that time. The patient was discharged to home the same day as the uncomplicated procedure.

PATHOLOGY OUTCOME

The final pathology was consistent with an intermediate-grade chondrosarcoma (2/3). The tumor was composed of lobules of large cells with ample eosinophilic cytoplasm and highly atypical nuclei in a bed of cartilaginous matrix. Binucleated and multinucleated cells were present. Mitoses were infrequent, and necrosis was not present. Immunohistochemical staining was positive for S-100 and focally, to NSE. HMB-45, cytokeratin CAM 5.2, and cytokeratin AE1/AE3 were all negative, consistent with a cartilaginous tumor.

The case was presented at the multidisciplinary tumor board, which included Radiation Oncology, Medical Oncology, Head and Neck Surgery, Head

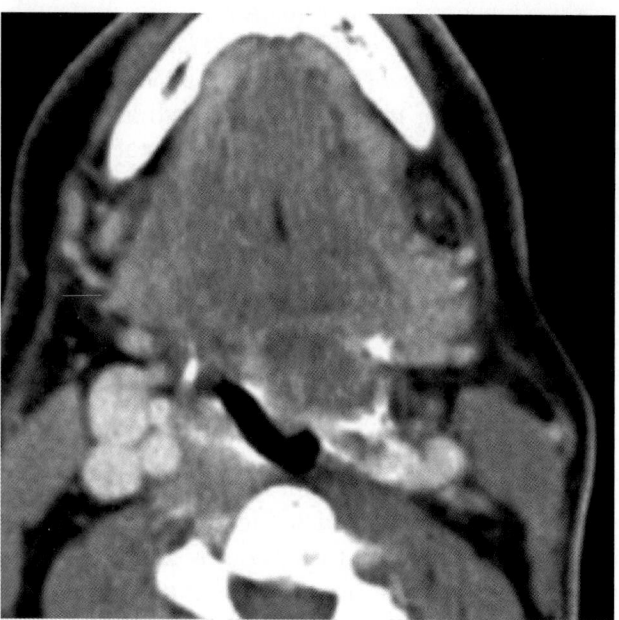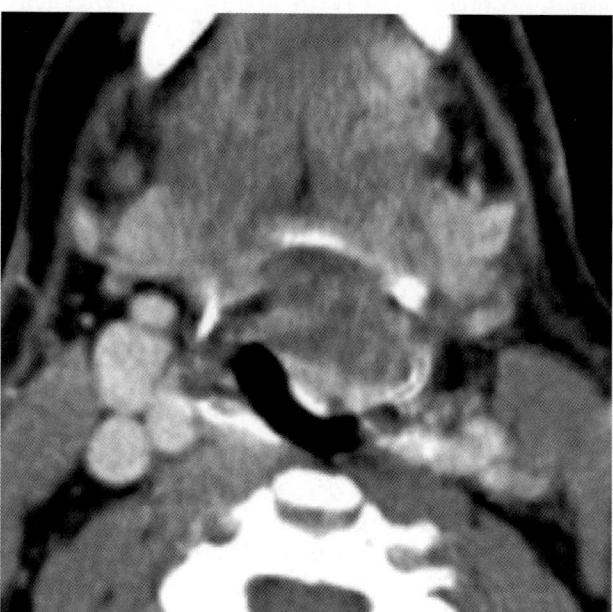

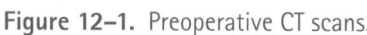

Figure 12–1. Preoperative CT scans.

and Neck Pathology, and Neuroradiology. The patient was seen by the members of the multidisciplinary team, which, in addition to the previously listed professionals, included Speech Pathology, Dentistry, Nutrition, Social Work, and Ambulatory and Inpatient Nursing. After discussion with the team and engagement in the decision with the family, a surgical excision was recommended with the possible need for postoperative intensification with radiation therapy.

The options for surgical resection included a transoral robotic surgical (TORS) approach versus transoral laser microsurgical approach versus an open surgical approach. Informed consent was obtained for a robotic supraglottic laryngectomy with possible transoral laser and possible open treatment if negative margins could not be obtained intraoperatively. Neck management was expectant based on the pathology.

TREATMENT

Surgical Treatment

The patient underwent a TORS laryngectomy with a partial left base of tongue resection. A size 4.5 laser-safe endotracheal tube was placed under visualization with a GlideScope. An FK (Feyh-Kastenbauer retractor) pharyngoscope was placed after surgical preparation and completion of a safety check, which demonstrated a deep and anterior larynx. Excellent visualization was afforded, and the scope was suspended from a Mayo stand. The Da Vinci surgical robot (Intuitive Surgical, Sunnyvale, California) was brought into the field. A two-person, "4-handed" approach was utilized, with the surgeon at the robotic console and an assistant providing retraction and suction at the head of the bed.

With the robot and assistant appropriately positioned, and excellent visualization afforded, the first cut was made through the midline epiglottis, and dissection began on the right down to the preepiglottic fat. The right false vocal fold was removed simultaneously with the ipsilateral epiglottis. Attention next turned to the primary tumor. Due to the size of the mass, further debulking was needed. Nonmarginal

blocks of tumor were resected and sent for permanent pathologic review until dissection could clearly identify the left epiglottis as the site of tumor origin. Cuts were then made into the preepiglottic fat on the left, with the dissection continuing to near the plane of the ipsilateral thyroid cartilage perichondrium. Posteriorly, cuts were made just anterior to the ipsilateral arytenoid, and the left false vocal cord was also removed with a more en bloc specimen from the left epiglottis. The epiglottic petiole was included. With the primary tumor removed, a cuff of the left tongue base was also removed. Hemostasis was maintained with cauterization, and the lingual artery was not appreciated due to the more medial nature of the cuff of tissue that had been removed from the base of tongue. All margins were negative both intraoperatively and on permanent final pathologic review. Given that the airway was excellent at the conclusion of the case, it was felt that overnight intubation in the surgical intensive care unit would be attempted, with plans to extubate the following morning with the goal of avoiding tracheostomy.

Initial Postoperative Care

The patient was extubated the morning of the first postoperative day (POD1), but he remained in the surgical intensive care unit (SICU) for an additional 24 hr on high-dose Decadron. He did begin clear liquid per oral on POD1, but had some coughing that appeared to resolve. On POD2, speech pathology (SLP) was consulted for a bedside swallow evaluation. In this setting, he was noted to have reflexive coughing when presented with some textures, although this improved with swallowing precautions. Specifically, he was instructed regarding position (seated at 90 degrees), chin tuck, effortful swallowing, and the supraglottic swallow sequence (swallow, clear throat, and reswallow). His diet was also modified to consist of nectar-thick liquids and pureed foods so as to improve his PO intake. These changes resulted in improved diet tolerance, and he was subsequently transferred to the head and neck surgery step-down unit for further observation. He had no further difficulties tolerating adequate PO throughout the remainder of his stay. He did suffer from nausea that required the addition of multiple medications and delayed his discharge, but he was ultimately discharged to home on POD5 with plans for follow-up within the week as an outpatient.

Postoperative Course

Mr. K's postoperative course was complicated by persistent coughing and an episode of bleeding that ultimately required readmission to the hospital and control of the bleeding under anesthesia on POD11 from the original surgery.

SLP Reevaluation

At the time of admission to the hospital, a repeat evaluation with SLP was requested. The patient was noted to be wary of coughing, which he attributed to a desire to avoid further bleeding. A modified barium swallow (MBS) was completed, and it demonstrated mildly reduced hyolaryngeal elevation with contrast bolus pooling in the pyriforms. (The epiglottis was noted to be surgically absent.) Penetration was noted with all consistencies, and frank aspiration was observed with both nectar-thick and thin liquids. He was also noted to fatigue over the course of the evaluation. Small-bore feeding tube placement was recommended, although prognosis for resumption of full PO was thought to be excellent with further healing. As he best tolerated applesauce, he was permitted to continue applesauce PO as tolerated with the above listed precautions. When he returned for follow-up SLP assessment with repeat MBS, he was noted to have persistent moderate to severe oropharyngeal dysphagia. He demonstrated reduced hyolaryngeal elevation, and repeated coughs were needed to fully clear boluses from the vestibule. Decreased hyolaryngeal elevation further contributed to decreased opening of the upper esophageal sphincter. He was noted to fatigue with the exhaustive effort of the swallow evaluation. The conclusion was a guarded prognosis for improvement. Recommendations included continued swallow precautions, as well as ice chips and sips of water to encourage aggressive swallowing practice (Frazier Water Protocol). Continued enteral nutrition was recommended, as was discussion regarding surgical placement of a gastrostomy tube

if he failed to demonstrate marked improvement at scheduled repeat MBS in 2 to 3 weeks.

When Mr. K was seen for follow-up the coming week, he had improved to the point where it was recommended the feeding tube be removed, which it was. He was able to maintain adequate PO intake. At his next follow-up 4 weeks after surgery, the recommendation to begin radiation in 3 weeks was put forth due to the intermediate grade of the tumor.

Postoperative Radiation Treatment. Radiation was initiated at 7 weeks following transoral resection of tumor, with plans to complete 6000 cGy of radiation in 30 fractions. This was completed as scheduled, with complications including Grade 2 mucositis and Grade 2 radiation dermatitis with dry, patchy desquamation as well as some persistent and expected dysgeusia. He maintained an oral diet throughout the treatment and immediately began to gain weight following completion of his treatment.

At the completion of radiation therapy, the patient was doing well, with some mild dysphonia, describing his voice as being "deeper" than it had been previously. From this point on, he was seen in serial follow-ups with the surgeon and a SLP with expertise in voice for stroboscopic assessment. Laryngeal stroboscopy demonstrated excellent healing following surgery and radiation, with expected tissue changes. He was able to quickly return to his daily activities and work with no restrictions. The patient did not want to pursue voice therapy, as he rated his voice changes as mild and not interfering with his daily vocal demands.

Treatment Course and Summary

As Mr. K approached 10 months from the completion of surgery, there were no reported complaints except mild persistent dysgeusia and occasional vocal fatigue resulting in hoarseness at the end of a long day (see Video 12–1). He was noted to have an excellent, healed surgical site without recurrent disease on laryngostroboscopy. This was evidenced by normal mucosa and no evidence of edema or thickened secretions on the exam. There was mild erythema that was thought to possibly stem from laryngopharyngeal reflux. As this persisted at his

12-month visit, lifestyle and dietary modifications were recommended. Omeprazole 40 mg daily was also prescribed, and he was noted to have excellent improvement at his next visit. CT neck and chest with contrast were obtained at the 12-month visit and were both interpreted as negative. Vibratory amplitude and mucosal wave were both noted to return to normal limits at subsequent follow-up examinations with laryngostroboscopy. The patient was most recently seen at 3 years following completion of his radiation therapy, and he has been doing well with no evidence of disease and continued excellent voice, speech, and swallow outcomes (Figure 12–2 and Video 12–2).

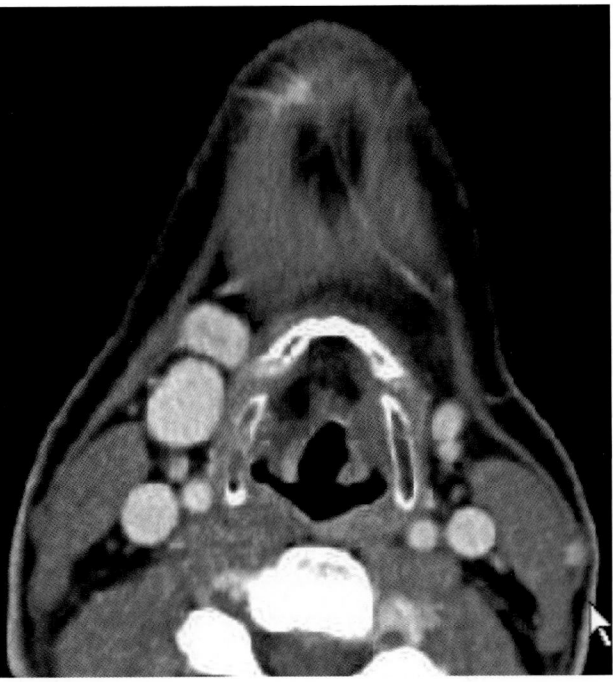

Figure 12–2. Postoperative CT scan.

REFLECTION AND ANALYSIS FOR FURTHER STUDY

1. One of the aspects that is rarely discussed in the literature is the level of pain that the patient may be experiencing as a result of the surgical procedure, the radiation treatment, or both. Since tolerance of pain and coping with pain are an individual response, what might you use as a clinician to assess and recognize the level of pain in your patients?

2. Fatigue is a critical factor to consider when introducing swallow exercise regimens to patients. How might fatigue be exacerbated by treatments for head and neck cancer?

3. Identify and explain three therapeutic approaches you might use to minimize the impact of fatigue on patients you are treating for dysphagia following treatment for head and neck cancer.

PART V

Laryngeal Cases

13

Management of SCCA In Situ in a Professional Performer

Adam T. Lloyd, Erin P. Silverman, and Brian C. Spector

HISTORY

This case describes a 65-year-old professional male actor referred to our otolaryngology practice by his primary care physician. The patient's chief complaint was an 8-week history of persistent hoarseness without complete aphonia. Prior to presentation, he completed a run of performances in a stage production where the character he portrayed required a markedly "rough" vocal quality. During rehearsals, he began to experience increased episodes of hoarseness and vocal fatigue, which persisted even after the show closed. In addition to hoarseness, other reported symptoms included recent-onset throat clearing and postnasal drainage. Past medical history was unremarkable with the exception of hypothyroidism (controlled with medication), hyperlipidemia, nasal fracture repair (1990), and tonsillectomy as a child. The patient was a nonsmoker and used alcohol rarely (less than 12 beverages per year). The patient did consume large amounts of caffeine (approximately one gallon of coffee) per day. He reported no prior history of voice impairment.

DIAGNOSTIC WORKUP

Diagnostic workup took place under the direction of our practice's Voice Care Team, consisting of otolaryngologists, speech-language pathologists, as well as singing and acting voice specialists. This patient was treated over a period of 5 months, beginning with an initial evaluation followed by multiple biopsy procedures.

Physical examination of the head and neck was unremarkable. As the patient's only complaint was hoarseness, the physician ordered a laryngostroboscopic examination for evaluation of laryngeal anatomy and physiology by a speech-language pathologist. This examination was completed at the patient's first appointment, as was a perceptual analysis of voice quality.

Initial Laryngostroboscopic Examination

Laryngostroboscopic examination is a procedure commonly used to assess vocal fold vibration in real time and during voicing maneuvers. The technique is also useful in differentiating among benign vocal fold lesions, invasive processes, vocal fold scarring, and functional disorders (Fleischer & Hess, 2006). Initial laryngostroboscopic examination was performed transorally using a 70-degree rigid laryngeal endoscope and revealed apparent leukoplakia versus fungal debris along the edge and middle surface of the right vocal fold as well as a small area of swelling along the edge of the left vocal fold. Mucosal wave and amplitude of vibration were mildly to moderately decreased on the left and significantly decreased on the right. There was also moderate supraglottic compression of the ventricular folds during phonation (Figure 13–1 and Video 13–1).

Perceptual Evaluation

Perceptual evaluation of vocal quality was completed by the speech-language pathologist using the Consensus Auditory Evaluation of Voice (CAPE-V). The CAPE-V allows for clinical assessment of multiple dimensions of vocal quality in adults with voice disorders (Karnell et al., 2007; Kempster et al., 2009; Zraick et al., 2011). These dimensions include the magnitude of overall severity, roughness, breathiness, strain, pitch, and loudness as well as the frequency with which these symptoms present (intermittent or consistent). The CAPE-V is a useful tool for documenting change in voice status over time, or as a result of treatment. The CAPE-V is used as a diagnostic tool in all dysphonia cases with this group of practitioners. Some vocal strain or *hyperfunction* was noted during conversation and was scored (30% intermittently). When asked to vocalize at higher pitch or falsetto levels, the patient demonstrated markedly increased vocal strain (70% consistent), significant roughness (85% consistent), and intermittent voice breaks.

INITIAL RECOMMENDATIONS

Given the patient was currently working as an actor, and contracted to perform in a stage production, a conservative treatment approach consisting of attention to vocal hygiene (including reducing caffeine intake), modified voice rest, and laryngeal massage was recommended (Behlau & Oliveira, 2009; Roy, 2008). The goal of treatment was to reduce hyperfunction within the extrinsic laryngeal musculature while imparting an "easy-onset" approach to voicing in order to minimize direct impact stress to the vocal fold edges. Nystatin (5 mL QID for 15 days) was prescribed to address the leukoplakia noted during initial laryngostroboscopy, and the patient was scheduled for follow-up in 2 weeks with microlaryngoscopy. Right vocal fold biopsy was tentatively planned for 3 weeks should no improvement be noted at follow-up.

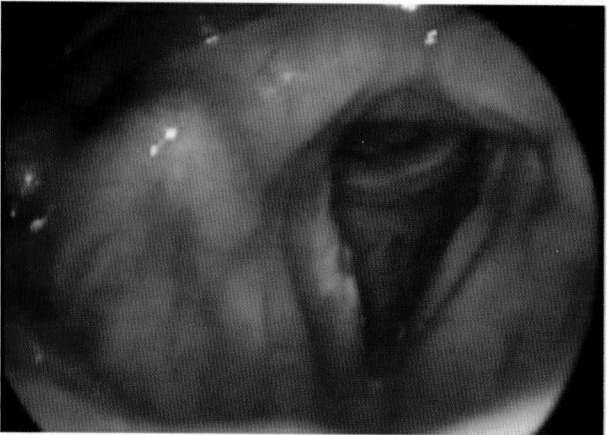
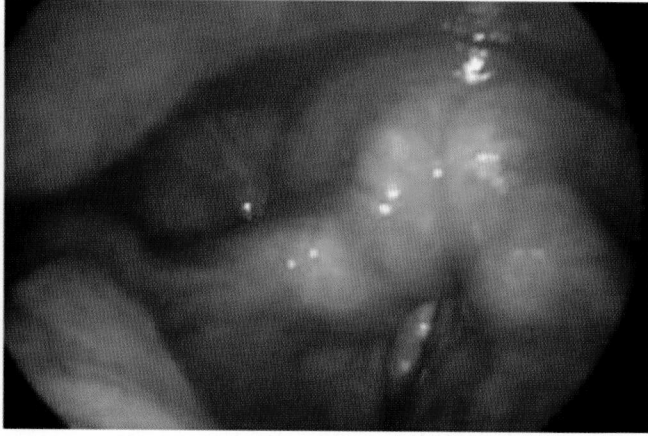

Figure 13–1. The initial laryngostroboscopic examination.

FOLLOW-UP

Two weeks later, during a follow-up visit with the otolaryngologist and speech pathologist, the patient reported that his hoarseness was mostly resolved. He noted that he was presently rehearsing 5 hr per day for a new production but had not experienced any voice difficulties. Perceptual evaluation of voice quality using the CAPE-V revealed continued roughness and voice breaks during high pitch phonation.

Repeat laryngostroboscopic examination was essentially unchanged: leukoplakia versus fungal laryngitis was noted along the middle third of the right vocal fold with extension to the vocal process as well as a small focal area within the left medial inferior vocal fold edge. As the patient was in the middle of a performance run, a conservative biopsy of only the areas of apparent leukoplakia was completed. Further intervention was deferred pending receipt of the pathology results.

RESULTS OF INITIAL BIOPSY

The microlaryngoscopy and biopsy was completed during the biopsy, adherent white debris on the right vocal fold was removed without mucosal incision. Pathology revealed superficial parakeratosis, and culture was pending. At the postoperative visit, the patient noted some hoarseness for a few days following biopsy, which was essentially resolved. Nystatin (5 mL QID for 10 days) was prescribed again, and the patient was instructed to follow-up in 4 weeks with a repeat videostroboscopic examination.

Follow-Up After Biopsy

Four weeks later the patient had completed the performance run and presented for follow-up. He denied dysphonia but did report frequent throat clearing and feeling as if he had increased mucus within his throat. A culture obtained from the previous biopsy was negative for fungal growth after 4 weeks. Perceptual evaluation of voice using the CAPE-V was significant for voice breaks, rough vocal quality, and increased vocal effort, particularly at higher pitches and during falsetto. Laryngostroboscopic examination was suggestive of reduced leukoplakia along the edge and surface of the right vocal fold. The patient was instructed to complete a 14-day course of Diflucan 100 mg QD but later switched to Nystatin (5 mL QID for 10 days) due to Diflucan and Lipitor causing possible rhabdomyolysis when taken together (Kahri, Valkonen, Backlung, Vuoristo, & Kivisto, 2005). Discussion of mucosal biopsy was tempered by the patient's desire to complete his theatrical commitments.

Six weeks later, the patient's symptoms and vocal quality remained unchanged. Laryngostroboscopic examination was also unchanged. Repeat direct microlaryngoscopy with biopsy was recommended with sampling of the epithelium for histologic review of tissue architecture. Given his status as a professional voice user and upcoming performance schedule, once again a conservative biopsy was completed and more invasive procedures deferred pending the pathology findings. Pathology revealed hyperkeratotic squamous mucosa with moderate to severe dysplasia. Clinically, the surface changes along the right vocal fold extended toward the anterior commissure, suggestive of residual disease. Given findings of dysplasia, microlaryngoscopy with microflap excision was recommended.

TREATMENT PLAN

Microlaryngoscopy with Microflap Excision of Dysplasia

The patient underwent direct microlaryngoscopy with microflap excision for right vocal fold dysplasia (Figure 13–2). Postsurgical pathology was consistent with squamous cell carcinoma in situ of the right true vocal fold, TisN0M0. The patient was given

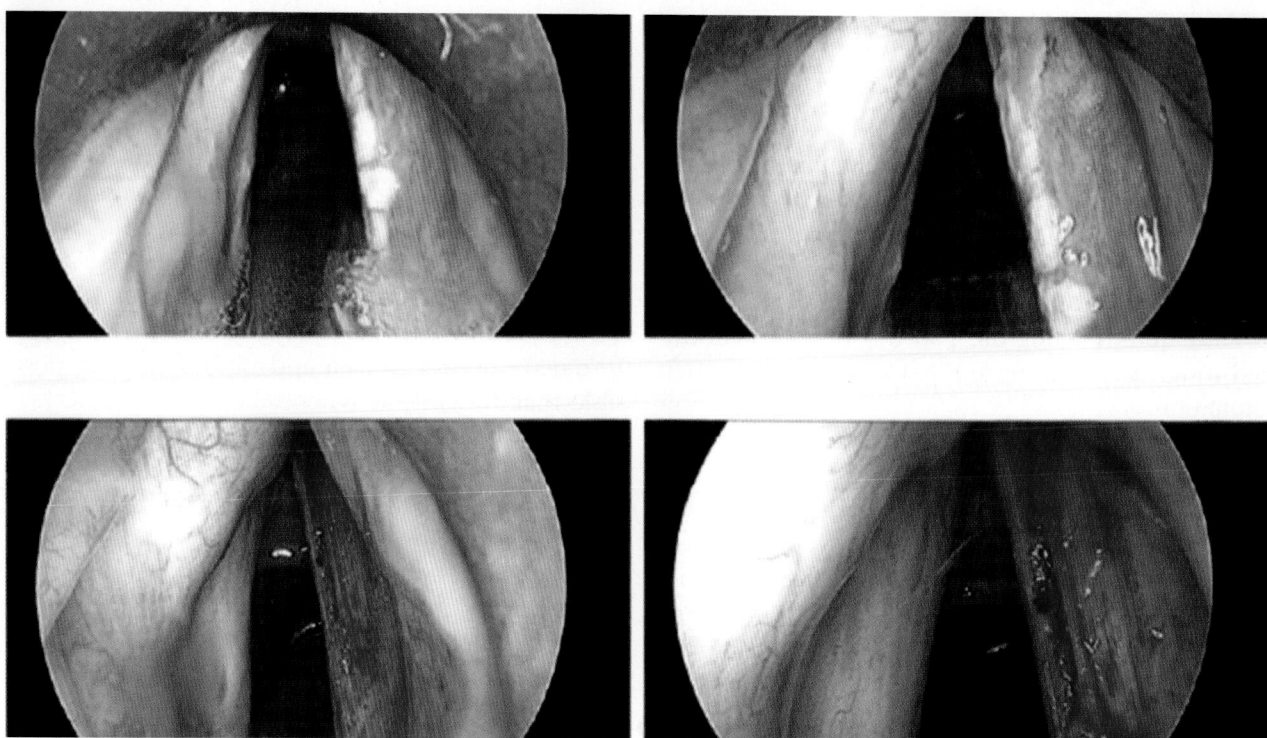

Figure 13–2. The microlaryngoscopy with microflap excision.

the option of surgical management versus radiation therapy. The potential impact of further surgical intervention on tissue dynamics, voice production, and long-term voice quality was discussed with the patient. This was compared to the similar characteristics of radiation therapy. The patient opted for radiation oncology consultation and subsequent treatment.

Adjuvant Radiation Therapy

The patient underwent 6 weeks of radiation therapy. He received 63 Gy in 28 fractions right and left lateral tangents of the larynx using image-guided radiation therapy (IGRT). And 6 MV photons were delivered. Throughout radiation therapy the patient complained of worsening hoarseness. Additional complaints included sore throat, dysphagia, and odynophagia, which was relieved with Magic Mouthwash. The patient was able to tolerate a regular diet throughout radiation and did not require a PEG tube.

POST RADIATION TREATMENT

Following completion of radiation therapy, the patient was evaluated jointly by otolaryngology and speech-language pathology. At this point his chief symptoms included sore throat, most noticeable during exhalation, and coughing. Although he reported experiencing partial voice loss during the last several weeks of radiation, these symptoms were improved. Increased thirst and mild xerostomia were noted; however, he denied difficulty swallowing aside from isolated instances of coughing on thin liquids and "sticking" while he was undergoing radiation therapy. All of these symptoms had reportedly resolved since treatment and no weight loss was evidenced as a result of radiation therapy.

Post treatment Laryngostroboscopy

Laryngostroboscopic examination revealed the vocal fold edges to be smooth and straight with no mass lesions present. The edge and surface of the vocal folds were slightly erythematous, with no irregular tissue noted. Mucosal wave was mildly decreased on the left and moderately decreased on the right (Figure 13–3 and Video 13–2).

Post treatment Perceptual Evaluation

Perceptual evaluation of vocal status using the CAPE-V revealed a lower speaking pitch (30% consistently decreased) compared to pretreatment baseline. Mild roughness (25% intermittent) and strain (15% inconsistent) were evident during the production of higher pitches and falsetto, although this was markedly improved compared to pretreatment status.

THERAPEUTIC RECOMMENDATIONS

The speech-language pathologist continued to emphasize increasing water while decreasing caffeine intake (the patient had continued to drink approximately a gallon of coffee per day). Vocal function exercises and resonant voicing strategies were introduced and practiced in order to help restore functional balance among respiration, phonation, and resonance during normal conversation and performance settings (Stemple, Lee, D'Amico, & Pickup, 1994; Verdolini-Marston, Burke, Lessac, Glaze, & Caldwell, 1995). The patient was instructed to perform these exercises three times per day and work toward carryover into his conversational voice usage. Nasonex was prescribed by the otolaryngologist for symptoms of postnasal drainage.

CONTINUED FOLLOW-UP

At his 5-month follow-up appointment with the otolaryngologist and speech pathologist, the patient reported that his hoarseness, cough, sore throat, and difficulty swallowing had resolved completely. The patient continued to experience an intermitted sensation of increased mucus within his throat.

PERCEPTUAL EVALUATION

Perceptual evaluation of voice revealed a vocal quality that was normal for his age and sex. Compared to pretreatment, his conversational pitch range was slightly

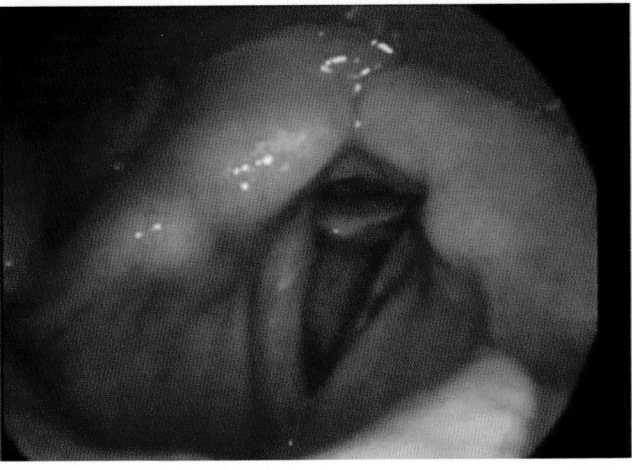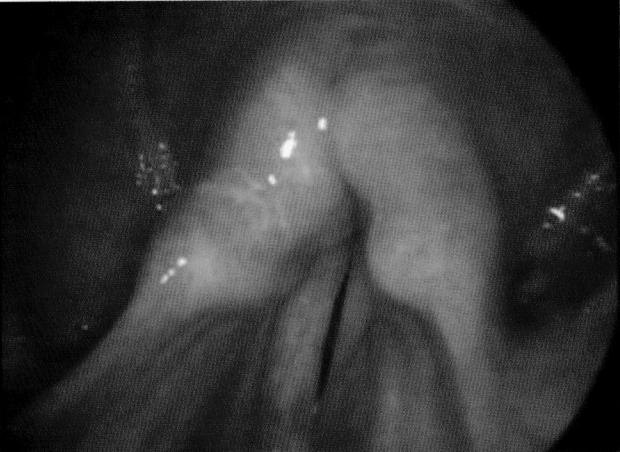

Figure 13–3. The first postoperative laryngostroboscopic examination.

decreased (30% consistently decreased). Production of falsetto was improved. Only mild roughness (15% intermittent) and strain (10% intermittent) were noted.

REPEAT LARYNGOSTROBOSCOPIC EXAMINATION

Laryngostroboscopic examination revealed smooth and straight vocal fold edges with no mass lesions. Some mild erythema along the surface of the right vocal fold was noted. Secretions were mildly increased in amount and consistency on the surface of the true vocal folds. When compared to the previous examination, erythema along the surface of the right vocal fold decreased. No evidence of reoccurrence was noted. Vibratory characteristics remained somewhat decreased on the right, but in general, vibration showed improvement (Figure 13–4 and Video 13–3).

RECOMMENDATIONS

Given the favorable outcome of improved vocal quality, it was recommended that the patient follow up with our practice in 2 months.

CONCLUSIONS

This case shows the multidisciplinary management of initially subtle voice change in a professional voice user. Given his career as an actor with a demanding performance schedule, the patient requested a conservative evaluation and treatment approach. Differential diagnosis of white surface changes included leukoplakia versus fungal laryngitis. Soon after beginning treatment with Nystatin and voice therapy, the patient noted improvement in symptoms although the vocal fold pathology persisted. Perceptually, the patient's voice continued to be rough, strained, with voice breaks during the production of high pitches. In spite of this, the patient noted improved vocal quality. This patient had no typical risk factors for laryngeal cancer; however, biopsy revealed a squamous cell carcinoma of the vocal fold mucosa. The patient responded very well to radiation therapy with mild dysphonia of limited duration during treatment. Other than a slight decrease in the patient's habitual pitch range, he had no persisting dysphonia symptoms following radiation treatment. He required voice therapy in order to resume his previous (elite) level of vocal function and was successful within a relatively short period of time. This case highlights the importance

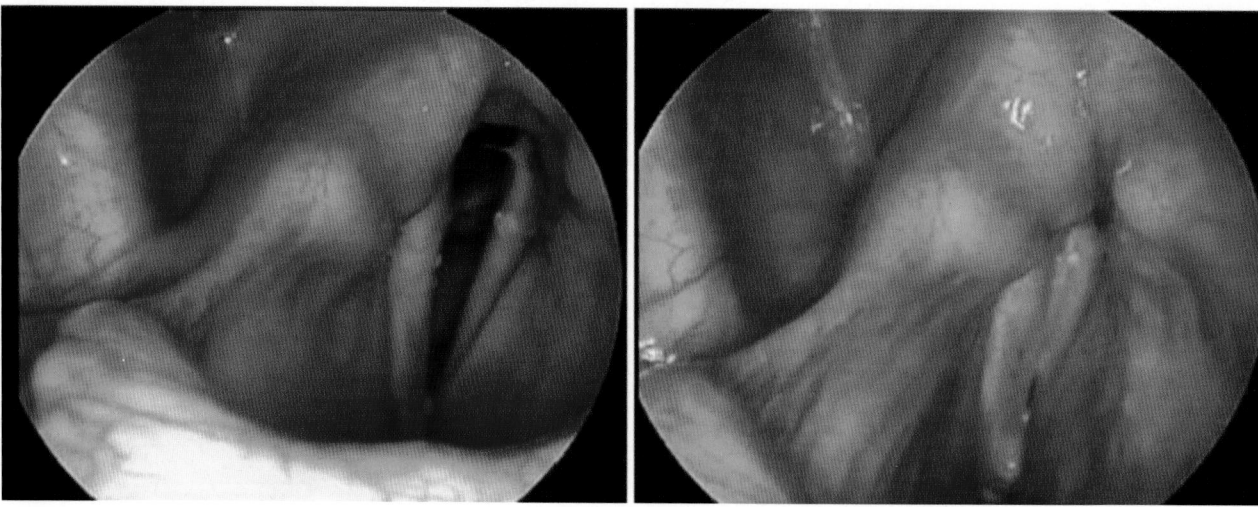

Figure 13–4. Still images of repeat laryngostroboscopic examination, 5 months post treatment.

of adapting treatment to the unique lifestyles and work schedules of the individual patient. In the current case, these factors delayed full evaluation and extensive biopsy. However, by continued close monitoring of suspicious vocal fold lesions and repeated, conservative biopsy, we were able to provide an effective, minimally disruptive and minimally invasive treatment, resulting in complete resolution of a potentially devastating condition.

REFLECTION AND ANALYSIS FOR FURTHER STUDY

1. Aside from the profession of this patient, an actor, what other professional classifications may necessitate a specialized approach toward treatment of vocal fold cancer?

2. Given the need for ongoing monitoring of subtle vocal quality changes in at-risk patients, what variables should a clinician emphasize when providing instruction to patients on self-monitoring?

3. How does the Vocal Function Exercise Program assist patients who have undergone vocal fold surgery or radiation regain vocal pitch range?

4. How might this patient's case been handled differently were he not an elite professional voice user?

REFERENCES

Behlau, M., & Oliveira, G. (2009). Vocal hygiene for the voice professional. *Current Opinion in Otolaryngology and Head and Neck Surgery, 17*(3), 149.

Fleischer, S., & Hess, M. (2006). The significance of videostroboscopy in laryngological practice. *HNO, 54*(8), 628.

Kahri, J., Valkonen, M., Backlund, T., Vuoristo, M., & Kivisto, K. T. (2005). Rhabdomyolysis in a patient receiving atorvastatin and fluconazole. *European Journal of Clinical Pharmacology, 60*(12), 905–907.

Karnell, M., Melton, S., Childes, J., Coleman, T., Dailey, S., & Hoffman, H. (2007). Reliability of clinician-based (GRBAS and CAPE-V) and patient-based (V-RQOL and IPVI) documentation of voice disorders. *Journal of Voice, 21*, 576–590.

Kempster, G. B., Gerratt, B. R., Verdolini Abbott, K., Barkmeier-Kramer, J., & Hillman, R. E. (2009). Consensus Auditory-Perceptual Evaluation of Voice: Development of a standardized clinical protocol. *American Journal of Speech-Language Pathology, 18*, 124–132.

Roy, N. (2008). Assessment and treatment of musculoskeletal tension in hyperfunctional voice disorders. *International Journal of Speech-Language Pathology, 10*(4), 195–209.

Stemple, J. C., Lee, L., D'Amico, B., & Pickup, B. (1994). Efficacy of vocal function exercises as a method of improving voice production. *Journal of Voice, 8*(3), 271–278.

Verdolini-Marston, K., Burke, M., Lessac, A., Glaze, L., & Caldwell, E. (1995). Preliminary study of two methods of treatment for laryngeal nodules. *Journal of Voice, 9*(1), 74–85.

Zraick, R. I., Kempster, G. B., Connor, N. P., Thibeault, S., Klaben, B. K., Bursac, Z., . . . Glaze, L. E. (2011). Establishing validity of the Consensus Auditory-Perceptual Evaluation of Voice (CAPE-V). *American Journal of Speech-Language Pathology/ American Speech-Language-Hearing Association, 20*(1), 14–22.

14

Management of Recurrent Laryngeal Cancer

Jeffrey J. Lehman, Vicki Lewis, Adam T. Lloyd, and Bari Hoffman Ruddy

MEDICAL AND SOCIAL HISTORY

The patient is a 57-year-old male Navy veteran, having served in Vietnam where he was stationed onboard a carrier. Prior to his illness, the patient was employed in marketing and sales. The patient had been married, but divorced during the course of his cancer treatment. He was initially seen by Otolaryngology in August 2003 with complaints of dysphonia and a burning sensation in the throat region. Past medical history was significant for hypertension (HTN), gastroesophageal reflux (GERD), diabetes mellitus-Type II with neuropathy, coronary artery disease, and hypercholesterolemia. The patient was a former smoker (having quit in 1999), previously smoking one pack of cigarettes per day for 45 years. The patient reported that he drank approximately 16 oz of beer or wine daily.

DIAGNOSTIC WORKUP

In August 2003, a flexible fiberoptic laryngoscopy and rigid laryngeal videostroboscopy were performed by the otolaryngologist and speech pathologist, respectively. These examinations revealed a polyp along the midmembraneous edge of the right vocal fold with no obvious ulceration. Mucosal wave and amplitude of vibration were significantly decreased on the right. Due to a desire not to interrupt his work in sales, the patient requested a conservative approach and refused surgery at the time. Treatment recommendations were modified voice rest, use of a low-impact voicing style and behavioral and dietary modifications to limit GERD. At follow-up in December 2003, a flexible laryngeal endoscopy was performed by the otolaryngologist revealed no change in the polyp on the right vocal fold. The patient requested another period of observation, and follow-up was scheduled for 1 month. At that time, if there was no improvement in appearance or symptoms, microlaryngoscopy with excisional biopsy would be carried out. The patient did not return for his follow-up appointment in January 2004.

In September 2006, the patient returned for evaluation of sore throat and severe dysphonia. At this time, he was evaluated by our group's physician assistant. Examination showed polypoid changes of the vocal folds with vocal fold erythema as well as erythema of the posterior laryngeal tissue and arytenoids. Zegerid 40 mg q.d. was prescribed, and the patient was instructed to return for a videostroboscopic examination. This was completed in early October and revealed a firm polypoid mass involving the right vocal fold. Portions of the polyp on the right side were papillomatous in appearance (Figure 14–1). At that time, a direct laryngoscopy with excisional biopsy was recommended.

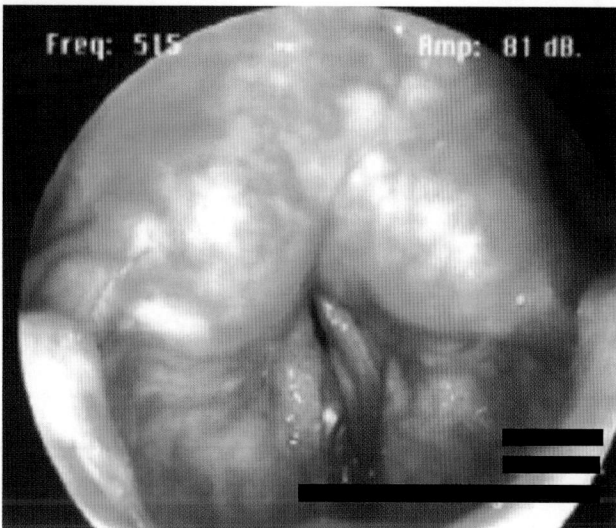

Figure 14–1. A still image from preoperative laryngostrobo-scopic examination.

Microlaryngoscopy With Biopsy

In November 2006, microlaryngoscopy with CO_2 laser debulking of right vocal fold mass was completed. Clinically, this was a T2 and would have required cordectomy for adequate surgical margins. In the interest of preserving the vocal fold, consultation with radiation oncology for definitive radiation therapy was recommended.

Pathology Findings

Invasive well-differentiated squamous cell carcinoma of the right vocal fold, T2N0M0.

TREATMENT

Radiation Therapy

The patient received 6300 cGy in 28 fractions, 225 cGy per fraction, with 6 MV photons via right and left lateral fields. Treatment initiated: 11/30/06 and completed 1/11/07. The patient tolerated treatment well and with mild-moderate pain reported.

The patient had a 6-pound weight loss but did not require percutaneous endoscopic gastroscopy (PEG) tube placement or swallowing rehabilitation.

POST TREATMENT

In April 2007, the otolaryngologist saw the patient for follow up. At that time, no evidence of tumor recurrence on flexible fiberoptic laryngoscopy was noted. In August 2007 the patient reported a 2-week history of increased GERD symptoms and hoarseness. Flexible fiberoptic laryngoscopy showed moderate erythema and edema of the supraglottic structures. A short steroid course was prescribed, along with a proton pump inhibitor (PPI). At the follow-up in September 2007, the patient complained of increasing dysphonia despite medical management. Flexible fiberoptic laryngoscopy revealed whitish discoloration on the superior vocal fold surface, with irregularity noted along the edge. Systemic antifungal therapy was prescribed to cover possible fungal laryngitis while the patient was set up for microlaryngoscopy.

DIAGNOSTIC WORKUP

Microlaryngoscopy With Biopsy

In mid-September 2007, the patient underwent microlaryngoscopy with biopsy of the right vocal fold. There was gross evidence of tumor affecting the right vocal fold, extending from the region of the vocal process of the arytenoid anteriorly to the anterior commissure. The right vocal fold had a stiffened appearance, and tumor appeared to extend into the ventricle. The tumor was staged as T3 due to vocal fold fixation, pending completion of a neck CT to assess for possible cartilage invasion.

Pathology Findings

The pathology findings showed moderately differentiated invasive squamous cell carcinoma. Postoperatively, a neck CT scan with contrast was completed, revealing a right vocal fold mass, without evidence of cartilage invasion (Figure 14–2). No pathologic adenopathy was seen. A CT scan of the chest revealed bibasilar infiltrates, consolidation, with bilateral pleural effusions. Extensive degenerative disease of the spine was noted. At the postop visit, the options of extended vertical hemilaryngectomy versus total laryngectomy were presented to the patient. Due to his desire to avoid a permanent stoma, as well as alaryngeal speech, the patient chose the partial laryngectomy option.

TREATMENT

Surgical Management

The patient underwent extended vertical right hemilaryngectomy with tracheotomy in late September 2007. The larynx was divided left of midline to include the anterior commissure in the specimen. When the larynx was opened, it was evident that the tumor extended to, but not across, the anterior commissure on the right side, and to the arytenoid vocal process posteriorly. Inferiorly, there was 5

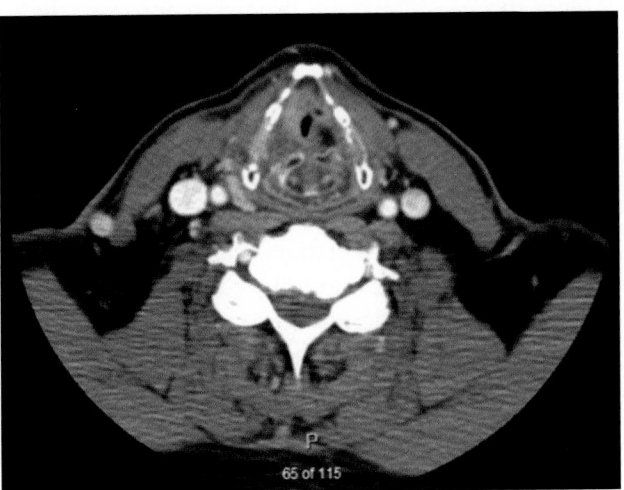

Figure 14–2. An image from the CT scan performed prior to the vertical right hemilaryngectomy.

mm of subglottic spread. The lesion did not cross to involve the false vocal fold. The anterior and posterior margins were negative on frozen section, and the inferior margin was grossly free of tumor. Reconstruction was performed with a thyrohyoid muscle rotation flap to create a surface on the right for the left vocal fold to contact during phonation.

Pathology Findings

Final pathology revealed invasive moderately differentiated squamous cell carcinoma. The tumor was 1.6 cm in greatest dimension, with 5-mm depth of invasion. Margins of resection were clear, although the anterior margin was 1 mm. There was no evidence of cartilage invasion.

POST TREATMENT

In October 2007, the patient was doing well with tracheostomy care and had been tolerating clear liquids by mouth. He was cleared to initiate full liquid diet with nonoral supplementation continued via nasogastric tube (NGT). One week later, swallowing was improved and the patient's NGT was removed. Continued follow-up was recommended for tracheostomy care and cancer surveillance. One month later, the patient reported improved vocal quality but consistent difficulty increasing vocal loudness as well as occasional coughing with intake of thin liquids. Flexible fiberoptic laryngoscopy revealed significant healing of the right hemilaryngeal reconstruction site. There was an anterior glottal gap where healing of the reconstruction flap appeared to have resulted in lateral retraction. The right arytenoid area mucosa remained edematous but did not impinge significantly on the laryngeal airway. There was no sign of recurrent tumor, and the left vocal fold appeared normally mobile. Radiesse injection by microlaryngoscopic approach was discussed as an option to medialize the anterior aspect of the reconstructed right vocal fold region; microlaryngoscopy would also allow closer examination of the anterior glottis to rule out tumor residual or recurrence. As this was being planned, the tracheostomy was left in place.

TREATMENT

Microlaryngoscopy and Tissue Defect Augmentation

The patient underwent microlaryngoscopy with Radiesse injection vocal augmentation in late November 2007. Some areas of granulation tissue were encountered throughout the reconstructed right hemilaryngectomy region, and a biopsy was submitted for permanent section pathology. A vocal fold-like ridge was located on the right side, slightly below the true glottic level, and was augmented by injection of 1 mL of Radiesse. Adequate laryngeal airway was preserved.

Pathology Findings

Granulation tissue and necrotic material were negative for malignancy.

POST TREATMENT

The patient followed up with the physician assistant at the otolaryngology practice in early December 2007. At this time he was doing well and tolerating capping of the tracheostomy tube over the preceding 2 weeks. Having patients incrementally increase the time that their tracheostomy tube is capped over a period of time has been shown to improve their candidacy for decannulation (Pandian et al., 2014). The patient was decannulated and an occlusive dressing was applied to the tract. A few weeks later the patient followed up with the otolaryngologist where he displayed modest improvements in vocal quality following injection augmentation. The patient reported continued difficulty, though slight, swallowing thin liquids. The patient was able to return to work.

By January 2008, the patient's voice was stronger, and he had resumed normal work activity. The patient noted that his swallowing had improved and he gained 9 pounds. Flexible fiberoptic laryngoscopy revealed significant reduction in edema of the right arytenoid area mucosa. The granularity in the reconstructed right hemilaryngeal region was noted to be resolved, and there was no evidence of residual or recurrent tumor. The left vocal fold mobility continued to appear normal, and airway patency was noted to be excellent. Monthly follow-up was recommended via alternating follow-up visits between the otolaryngologist and radiation oncologist.

In August 2008, the patient was seen for follow-up after having missed two scheduled follow-ups since his visit in January. The patient indicated that his voice was serviceable. There was no evidence of tumor recurrence 1-year post salvage vertical hemilaryngectomy. Continued bimonthly follow-ups were recommended with otolaryngologist and radiation oncologist.

POST TREATMENT: NEW COMPLAINTS

In January 2009, the patient developed swelling in the region of old tracheostomy tract. During the physical examination by the otolaryngologist, swelling and erythema were noted, and the area was tender on palpation. Aspiration with an 18-gauge needle was completed, and 2 mL of pus was obtained with noted reduction in swelling. A #15 blade was used to more widely incise and drain the area in an office-based procedure. Antibiotics were prescribed, and follow-up in 2 days was recommended. Two days later a flexible fiberoptic laryngoscopy revealed a small amount of crusted secretions within the region of the right hemilaryngeal reconstruction. The left true vocal fold remained fully mobile, and there was no visible evidence of tumor recurrence. The airway was adequate, and it appeared as if the neck abscess was responding well to incision and drainage and antibiotic therapy. The patient was instructed to continue oral antibiotics and follow-up in 2 weeks. Two weeks later the patient's voice was stable, and the superficial abscess in the region of the tracheostomy tract was resolved.

One month later the patient returned with complaints of pain and erythema of the neck. Left peritracheal cellulitis was noted. Antibiotics were again prescribed, and follow-up in 1 week was scheduled. At follow-up the patient was doing better. The trach tract appeared crusted but healed. There was a concern regarding a possible tracheocutaneous fistula, and plans were made for continued monitoring of this site. There was no visible sign of tumor recurrence on head and neck exam.

In March 2009 no further swelling of the peritracheal region was evident. There was some continued leakage of mucoid secretions noted from the old tracheostomy site, consistent with a tracheocutaneous fistula. Surgical intervention was recommended for excision and closure of the old tracheostomy tract, as well as microlaryngoscopy with biopsy to rule out recurrent cancer.

DIAGNOSTIC WORKUP

Imaging

A CT scan of the neck was performed and compared to that from September 2007. This revealed multiple interval changes relative to the previous CT scan in 2007, including postsurgical changes. There was asymmetric lobulated and in some locations ill-defined enhancing soft tissue attenuation. This straddled both sides of the dysmorphic left thyroid cartilage and appeared to involve portions of the medial margins of the bilateral strap muscles, while extending caudally in to the subglottic airway on the left side. Findings were suggestive of posttherapeutic granulation tissue versus recurrent neoplasm/squamous cell carcinoma with associated cartilaginous destruction and paraglottic spread (Figure 14–3).

Microlaryngoscopy and Biopsy

The patient underwent microlaryngoscopy with biopsy along with excision and closure of tracheostomy tract in late March 2009. There was a small hyperkeratotic prominence in the midportion of the reconstructed right vocal fold region. The draining tracheostomy tract connected to a deep cavity lined with abnormal tissue that was granular in appearance. A specimen of this tissue was submitted for frozen section with the resultant analysis significant for squamous cell carcinoma. The tumor cavity was located anterior to the thyroid and cricoid cartilages

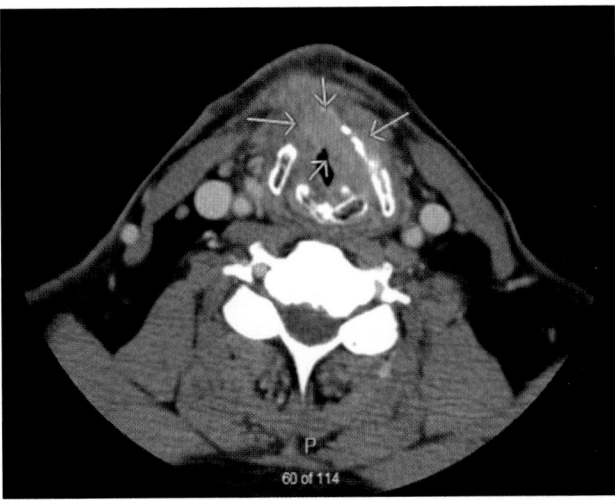

Figure 14–3. An image from the CT scan performed prior to the total laryngectomy.

but did not appear to extend inferiorly beyond the first tracheal ring.

Pathology Findings

Squamous cell carcinoma of the vocal fold and tracheostomy tract with invasion of overlying soft tissue was found. Because this represented a T4 recurrence, total laryngectomy was presented as the only viable option, and the potential for a myocutaneous flap reconstruction was also anticipated.

Preoperative Laryngectomy Counseling

One day following biopsy, the patient presented to the Voice Care Center to meet with the speech pathologist for preoperative laryngectomy counseling. The focus of the evaluation was to educate the patient regarding the anatomic changes associated with a total laryngectomy, and postsurgical voicing options were reviewed. Voicing options following surgery were reviewed with the patient including electrolarynx, esophageal speech, and tracheoesophageal voice production with a voice prosthesis (as a secondary surgical procedure). Postoperative changes in swallowing function were discussed along with water safety precautions (Keith, Linebaugh,

& Cox, 1978; McColl, Hooper, & Von Berg, 2006). The patient was also educated local laryngectomee support groups.

TREATMENT

On the first day of April 2009, the patient underwent total laryngectomy, total thyroidectomy, reconstruction with pectoralis major myocutaneous flap, and central compartment neck dissection. There was a large erosive tumor affecting the anterior commissure region, with subglottic extension to the left, and invasion through the anterior laryngeal framework into the overlying prelaryngeal soft tissues.

POST TREATMENT

The patient underwent a Gastrografin swallow study following total laryngectomy on postoperative Day 15 to rule out a leak and determine if it was safe to initiate a PO diet. The contrast media Gastrografin was selected, as barium could be detrimental to healing if there was a postsurgical fistula. The Gastrografin swallow study was negative for leak; the nasogastric feeding tube was removed, and full liquid diet was initiated (Ward & Corina, 2014). At 2 weeks postop, the patient returned to clinic, and excellent healing of the flap, neck, and stomal area was evident. The stoma was clean and patent. There was no evidence of pooled secretions in the hypopharynx or upper esophageal areas on indirect exam. Use of the electrolarynx with intraoral adapter was initiated postoperative Day 2; use of the intraoral adapter was extended beyond the immediate postoperative healing phase due to edema of the neck. Once edma was improved, neck placement of the electrolarynx improved speech intelligibility.

At follow-up in December 2009, the patient demonstrated independent use of the electrolarynx and had good intelligibility. Since he last presented to Otolaryngology, the patient was diagnosed with coronary artery disease (CAD), and a coronary artery bypass graft (CABG) was being considered

by the patient's cardiologist. The possibility of tracheoesophageal puncture (TEP) for voice restoration was discussed with the patient and was tentatively planned for after completion of and recovery from the CABG.

The patient followed up in February 2010. There was no evidence of local or regional tumor recurrence on head and neck exam. At that time, the patient reported that he had received a second opinion regarding his CAD and was told that he did not need to undergo a CABG. The patient expressed continued interest in pursuing TEP. The otolaryngologist recommended a speech pathologist consult along with follow-up CT scan of the neck. The patient was scheduled for a follow-up with the otolaryngologist in March 2010 but did not show for the visit and did not schedule with the speech pathologist for further assessment for TEP.

POST TREATMENT: NEW COMPLAINTS

In late 2010, the patient developed unstable anginal syndrome. The patient underwent CABG × 3 in December 2010. In February 2011, the patient developed a sternal wound infection and underwent initial débridement by his cardiothoracic surgeon after which he was seen by a general/plastic surgeon for definitive repair. This included sternal wound débridement, repair of sternotomy separation with Stryker titanium reconstruction plate, repair of sternal wound with vertical rectus abdominis myocutaneous flap, and usage of right pectoral myocutaneous flap for sternal wound closure. Due to his complicated recovery, the patient postponed tumor follow-up and consideration for TEP.

In November 2011, the patient presented to the gastroenterologist with reports of dysphagia with solids. Videofluoroscopic examination of swallowing revealed a 3.8-mm stricture of the upper esophagus that was 2.5-cm long. At that time, a balloon dilator of 8 mm was used and could not be passed into the esophagus. In December 2011 a balloon dilator of 9 mm was used and again could not be passed through the esophagus. The gastroenterologist recommended follow-up with the otolaryngologist for dilatation under anesthesia. The gastroenterologist discussed with the patient the likely need for multiple dilation procedures to get the upper esophagus to a 10 to 11 mm opening. Upper esophageal stricture following radiation is common among this population and often requires serial dilation treatments to obtain a normal opening of the upper esophagus, which can distend to approximately 2 cm in the anterior-posterior dimension and up to 3 cm laterally to accommodate a swallowed bolus (Farwell et al., 2010; Long & Orlando, 2002).

In February 2012, the patient returned to the otolaryngologist for evaluation and treatment of upper esophageal stricture. At that time, the patient indicated that he had to crush his pills and was consuming primarily pureed foods. A videofluoroscopic swallow study was recommended and revealed a marked stricture between C4-5, which interrupted bolus flow. The patient was able to achieve passage of solid bolus only with repeat swallows and liquid washes.

TREATMENT

The patient underwent esophageal dilation using soft tapered tip bougies with mitomycin C application in April 2012. Mitomycin C is an antifibrotic agent, which has been used to prevent recurrence of anatomic strictures (Annino & Goguen, 2003). The patient was successfully dilated to 40-French (13.33 mm). The patient underwent a repeat dilation with mitomycin C application to the esophageal inlet/hypopharyngeal juncture in July 2012. At this time, the dilation progressed to 60-French (20 mm).

In August 2012, the patient reported no dysphagia symptoms. Follow-up with speech pathology was recommended for a preoperative TEP consult with possible esophageal insufflation testing to determine candidacy for secondary tracheoesophageal puncture (TEP) with placement of a voice prosthesis. Preoperative assessment reduces complications and increases the success rates of tracheoesophageal (TE) voice restoration by identifying unsuitable candidates for the procedure. The appropriateness of a patient for TE voice restoration is based on medical, psychologic, structural, and physiologic factors. Predictive testing, like esophageal speech and insuf-

flation testing, can help to identify patients with structural or physiologic abnormalities. Early recognition and management of abnormalities can shorten the recovery time to achieve functional communication (Gress, 2004). Four weeks later the patient met with the speech pathologist. The patient expressed a desire to pursue hands-free voice production and to have a more natural sounding/less robotic voice. The Blom-Singer Insufflation Test Set was utilized. Following insertion of the catheter via the naris to the 25-cm mark, indicating the length of insertion necessary to reach the upper esophagus, air was directed from the stoma into the catheter to direct it into the upper esophagus. Upon exhalation with occlusion of the stomal attachment, no audible vibration was evident; however, there was audible passage of air noted. This finding was thought to indicate possible temporary postesophageal dilation edema at the site of the pharyngoesophageal (PE) segment resulting in poor vibration of the PE segment versus a more stable issue of lack of vibratory function of the PE segment. Repeat esophageal insufflation testing was recommended in 4 weeks to determine if there was improvement in audible vibration as the patient recovered further from esophageal dilation.

In October 2012, the patient presented for follow-up with otolaryngologist and speech pathology as recommended. The patient reported that he had been sensing tightness during swallowing for the past 4 weeks. During this office visit, the patient exhibited spontaneous production of audible esophageal voice production without the use of esophageal insufflation. The tone quality was noted to be quite good with no significant strain evident, and loudness was adequate. Based on this finding, repeat esophageal insufflation testing was deferred. Repeat esophagoscopy and dilation as well as secondary tracheoesophageal puncture (TEP) with placement of a voice prosthesis were scheduled, and the patient's speech pathologist at the VA was contacted and updated regarding these plans.

In November 2012, the patient underwent repeat rigid esophagoscopy with dilation. Significant stenosis was evident with a lumen of approximately 18-French (6 mm) in diameter and dilation was successful to 50-French (16.67 mm). TEP was determined not to be prudent at that time due to the degree of esophageal stricture. Two months later, the patient reported improved swallowing function at follow-up. A repeat dilation with application of mitomycin C was performed in January 2013. Dilation progressed from 22-French (7.33 mm) up to 60-French (20 mm). The patient was able to resume a normal diet without crushing his pills. Again a repeat dilation with application of mitomycin C was performed in February 2013. The patient was successfully dilated to 60-French (20 mm), and the degree of stricture visualized was significantly less than that noted during previous dilation procedures.

In March 2013, the patient underwent rigid esophagoscopy with tracheoesophageal puncture. There was mild stenosis noted at the lower hypopharyngeal/upper esophageal juncture. The scope was easily passed through this area. The posterior tracheal wall was punctured utilizing the needle introducer from the Blom-Singer TE puncture kit from InHealth Technologies, and a 16-French (5.33 mm) catheter was placed in the TE tract. The day after surgery the catheter that was placed in the patient's TE tract became dislodged. The patient was seen emergently by the speech pathologist and otolaryngologist; he presented to the office with an open TE tract. Examination revealed that the tract was open as there was saliva coming through the puncture site when the patient swallowed his secretions. The patient's TE tract was successfully dilated from an 8-French (2.67 mm) to a 16-French (5.33 mm) diameter with successive placement of increasingly larger diameter catheters. A 16-French (5.33 mm) red rubber catheter was left in place as a stent.

The patient was scheduled to see the speech pathologist a week later for removal of the catheter and placement of a voice prosthesis. This was completed successfully, and the patient progressed from use of a low-pressure voice prosthesis to placement of an indwelling voice prosthesis as his tract length stabilized. The patient continues to follow up for routine voice prosthesis changes.

SUMMARY

This case presentation, which spans a time period of 10 years, outlines a patient's progression through several medical and surgical interventions and associated complications, along with an overlay of compliance and psychosocial issues that are not uncommon in this patient population. Cancer recurrence occurred on two occasions, requiring decision making regarding intervention options to target functional outcomes while targeting a cure. Eventually, the patient required total laryngectomy, which was completed 6 years following the initial diagnosis of a right-sided vocal fold mass. Further interventions, including esophageal dilation and tracheoesophageal puncture (TEP) with placement of a voice prosthesis, were completed to maximize swallowing and communication function. There are many teaching points regarding decision making for medical and surgical intervention outlined in this case. And, most importantly, this patient has been cancer free since his total laryngectomy surgery nearly 6 years ago with swallowing function that allows for intake of a regular consistency diet with thin liquids and excellent voice production with TEP.

REFLECTION AND ANALYSIS FOR FURTHER STUDY

1. Describe precautions you would give to a patient undergoing a TEP procedure.
2. How do partial and total laryngectomy procedures vary with regard to risks, benefits, and anatomic alteration?
3. What dietary/swallowing recommendations are appropriate for patients who undergo repeat esophageal dilations?

REFERENCES

Annino, D. J., & Goguen, L. A. (2003). Mitomycin-C for the treatment of pharyngoesophageal stricture after total laryngopharyngectomy and microvascular free tissue reconstruction. *Laryngoscope, 113*(9), 1499–1502.

Farwell, D. G., Rees, C. J., Mouadeb, D. A., Allen, J., Chen, A. M., Enepekides, D. J., & Belafsky, P. C. (2010). Esophageal pathology in patients after treatment for head and neck cancer. *Otolaryngology-Head and Neck Surgery, 143*(3), 375–378.

Gress, C. D. (2004). Preoperative evaluation for tracheoesoph-ageal voice restoration. *Otolaryngologic Clinics of North America, 37*(3), 519–530.

Keith, R. L., Linebaugh, C. W., & Cox, B. G. (1978). Presurgical counseling needs of laryngectomees: A survey of 78 patients. *Laryngoscope, 88,* 1660–1665.

Long, J. D., & Orlando, R. C. (2002). Anatomy, histology, embryology, and developmental abnormalities of the esophagus. In M. Feldman, L. S. Fieldman, & M. H. Sleisenger (Eds.), *Gastrointestinal and liver diseases* (pp. 551–560). Philadelphia, PA: W.B. Saunders.

McColl, D., Hooper, A., & Von Berg, S. (2006). Preoperative counseling in laryngectomy. *Contemporary Issues in Communication Sciences and Disorders, 33,* 147–151.

Pandian, V., Miller, C. R., Schiavi, A. J., Yarmus, L., Contractor, A., Haut, E. R., . . . Bhatti, N. I. (2014). Utilization of a standardized tracheostomy capping and decannulation protocol to improve patient safety. *Laryngoscope, 124*(8), 1794–1800.

Ward, E. C., & Corina, J. V. (Eds.). (2014). *Head and neck cancer: Treatment, rehabilitation, and outcomes* (2nd ed.). San Diego, CA: Plural.

15

Team Approach in Treating Laryngeal Cancer Resulting in Total Laryngectomy

Jennifer Craig, Kyle Mannion, and C. Gaelyn Garrett

HISTORY

Patient S is a 64-year-old Englishman with medical history remarkable for well-controlled hypothyroidism, hypertension, benign prostate hypertrophy, arthritis, and gastroesophageal reflux disease (GERD), with excellent health maintenance.

Medical History

In early 2008, Patient S presented to his primary care physician (PCP) for a routine check-up. He had a remote smoking history (as a teenager) but had not used any tobacco products since then. Patient S noted enjoying approximately one alcoholic beverage a week but denied any history of excessive use or other abuse of illicit substances. He reported a troublesome 12- to 18-month history of persistent hoarseness to his PCP who promptly referred him to a local otolaryngologist.

Shortly thereafter in May 2008, Patient S presented to the Vanderbilt Voice Center for a second opinion; his local ENT physician had biopsied a lesion on his left true vocal fold. Pathology revealed "severe dysplasia, concerning for carcinoma in situ." During his visit to the Vanderbilt Voice Center, flexible transnasal endoscopy revealed a lesion

at the posterior portion of the left true vocal fold (Figure 15–1). At the time, it was unclear whether this represented a new lesion or healing tissue at the operative site. The patient was offered an additional biopsy or close monitoring of this area for change. Patient S decided to follow up with his local ENT who performed the original biopsy.

Social History

Patient S was a well-educated chief financial officer and financial planner with proficiency in both English and French. His voice was particularly important to him, as clear, concise communication was important to his success as a businessman.

DIAGNOSTIC WORKUP

Visual Examination

In August 2008, Patient S again returned to the Vanderbilt Voice Center for another opinion. He underwent an additional biopsy 2 months prior with his local ENT, which revealed carcinoma in situ of the left true vocal fold. He met with a radia-

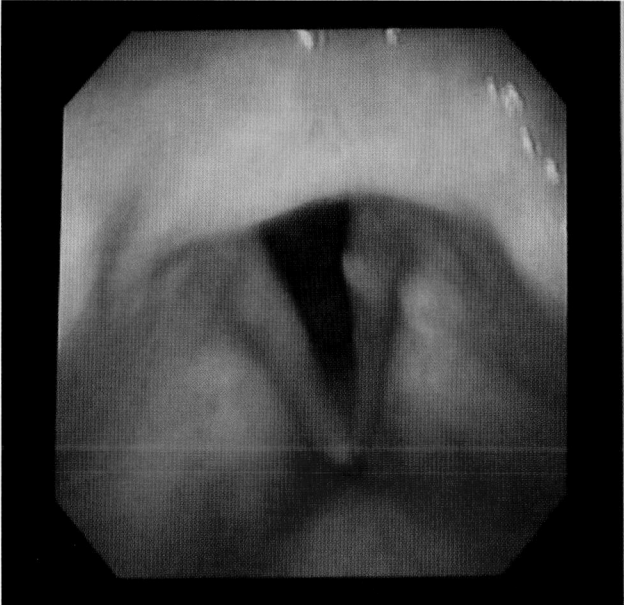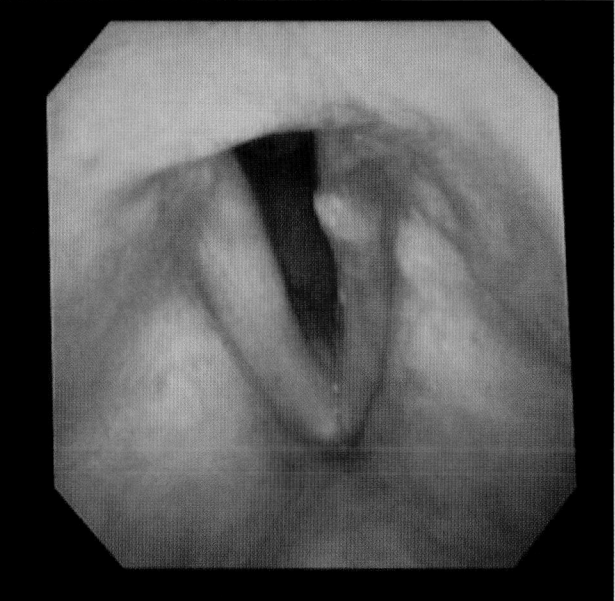

Figure 15–1. Bilateral true vocal fold abduction with evidence of left true vocal fold lesion, May 2008.

tion oncologist but wanted to explore the option of laser excision of the lesion, with the ultimate goal being functional voice preservation. Voice evaluation with laryngostroboscopy was completed during this visit, revealing a persistent lesion on the posterior aspect of the left true vocal fold (Figure 15–2; Video 15–1).

TREATMENT PLAN

Patient S was again presented with the options of (a) close observation, (b) radiation therapy, and (c) repeat direct microlaryngoscopy (DML) with biopsy with appropriate risks and benefits discussed in detail. Patient S reiterated his goals of functional voice preservation; he planned on retiring in a little over 2 years.

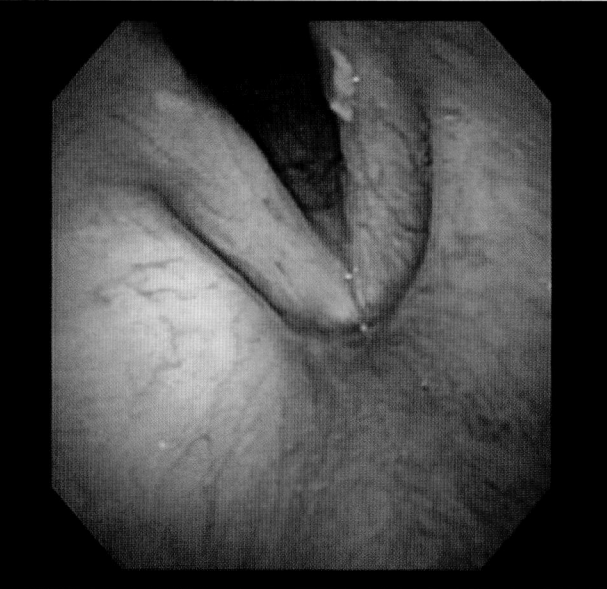

Figure 15–2. Bilateral true vocal fold abduction with evidence of left true vocal fold lesion, August 2008.

Surgical Management

Patient S was encouraged to and elected to undergo DML with biopsies, this time at Vanderbilt Medi-

cal Center, as this was considered to fully assess the character of the lesion. Pathology at that time revealed "squamous cell carcinoma in situ. The edges of these small biopsies appear to be free of any involvement by in situ carcinoma." Intraoperative photos are available in Figure 15–3.

Postoperative Treatment Plan

Per recommendations, Patient S presented for his routine follow-up 2 weeks later. He was recommended to follow up again in 2 months, but presented just 4 weeks later with complaints of globus sensation that began shortly after his last visit. He denied any dysphagia, odynophagia, otalgia, or voice change, simply a "fullness." Flexible transnasal endoscopy completed by the laryngologist revealed an area at the posterior aspect of the left true vocal fold, concerning for persistent lesion versus granulation. Globus sensation was attributed to compensatory muscle tension dysphonia and/or GERD. He was treated with an increase in PPI and considerations for voice therapy made, should his symptoms not resolve. One month later, Patient S's symptoms resolved; while his voice quality remained moderately rough by clinical standards, he noted significant improvement in functionality and even an ability to sing. Additionally, he had no evidence of disease on exam. A routine follow-up visit was recommended in 2 months.

FOLLOW-UP ASSESSMENT

At Patient S's follow-up in March 2009, despite a lack of changes in voice quality or any other new complaints, changes were appreciated on the anterior infraglottic and posterior aspects of the left true vocal fold during indirect laryngoscopy completed by the physician. Given his history, repeat DML was completed shortly thereafter, revealing squamous cell carcinoma in situ (Figure 15–4). Biopsies were submitted for HPV testing, as observations during the procedure indicated a "significant area of hyperkeratosis . . . lesion was leukoplakia with the anterior portion having a papillomatosis appearance. There were also separate smaller foci of papillomatosis lesions. . . . " The physician and patient discussed further treatment options at length. Patient S elected to undergo an in-office pulsed-dye laser (PDL) procedure. At his 2-week follow-up, Patient S was very pleased with his mildly rough voice quality—he again was able to sing. However, another lesion was appreciated on the infraglottic anterior aspect of the left true vocal fold.

Over the next year and a half, this pattern would repeat itself. Patient S presented for follow-up, and suspicious appearing lesions were appreciated. Treatment options, including formal DML with biopsy and excision, were discussed at length

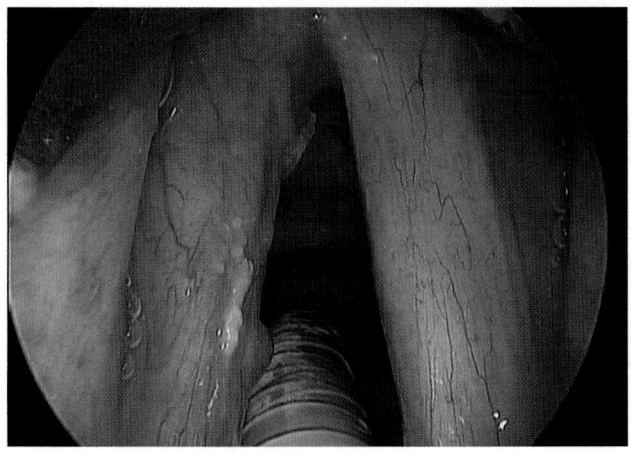

Figure 15–3. Preoperative image of the bilateral true vocal folds, October 2008.

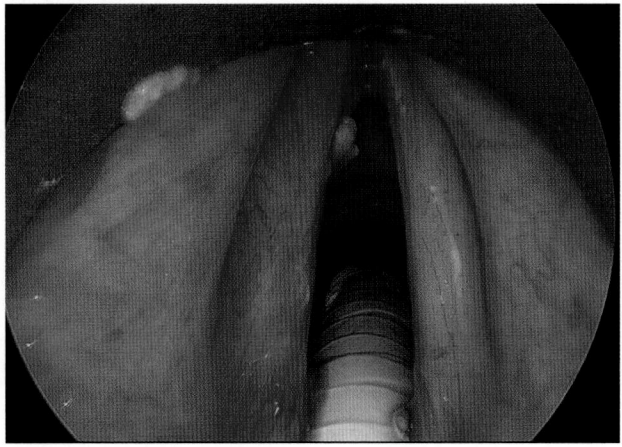

Figure 15–4. Preoperative image of the left true vocal fold with carcinoma in situ, March 2009.

each time. Ultimately, Patient S elected to continue with PDL treatment to remove presumed carcinoma in situ or other suspicious-appearing lesions on the left true vocal fold, as his voice quality with this procedure was optimal after healing (relative to presurgical intervention, not prediseased baseline). The lesions appreciated during follow-up gradually became more and more concerning, and the patient's voice quality slowly deteriorated. Although his Voice Handicap Index scores hovered around the mild-moderate range (Jacobson et al., 1997) at each visit, increasing roughness and pitch breaks were appreciated by clinicians. In July 2010, Patient S presented with worsening

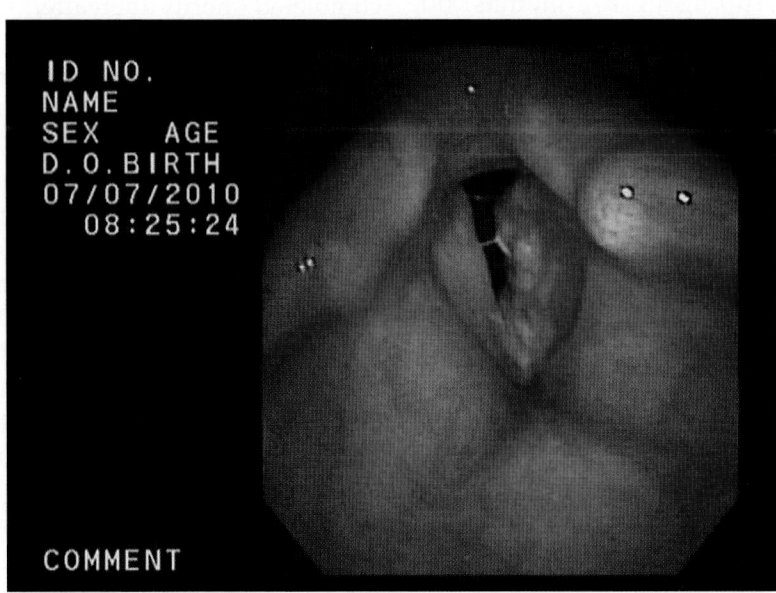

Figure 15–5. Left true vocal fold thickening.

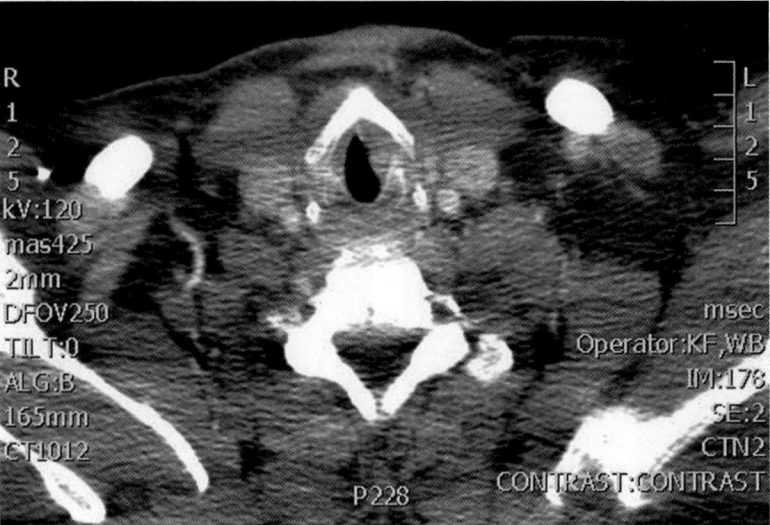

Figure 15–6. CT scan of the neck.

vocal quality and persistent, untreated cough for 2 to 3 weeks.

Laryngostroboscopy revealed increased thickness with significant decrease in mucosal wave of the left true vocal fold (Figure 15–5, Video 15–2). CT scan of the neck indicated an "asymmetric fullness of the mid portion of the left true vocal fold (Figure 15–6)." DML with biopsy revealed "the left vocal fold involved with an irregular exophytic but broad-based thickening. There appeared also to be a possible ulceration. There was more bulky involvement toward the anterior commissure with some abnormal change of the right anterior vocal fold." Left true vocal fold biopsy revealed "invasive squamous cell carcinoma, moderately-differentiated. Examination of deeper sections reveals areas diagnostic of stromal invasion."

FURTHER TREATMENT CONSIDERATIONS

Patient S and his physician had an extensive discussion regarding treatment options at this point for his T1b invasive squamous cell carcinoma. He elected to pursue radiation therapy with the hopeful goal of organ and voice preservation (Jones, Fish, Fenton, & Husband, 2004). He noted side effects of a mild sore throat and further dysphonia. Follow-up with the laryngologist was recommended 1 month after completion of radiation treatment.

POSTRADIATION OUTCOME

Two and a half months after complete of radiation therapy, Patient S presented for follow-up with his physician. His lag in follow-up was attributable to a hip replacement in October. Severe dysphonia characterized by rough, breathy, and strained quality with aphonic breaks and pitch breaks were appreciated by the speech pathology team, and an exophytic white lesion with surrounding erythema was appreciated along the superior surface of the left true vocal fold. The mobility of the left true vocal fold also appeared impaired (Figure 15–7; Video 15–3). A neck CT with contrast was obtained

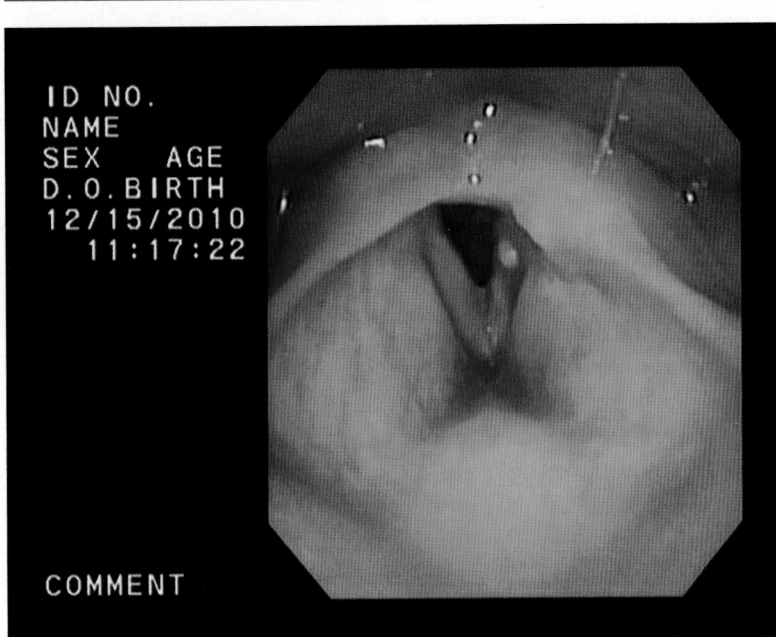

Figure 15–7. Bilateral true vocal fold abduction, December 2010.

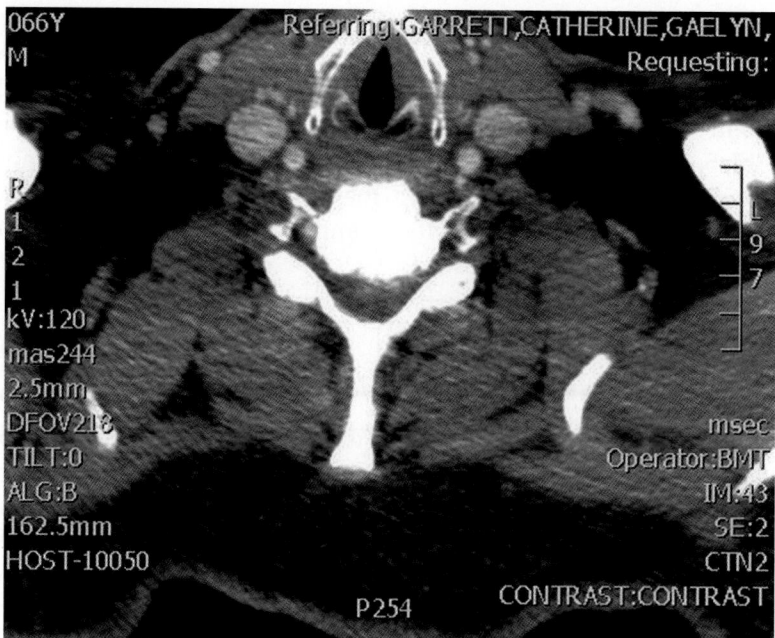

Figure 15–8. CT scan of the neck, December 2010.

with findings that included a "mild stable asymmetric fullness of the left true vocal cord. No pathologic appearing adenopathy within the neck [was] seen" (Figure 15–8).

The apparent persistence of disease with continued growth versus postradiation effects was immediately concerning to the treating laryngologist, who quickly referred Patient S to the Head and Neck Surgery team at the John S. Odess Otolaryngology and Head and Neck Surgery Clinic at Vanderbilt University for consideration of more aggressive surgical intervention. Further biopsies were recommended, with the understanding that should they come back negative, additional biopsies would likely be necessary over the next year. Fortunately, his biopsy in February 2011 was negative for dysplasia or malignancy (Figure 15–9). However, frequent follow-up was recommended to monitor the healing tissue and determine the need for additional biopsies. At a second follow-up in April 2011, Patient S complained of a tickle in his throat, and though his voice quality remained stable, his left vocal fold had further reduced mobility and an irregular, nodular appearance, warranting additional biopsy. Patient S requested to postpone this biopsy for at least a

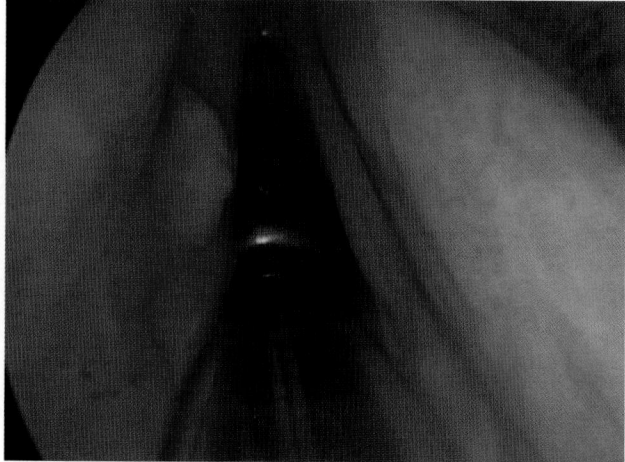

Figure 15–9. Bilateral true vocal fold abduction with no evidence of dysplasia, February 2011.

month, as he was planning several trips with his family. At his next follow-up, flexible laryngoscopy completed by the treating surgeon revealed "edema of the supraglottis involving the false vocal fold and arytenoids . . . increased change of the left true vocal cord with some leukoplakia anteriorly in addition to the erythema posteriorly . . . airway still widely patent." Again, additional biopsy was strongly recommended, and cautions against waiting were made. Patient S elected to discuss further treatment options with his radiation oncologist and decide shortly thereafter how to proceed.

Within the next 11 days, Patient S lost his voice entirely and presented to his local emergency department with airway distress. He was transferred to Vanderbilt and underwent biopsies with an emergency tracheotomy. Surgical pathology revealed "reactive cellular changes and underlying necrosis" of the right true vocal fold and "invasive squamous cell carcinoma, well differentiated with associated necrotic debris" of the left true vocal fold. Operative notes indicated "extensive erosion within the larynx with fixation of the left true vocal cord and arytenoid with mucosal changes extending back onto the arytenoid on the left side itself . . . nodes negative."

EMERGENCY SURGERY RESULTS

Five days later, Patient S underwent total laryngectomy with left neck dissection, left thyroidectomy, and cricopharyngeal myotomy. Given the near-emergent nature of this surgery, preoperative laryngectomy counselling was not completed. A nasogastric tube was placed in the operating room. A laryngectomy tube was not recommended, as his stoma was widely patent without surrounding edema.

SLP CONSULTATIONS

Alaryngeal communication was introduced the following day with a Servox electrolarynx and intraoral adapter. Initially, early termination, clenched jaw, imprecise tongue movements, and reduced labial movements were appreciated. Intelligibility was initially less than 20%, but Patient S demonstrated an excellent motivation to improve his communication. He demonstrated a moderate level of intelligibility with the electrolarynx by his discharge from the hospital 4 days later. Home health was recommended to further manage communication skills with the electrolarynx and tube feedings.

At his follow-up 2 weeks later, Patient S was tolerating soft solids and thin liquids without difficulty. The NG tube had been removed 3 days prior. His anosmia subsided, though dysgeusia persisted. Pulmonary rehabilitation was initiated; Patient S preferred use of a LaryTube and LaryClips as housing for his heat moisture exchanger (HME) versus adhesive baseplates. Preoperative counseling and education for tracheoesophageal puncture and prosthesis were provided; Patient S was eager to pursue TEP communication.

ANOTHER COMPLICATION

Prior to completion of his secondary puncture for TE communication, Patient S presented to his local hospital emergently for an oropharyngeal bleed from the left lingual artery, losing approximately 150 mL of blood. He received four units of packed red blood cells and 3 L of crystalloid and was transferred to Vanderbilt where embolization of branches of bilateral lingual arteries was completed. A four-vessel CT angiogram of the neck revealed no vascular injury or extravasation. A chest x-ray suggested left basilar consolidation, consistent with pneumonia and bibasilar atelectasis.

EXPLORATORY SURGERY

He was taken back to surgery 2 days later to further investigate mucosal breakdown as the source of arterial erosion. Operative notes indicated a 10-mm area of dehiscence of the midline closure on the anterior wall of the neopharynx. There was no definable pocket or fistula tract extending from this area of dehiscence of the mucosal closure. The next day, Patient S was discharged from Vanderbilt under NPO status with dobhoff feeding tube (DHT) and scheduled for follow-up with his head and neck surgeon 3 weeks later with an esophagram.

The results of the esophagram 3 weeks later revealed "a normal appearing esophagus without evidence of structure, mass, ulceration or fistula." From an otolaryngology standpoint, Patient S was back on a favorable healing course: he was communicating well with his electrolarynx and was ready for TEP placement. However, the esophagram also revealed a concerning area of increased opacification in the left lung base. Follow-up CT of the chest indicated a soft tissue mass, micro- and macrolobulated, in the left posterior sulcus measuring 6.3 × 4.3 × 5.4 (height) cm, which appeared malignant. Cytopathology from fine-needle aspiration returned "Few groups of moderately atypical cells in a background of mucinous/myxoid matrix."

This finding, especially in the abbreviated time frame from his most recent discharge from the hospital, came as quite a surprise to Patient S At his visit to his thoracic surgeon he stated, "I feel too good to have this many problems." Ultimately, Patient S was diagnosed with T3N0 colloid adenocarcinoma. Initial concern for surgical intervention existed, as physiologic reserve base was not able to be determined because pulmonary function tests were precluded by laryngectomy. However, Patient S remained physically active, exercising between 30 and 60 minutes per day. His surgeon deemed him an appropriate candidate based on these grounds. In December 2011, Patient S successfully underwent left video-assisted thoracoscopic surgery and resection of his cancer, esophagoscopy, and tracheoesophageal puncture with placement of catheter during a single course of anesthesia. His hospital course was uneventful.

TEP PLACEMENT AND OUTCOMES

One week later, Patient S underwent initial placement of a 16 Fr 12-mm indwelling tracheoesophageal prosthesis. Use and maintenance of the prosthesis was reviewed. Strong voicing was established, but inadequate seal of adhesive baseplate subverted continuous speech. Adhesive skin prep pads were employed as well as a more durable adhesive baseplate. Using these different setups, he was able to achieve tracheoesophageal speech without air escape from under the baseplate.

His next several sessions were fairly routine: refitting a prosthesis, troubleshooting adequate seal of a baseplate, and managing pulmonary rehabilitation while intermittently coordinating his cancer surveillance appointments. He remained cancer free, but Patient S frequently had the same complaints during his prosthesis changes. Adhesive baseplates either irritated his skin or would not adhere for longer than a few hours. Additionally, his prostheses were leaking more and more frequently, with an average life span of the prosthesis going from approximately 2 months to less than 3 weeks secondary to yeast and biofilm formation. He had been on antireflux medication throughout his entire course, and there was no evidence of granulation tissue that may have suggested an increase in reflux. He was placed on Nystatin and use of probiotics was recommended to improve the life of the prosthesis (Rodrigues, Banat, Teixeira, & Oliveira, 2007). These measures proved beneficial, as Patient S's prostheses began to last slightly longer than 2 months again. He was also placed in a LaryButton with LaryClips as housing for his HME; his voicing was excellent, and this combination was the most satisfactory to Patient S.

Although Patient S was very compliant to recommendations pertaining to extending the life of his prostheses, again they began to fail more and more frequently. Over the next year, he underwent 10 prosthesis changes despite his diligence to care. Expenses directly from traveling to the clinic for prosthesis replacement were mounting and becoming burdensome to him and his family, not to mention the cost of the care itself. The decision was made to transition Patient S to a non-indwelling prosthesis, which would directly reduce his cost of care and need for frequent travel to our clinic. Patient S and his wife, daughter, and inquisitive young grandson all participated in the visit, each independently removing and placing the non-indwelling prosthesis. Each individual affirmed a high comfort level and independence with this prosthesis. Over the next several months, communications with Patient S largely revolved around his satisfaction with the non-indwelling (NID) prosthesis.

To date, Patient S remains cancer free and an excellent alaryngeal communicator using his NID prosthesis with LaryButton and LaryClips.

DISCUSSION AND CONCLUSION

Best treatment for T1 and T2 glottic cancer is a highly debateable topic. Research shows that survival rates with surgical intervention and radiation therapy are comparable, but functional outcomes remain contested. Management of disease must be balanced with patient goals. Often these goals will change with the progression of disease. Regardless, a team approach inclusive of the patient's family, laryngologist, head and neck cancer surgeon, and speech-language pathologist must be incorporated to provide the patient with the best outcomes. The case of Patient S details the unpredictable nature of carcinoma in situ and its persistence despite diligent patient pursuit of treatment and frequent medical intervention. It also suggests that decreased coping skills and fear lead to shifts in timely treatment, necessitating more drastic intervention including total laryngectomy. Fortunately for Patient S, his supportive family and surrounding medical team fostered positive outcome and quality of life through his treatment for laryngeal cancer.

Consider Patient S's case representative of several patients with T1 or T2 glottic cancers: What treatment modality would cure his cancer and provide superior voice outcomes to allow him to fulfil his functional goals? Five-year survival rates for both T1 and T2 (N0) cancers are comparable when treated with radiation therapy and endoscopic excision (Cohen, Garrett, Dupont, Ossoff, & Courey, 2006; Loughran, Calder, MacGregor, Carding, & MacKenzie, 2005; Warner et al., 2014). While survival rates for surgical and nonsurgical therapy are well established, research detailing functional outcomes is more sparse. A large majority of this research is retrospective in nature, understandably given its level of difficulty to conduct. Factors that further complicate prospective research design include surgeon preference toward treatments, treatment variability by geographic location (Jones, Fish, Fenton, & Husband, 2004), and consideration toward patient preference. Some studies provide contradictory results in perceptual voice outcomes (Cohen et al., 2006). Furthermore, patients with similarly staged tumors remain a heterogenous group, making outcome measurements challenging. Some studies even

compare voicing outcomes among patients that received radiation and those that underwent partial laryngectomy (Jones et al., 2004); it is no surprise that voicing outcomes were superior in the radiation group.

Patient S's case highlights the necessity of tailoring treatment regimens and the unique nature of decision-making processes that are not always reflected in the research. For his particular case, surgeon expertise and lesion location without invasion of the anterior commissure or crossing of midline made surgical removal of the lesion reasonable. The vocal ligament was preserved in each of the interventions and unaffected mucosa relatively spared, allowing for adequate vibration of the fold and optimal voice outcomes. Furthermore, beginning Patient S's treatment with surgical intervention allowed for more treatment options as his cancer persisted. That is, had his treatment started with radiation, he would not have been a candidate for additional radiation treatments in the future. It was unfortunate and unexpected that his disease seemed to flourish in the face of radiation.

Patient S's eagerness to pursue treatment in the early stages of his diagnosis was interestingly offset by his decision to delay intervention, which ultimately contributed to his need for total laryngectomy. When he was first advised to pursue repeat biopsy after radiation, his disease was still felt to be amenable to partial laryngectomy. Recall that Patient S regularly presented for close monitoring of his cancer shortly after his diagnosis until his completion of radiation, at which point his follow-up appointments and recommended biopsies were delayed by several weeks to months at a time. Patient S frequently cited personal reasons for postponing intervention, though one must question his acceptance of the disease and coping skills as the gravity of its suggested treatment escalated to more and more invasive procedures. Research suggests that increased duration from diagnosis to the effect of treatment allows for greater implementation of coping strategies (Babin et al., 2008). To be clear, this does not mean duration from diagnosis to the treatment itself, but rather the effects of the treatment, which Patient S's case supports. As time progressed after his laryngectomy, he demonstrated increased coping skills and currently demonstrates relatively preserved quality of life. Babin and colleagues also noted that health-related quality of life alteration is minimal in head and neck cancer patients who fail organ-preservation therapies and must ultimately undergo TL. Furthermore, these researchers did not correlate loss of speaking abilities and permanent stoma to decreased quality of life. They again attributed this to the length of time allowed for implementation of coping strategies. Patient S's treatment course lasted nearly 3 years prior to his laryngectomy. Though his laryngectomy was not necessarily predictable at the initial staging of cancer, it is arguable that implementation of coping mechanisms were initiated several years before his laryngectomy.

Several studies link socioeconomic status to quality of life outcomes in head and neck cancer patients. Babin et al. (2008) demonstrated that patients with a higher SES, education level, and fewer comorbidities tended to have a higher quality of life postoperatively than their similarly diagnosed counterparts. Patients with lower SES tend to have poorer access to quality health care, receive a later diagnosis, and subsequently have more advanced stage of disease, increased disability, and poorer healing (Demiral, Şen, Demiral, & Kınay, 2008). While approximately 90% of T1 cancers respond favorably to conservative management, it is arguable that Patient S's outcome in treatment for his initial T1b laryngeal cancer was representative of the ~10% of patients who do not respond to initial conservative management. However, this was not a result of his SES, education, or access, but rather a delay in seeking recommended treatment as his disease progressed. He remained convinced of the typical outcome of a T1 cancer. Indeed, Patient S's demographics may be considered positive predictors to his current quality of life as a laryngectomee: he is largely independent in his daily maintenance of his stoma and TEP, he is disease free, and he continues to be independent in his activities of daily living. In essence, these predictive factors made him the optimal candidate for a laryngectomy.

Despite the anomalies in his case leading up to the laryngectomy, Patient S's recovery of voicing and swallowing following laryngectomy was quite remarkable. His goals of reliable communication were met with both tracheoesophageal speech and electrolaryngeal communication. To promote relative ease and independence with voicing and tracheoesophageal prosthesis (TEP) maintenance, Patient S was transitioned to a self-maintained non-indwelling (NID) TEP. The NID prosthesis was selected as the best, most cost-effective option after frequent prosthesis failure secondary to biofilm formation and *Candida* colonization (Rodrigues et al., 2007). Patient S was an excellent candidate for this type of prosthesis given his excellent manual dexterity, visual acuity, location of puncture site, and quick implementation of recommendations from his clinicians (Leder & Sasaki, 1995). Furthermore, the option of self-maintenance reduced the burden of cost dramatically with regard to prosthesis, appointment, and travel as compared to a clinician-managed prosthesis (Rodrigues et al., 2007).

Patient S's case brings up several relevant topics in the treatment of head and neck cancer. His initial presentation was that of a glottic carcinoma in situ, which quickly exemplified the unpredictable nature of this type of malignancy. The debate of whether T1 or T2 glottic carcinomas should be treated with surgery or radiation should not be generalized across patients, but rather decided on a case-by-case basis, as a physician-patient alliance is established and patient goals are considered. Patient S also demonstrates the variable patterns of human behavior when faced with the diagnosis of cancer and increasingly difficult treatments. Patient S's surrounding team, his family, physicians, and clinicians, provided him with positive support throughout his treatment course and continuously kept his goals at the forefront of his treatment.

REFLECTION AND ANALYSIS FOR FURTHER STUDY

1. Generate examples of possible patient goals at early, mid-, and late-disease stages.
2. How would a treatment plan differ for a patient with high levels of family support versus one with low levels of family support?
3. Think of as many reasons as possible why someone would delay treatment for a potentially life-threatening condition? What can we do, as a profession, to lessen the likelihood that this happens?

REFERENCES

Babin, E., Sigston, E., Hitier, M., Dehesdin, D., Marie, J. P., & Choussy, O. (2008). Quality of life in head and neck cancers patients: Predictive factors, functional and psychosocial outcome. *European Archives of Oto-rhino-laryngology, 265*(3), 265–270.

Cohen, S. M., Garrett, C. G., Dupont, W. D., Ossoff, R. H., & Courey, M. S. (2006). Voice-related quality of life in T1 glottic cancer: Irradiation versus endoscopic excision. *Annals of Otology, Rhinology & Laryngology, 115*(8), 581–586.

Demiral, A. N., Şen, M., Demiral, Y., & Kınay, M. (2008). The effect of socioeconomic factors on quality of life after treatment in patients with head and neck cancer. *International Journal of Radiation Oncology, Biology, Physics, 70*(1), 23–27.

Jacobson, B., Johnson, A., Grywalski, C., Silbergleit, A., Jacobson, G., Benninger, M., & Newman, C. (1997). The Voice Handicap Index (VHI): Development and validation. *American Journal of Speech-Language Pathology, 6*, 66–70.

Jones, A. S., Fish, B., Fenton, J. E., & Husband, D. J. (2004). The treatment of early laryngeal cancers (T1–T2 N0): Surgery or irradiation? *Head & Neck, 26*(2), 127–135.

Leder, S. B., & Sasaki, C. T. (1995). Incidence, timing, and importance of tracheoesophageal prosthesis resizing for successful tracheoesophageal speech production. *Laryngoscope, 105*(8), 827–832.

Loughran, S., Calder, N., MacGregor, F. B., Carding, P., & MacKenzie, K. (2005). Quality of life and voice following endoscopic resection or radiotherapy for early glottic cancer. *Clinical Otolaryngology, 30*(1), 42–47.

Rodrigues, L., Banat, I. M., Teixeira, J., & Oliveira, R. (2007). Strategies for the prevention of microbial biofilm formation on silicone rubber voice prostheses. *Journal of Biomedical Materials Research Part B: Applied Biomaterials, 81*(2), 358–370.

Warner, L., Chudasama, J., Kelly, C. G., Loughran, S., McKenzie, K., Wight, R., & Dey, P. (2014). Radiotherapy versus open surgery versus endolaryngeal surgery (with or without laser) for early laryngeal squamous cell cancer. *The Cochrane Library, 12*, CD002027.

16

Eliminating Aspiration Risk Through Total Laryngectomy: A Surgical Approach Requiring Laryngectomy

Linda Stachowiak

HISTORY

Mr. A was 38 years of age in 2000 when diagnosed with T4N0M0 squamous cell carcinoma of the larynx (SCCA).

Medical History

At the time of our visit to the otolaryngology unit, the patient presented with a tracheostomy that was completed after chemoradiation. He was subsequently decannulated approximately 6 months after the initial tracheostomy. The patient's past medical history (PMH) was significant for

- 5/2007 transitional cell bladder cancer s/p transurethral resection;
- 9/2008 recurrent bladder cancer s/p transurethral resection;
- 2/2009 recurrent bladder cancer s/p transurethral resection;
- 4/2009 renal transitional cell cancer s/p R nephrectomy;
- 7/2009 recurrent bladder cancer s/p transurethral resection;

- 9/19/11 right true vocal fold lesion, biopsied as dysplasia;
- multiple recurrent pneumonias;
- hypertension (HTN);
- coronary artery disease (CAD);
- chronic obstructive pulmonary disease (COPD);
- obstructive sleep apnea (OSA)-CPAP at night;
- hypothyroidism;
- pain;
- myocardial infarction (MI) 1999 with multiple stent placements; and
- 75 pack-year history of smoking, quit 2000.

Social History

This patient attended 2 years of college and owned his own contracting business. He reported that despite his several-year history of aphonia, he had been successfully working and earning an income. He lived with his wife of 32 years. They have two adult children. He was a grandfather with one additional grandchild on the way. He reported that he had always been very active and that, the month prior to his diagnosis and hospitalization, he was hiking in Alaska.

ASSESSMENT

Mr. A transferred to our hospital from another local hospital where, for the previous 5 days, he was treated for aspiration pneumonia. When first assessed at our facility, Mr. A continued to have a small, persistent unhealed tracheostomy site (12 years later), and he demonstrated considerable aphonia and stridor. The transfer hospital unit had completed a modified barium swallow (MBS) study that reportedly identified significant aspiration risk with a recommendation to withhold oral feeding (or NPO status) in favor of an alternate means of nutrition.

The admitting head and neck surgeon at our hospital consulted the speech pathology oncology staff to perform a repeat MBS upon transfer. On September 21, 2012, the MBS noted a severe pharyngeal stage dysphagia with high risk of aspiration. A portion of the MBS video can be viewed as Video 16–1.

RESULTS OF THE MBS EVALUATION

The patient's larynx was fixed and nonfunctional, with significant changes to the laryngeal anatomy that were difficult to interpret. He had no discernable epiglottis and exhibited aspiration before, during, and after the swallow, some of which was silent and at other times was audible. The patient aspirated on all consistencies, despite the implementation of various postural strategies and airway protection maneuvers. Due to the patient's history of recurrent pneumonias, combined with the severity of his chronic dysphagia and increase in airway compromise, the head and neck surgeon felt that a percutaneous endoscopic gastrostomy (PEG) and tracheostomy tube placement were needed in order to optimize his medical status and prepare him for a total laryngectomy.

PREOPERATIVE SPEECH PATHOLOGY INTERVENTION

On September 25, Inpatient Speech Pathology preoperative laryngectomy teaching was initiated and included education on alterations in anatomy and physiology associated with the surgery and its subsequent effects on activities of daily living including communication, showering, nose blowing, lifting, smelling, and defecating. Mr. A and his wife were introduced to three forms of alaryngeal communication: esophageal speech, electrolarynx, and tracheoesophageal speech. They were also educated on various supplies that would be recommended for use after surgery, including a medical alert bracelet identifying him as a "neck breather," shower shield and various stoma covers/heat moisture exchangers.

On September 26, Mr. A and his wife attended a laryngectomy support group to further prepare him for his upcoming surgery while providing an opportunity to meet others who have gone through the surgery and successful rehabilitation. The surgery was scheduled for 5 weeks out where the consensus of the medical team was that the patient would be medically optimized.

On September 28, Speech Pathology inpatient Passy-Muir evaluation was completed. Although the patient demonstrated persistent dysphonia, he appreciated the ability to communicate without having to use his finger to manually occlude his newly placed tracheostomy tube. The patient was subsequently discharged home.

Hospital Admission Timeline Prior to Surgery

On October 29, Mr. A was admitted with abnormal bloodwork, including anemia, and required transfusion with two units of packed red blood cells (pRBCs) prior to surgery.

SURGICAL TREATMENT

Due to the recent bout of pneumonia and abnormal labwork that included anemia, the plan was to preadmit him to be medically optimized for surgery. Mr. A was educated that the surgery was a possible 10- to 12-hr procedure, and that he may consider presurgical transfusion as his hemoglobin (Hg) was 8.4 during preadmission testing. He was advised to stop his Clopidogrel 1 week prior to surgery, though he may continue ASA 81 mg. His levothyroxine was also increased to 150 mcg from 100 given recent testing of his thryoid simulating hormone (TSH) level. Mr. A was consuming six to seven cans of Isosource 1.5 per day via PEG. He had been cleared by cardiology for surgery after performing an electrocardiogram (EKG) and echocardiogram. On November 1, the patient underwent a total laryngectomy, exploration of great vessels of the right neck, including carotid artery and jugular vein reconstructed with an anterolateral thigh free flap.

Postoperative Speech Pathology Intervention

On November 13, the speech pathologist began working with the patient and his wife on laryngectomy tube care. This included removal, cleaning, and replacement with trach ties. Mr. A had very limited tongue mobility (unplanned finding) with only slight tongue lateralization noted. Mr. A continued to have his tongue lie on his lower lip due to edema and was therefore unable to completely close his mouth. The patient was not a candidate for an electrolarynx at this time. He had been writing to communicate and was beginning to explore some text-to-speech applications on his iPad.

On November 16, the speech-language pathologist once again saw Mr. A for laryngectomy tube care and initial instruction on sterile saline tracheal lavage. The patient was discharged home on November 20, but he was soon readmitted, on November 22, with complaints of nausea, vomiting, failure to thrive, and a mild wound separation on the left side of the neck.

On November 18, significant postsurgical edema was noted, which appeared slow to resolve and consequently further delayed the initiation of electrolarynx training. The patient also had a bulky anterolateral thigh (ALT) free-flap reconstruction with a #6 Shiley cuffed tracheostomy tube sutured in place that prohibited laryngectomy tube placement. The plan at that time was to check the patient intermittently during hospitalization to check for decreases in tongue edema, allowing for training use of an intraoral electrolarynx. In the meantime, Mr. A was effectively communicating by writing or the use of his iPad with a program that verbalizes his typed messages.

Mr. A was taken back to surgery for a local wound débridement of left neck and right neck wound breakdown with the reapproximation of the skin. The patient was sent to begin hyperbaric oxygen treatment (HBO) on November 26, to assist with wound healing by increasing tissue oxygenation, thereby stimulating angiogenesis and fibroplasia (Dequanter, Jacobs, Shahla, Paulus, Aubert & Lothaire, 2013). Surgical repair plus HBO was successful, and 2 weeks later as an inpatient, a leak test was completed revealing no leak in the lateral, oblique, or anteroposterior planes (see Video 16–2).

However, postsurgically the patient continued to demonstrate significant oropharyngeal deficits including significantly limited tongue mobility, reduced base of tongue propulsion, reduced pharyngeal constriction resulting in difficulty with AP bolus transit, anterior spillage of liquids, oral stasis, and pharyngeal stasis. The patient had no risk of pulmonary aspiration due to surgical alterations to his neck anatomy coupled with adequate healing. The therapeutic focus was therefore facilitating adequate intake through swallowing rehabilitation to compensate for his oropharyngeal deficits. Until these deficits were able to be rehabilitated, he would require continued use of his PEG tube for primary nutritional support.

SPEECH PATHOLOGY INTERVENTION PLAN

In mid-November, speech pathology initiated swallowing rehabilitation. The patient was started on a clear liquid diet and trained on use of a posterior head tilt and upright positioning for optimum bolus clearance. At this time he did best with small amounts of liquid placed posteriorly via teaspoon or via squirt bottle. The patient was discharged home December 1.

By 6 weeks post surgery, the patient had received 11 out of a planned 45 HBO treatments. At this time he exhibited limited tongue mobility that had subsequently limited any training in alaryngeal communication, and the patient was solely communicating by writing. As tongue mobility improved, he was gradually able to advance his diet. Initially this was limited to a thin purée diet that can be taken through his squirt bottle due to the extent of his oral stage deficits. The patient continued to wear his 10/55 laryngectomy tube in the stoma. He was required to wear this continually all day and night due to the bulkiness of his free-flap reconstruction and the need for the tube to maintain stomal patency. Mr. A's issues with wound healing persisted at 3 months post surgery whereupon he had received 31 out of a planned 45 treatment sessions. At this time, the focus of speech therapy was on three main areas: communication, swallowing, and laryngectomy care (Table 16–1). As his wound continued to heal, this focus was extended to include additional goals (Table 16–2). By April he was able to take adequate amounts of food PO, and subsequently his PEG was removed on April 9, 2013 (see Video 16–3).

The patient underwent a secondary tracheo-esophageal voice prosthesis (TEP) on May 20 with placement of a 17 Fr 10-mm indwelling voice pros-thesis. Speech therapy continued to focus primar-ily on swallowing, and treatment was expanded to include instruction in the use/maintenance of the newly placed trachea-esophageal puncture (TEP). The patient's extensive reconstruction, com-bined with his limited tongue mobility, resulted in a severely dysarthric, deep, and hollow vocal qual-ity. Initially, he used a combination of TEP voicing supplemented by his iPad and text-to-talk apps to maximize communicative effectiveness. As he became more effective with TEP voicing, he found less need to augment his verbal attempts with his iPad (see Video 16–4).

SUMMARY

This patient's nonfunctional larynx placed him at sig-nificant risk for aspiration and pulmonary infection.

Table 16–1. Initial Therapy Focus

Communication	Swallowing	Laryngectomy Care
✓ Augmentative communication: iPad with text to talk apps ✓ Improve tongue mobility via lingual range of motion (ROM) and strengthening exercises ✓ Increase patient's ability to wear his upper and lower dentures to maximize articulation ✓ Improve trismus with some simple jaw stretches	✓ Increase diet consistency while decreasing PEG tube dependency ✓ Strategies to improve oral efficiency (posterior head flexion, small bowled spoon, etc.)	✓ Laryngectomy care ✓ Lavaging the stoma with sterile saline ✓ Heat moisture exchanger education

Table 16–2. Expanded Therapy Focus

Communication	Swallowing	Laryngectomy Care
✓ Introduction to an electrolarynx ✓ Insufflation testing to assess candidacy for a secondary tracheoesophageal voice prosthesis (TEP)	✓ Continue to increase oral efficiency with various postural strategies ✓ Assist in weaning the patient from the PEG tube	✓ Introduction to taped peristomal attachments ✓ Introduction to an intraluminal devices

Consequently, 12 years after his initial chemoradiation treatment for his laryngeal cancer, he elected to undergo a total laryngectomy with free-flap reconstruction. The patient experienced multiple postsurgical complications including severe edema, poor wound healing requiring extensive HBO treatments, and extremely limited tongue mobility resulting in reduced speech intelligibility and severe oropharyngeal dysphagia. The patient was very motivated to attend therapy and continually strived to improve both his swallowing as well as his communication abilities. Mr. A had a very strong support system as well, which had a significantly positive effect on the rehabilitation process. Mr. A has reintegrated successfully back into society despite significant functional deficits.

REFLECTION AND ANALYSIS FOR FURTHER STUDY

1. The focus of this patient's postsurgical swallow therapy was not on preventing aspiration, as his surgery resulted in complete separation of his respiratory and gastrointestinal tracts. What are the benefits of resuming PO following total laryngectomy even when nutritional support is met via nonoral means? In your response, focus not only on physical advantages but also psychosocial and emotional aspects.

2. The creation of a multidisciplinary team takes considerable effort and the development of mutual respect for the roles of each professional medical provider. The field of speech-language pathology is relatively new compared to that of the physician and nurse practice model. Imagine having a conversation with a treating physician and you are working to explain the critical nature of preservation of voice and swallow function. Provide an example of the dialogue that you would have in this position, making your case that these two functions (voice and swallow) are critical and have a high impact on a patient's quality of life.

REFERENCES

Dequanter, D., Jacobs, D., Shahla, M., Paulus, P., Aubert, C., & Lothaire, P. (2013). The effect of hyperbaric oxygen therapy on treatment of wound complications after oral, pharyngeal and laryngeal salvage surgery. *Undersea and Hyperbaric Medicine, 40*(5), 381–385.

Hutcheson, K. A., Lewin, J. S., Barringer, D. A., Lisec, A., Gunn, G. B., Moore, M. W., & Holsinger, F. C. (2012). Late dysphagia after radiotherapy-based treatment of head and neck cancer. *Cancer, 118*(23), 5793–5799.

Theunissen, E. A., Timmermans, A. J., Zuur, C. L., Hamming-Vrieze, O., Paul de Boer, J., Hilgers, F. J., & van den Brekel, M. W. (2012). Total laryngectomy for a dysfunctional larynx after (chemo)radiotherapy. *Archives of Otolaryngology-Head and Neck Surgery, 138*(6), 548–555.

PART VI

Less Common Cases

17

Management of Nasopharyngeal Carcinoma

Jeffrey E. Baylor, Christian E. Soto, and Vicki Lewis

INTRODUCTION

This case outlines the evaluation, diagnosis, and treatment of nasopharyngeal carcinoma in a Southeast Asian male. The etiology of nasopharyngeal carcinoma is not completely understood. This particular type of head and neck cancer is typically rare throughout most of the world but is known to have a higher incidence in certain portions of the population which include Southeast Asia, China, parts of Africa, and the Arctic (Chang et al., 2006). Epidemiological factors that have been found to contribute include elevated antibodies for the Epstein-Barr virus, family history of nasopharyngeal cancer and a diet rich in salt-preserved fish. Additionally, consumption of preserved foods, lack of intake of fresh fruits and vegetables, and chronic respiratory infections are considered to be moderate risk factors (Chang & Adami, 2006). Nasopharyngeal cancer is typically treated with radiation therapy; however, chemotherapy may also be used in treatment. The field of radiation for this type of cancer is typically large and is adjacent to many critical structures including the brain, eustachian tubes, and the parotid glands.

HISTORY

The patient, a 40-year-old Cambodian male initially presented to an otolaryngologist with a new-onset, progressive history of right-sided hearing loss, right-sided epistaxis, and right-sided nasal congestion that began 2 weeks prior to his appointment. The patient reported right-sided jaw pain and a 9-lb weight loss over the course of 3 weeks with a decrease in appetite. Past medical history at that time included seasonal allergies for which he used multiple nasal sprays without noted improvement. The patient also reported some symptoms of heartburn/indigestion. The patient denied any history of prior ear surgery, skull trauma, or noise exposure.

Social History

There was no history of alcohol use, but the patient was a former smoker. He reported smoking one pack of cigarettes per week and quit 3 to 4 years prior to his otolaryngology consultation.

DIAGNOSTIC WORKUP

Otolaryngology assessment included physical examination and nasopharyngoscopy. On physical examination, temperature, heart rate, and blood pressure were within normal limits. Vocal quality was normal. Face was symmetric with normal facial strength and normal salivary glands noted. The external auditory canals were normal. On the right side there was a serous middle ear infusion evident with no acute infection; on the left side, the tympanic membrane was clear and intact. Tuning fork testing revealed a Weber that lateralized to the right. Rinne testing was bone conduction greater than air on the right and air greater than bone on the left. The external nose was normal. There was no active epistaxis or crusted blood evident on anterior rhinoscopy. Nasopharyngoscopy showed an exophytic mass on the right side of the nasopharynx engulfing the view of the eustachian tube orifice and extending into the nasal cavity. The mass did not appear to cross midline and did not extend into the oropharynx. No abnormalities were noted at the base of tongue or the epiglottis. Lips, teeth, and gums were normal. Neck exam showed no evidence of lymphadenopathy, masses, or thyromegaly.

An audiogram was completed that revealed a right-sided mild conductive hearing loss with normal hearing on the left side (Figure 17–1). Auditory discrimination was 100% bilaterally. Tympanogram was Type B on the right (indicating a middle ear effusion), and Type A on the left (indicating a well-aerated middle ear).

Impressions from the initial consultation were (a) right nasopharyngeal mass concerning for nasopharyngeal carcinoma and (b) right-sided serous otitis media as a result of the nasopharyngeal mass obstructing the eustachian tube orifice. At that time, a computed tomography (CT) scan of the neck with contrast was ordered to evaluate the extent of the mass and to look for any evidence of metastasis. Also, surgical scheduling for nasal endoscopy with biopsy and right tympanostomy tube placement was initiated.

Imaging Findings

Computerized topography (CT) scan of the neck was completed 5 days following the initial otolaryngology consultation which showed an abnormal enhancing soft tissue mass identified with its epicenter at the skull base on the right side (Figure 17–2). This finding was considered to be most consistent with an underlying nasopharyngeal cancer, probably extending into the skull base, as well as the pterygopalatine fossa.

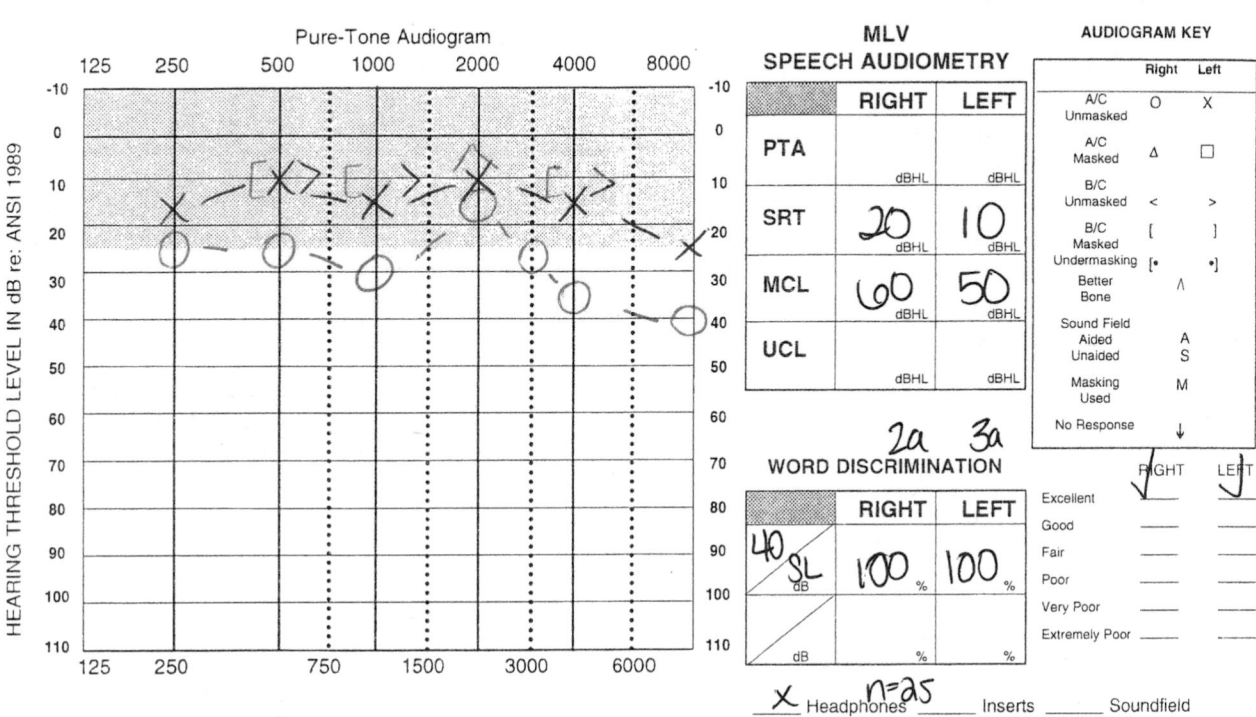

Figure 17–1. Initial audiogram.

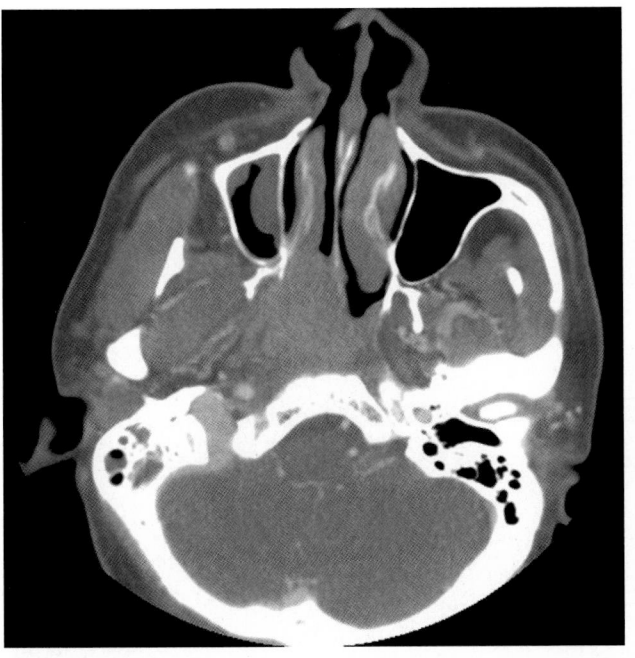

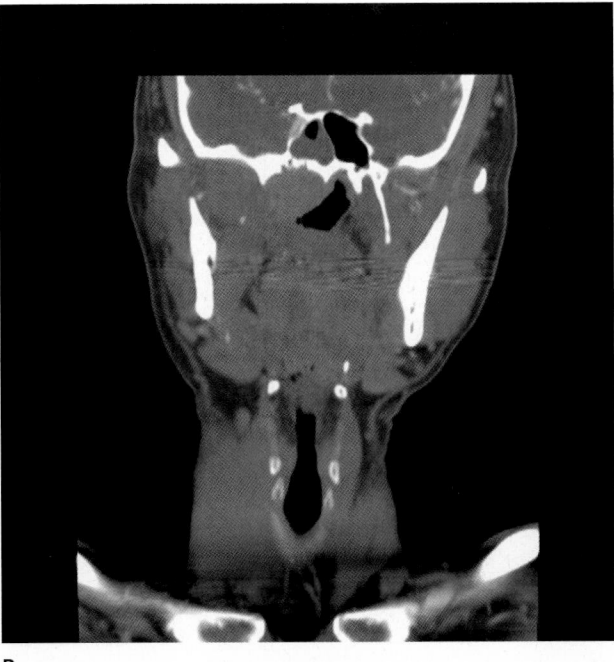

A   B

Figure 17–2. Initial CT scan images depicting enhancing soft tissue mass identified with its epicenter at the skull base on the right side.

A positron emission tomography (PET) scan was recommended for further characterization of the suspected aggressive underlying neoplastic process. The PET scan was completed following the CT scan (Figure 17–3), and impressions were as follows: (a) Marked hypermetabolism was noted in the mass in the posterior aspect of the right nasal cavity and in the right side of the nasopharynx. (b) Mild to moderate hypermetabolism was noted in Level II lymph nodes, bilaterally, nonspecific. This was noted by the radiologist to be representative of inflammation or perhaps metastatic disease. (c) Asymmetrical enhancement was noted in the parapharyngeal area. Hypermetabolism was greater on the left, with an SUV measured at 9.8 versus 5.4 on the right. Per the radiologist's report, hypermetabolism in the parapharyngeal region may represent reactive lymphadenopathy but could also indicate metastatic disease. (d) Minimal hypermetabolism was noted in the right axilla, nonspecific, probably representing inflammation. (e) Minimal hypermetabolism was noted in at least two right Level III lymph nodes, also nonspecific. (f) Normal distribution was noted in the thorax.

Surgical Biopsy

The patient underwent a nasal endoscopy with biopsy of the nasopharyngeal mass with right tympanostomy tube placement 2 days following his initial otolaryngology consultation. Findings included an exophytic, friable nasopharyngeal mass and right serous otitis media. Pathology findings showed an undifferentiated, nonkeratinizing nasopharyngeal carcinoma. The patient was seen for postoperative follow-up 7 days following the biopsy. Some intermittent active bleeding of the operative site was evident. Radiation oncology consultation was facilitated at that time.

Radiation Oncology Consultation

The patient was seen by radiation oncology 1 day following his first postoperative otolaryngology visit. During the radiation oncology consultation, the patient reported that his ear pain and right-sided

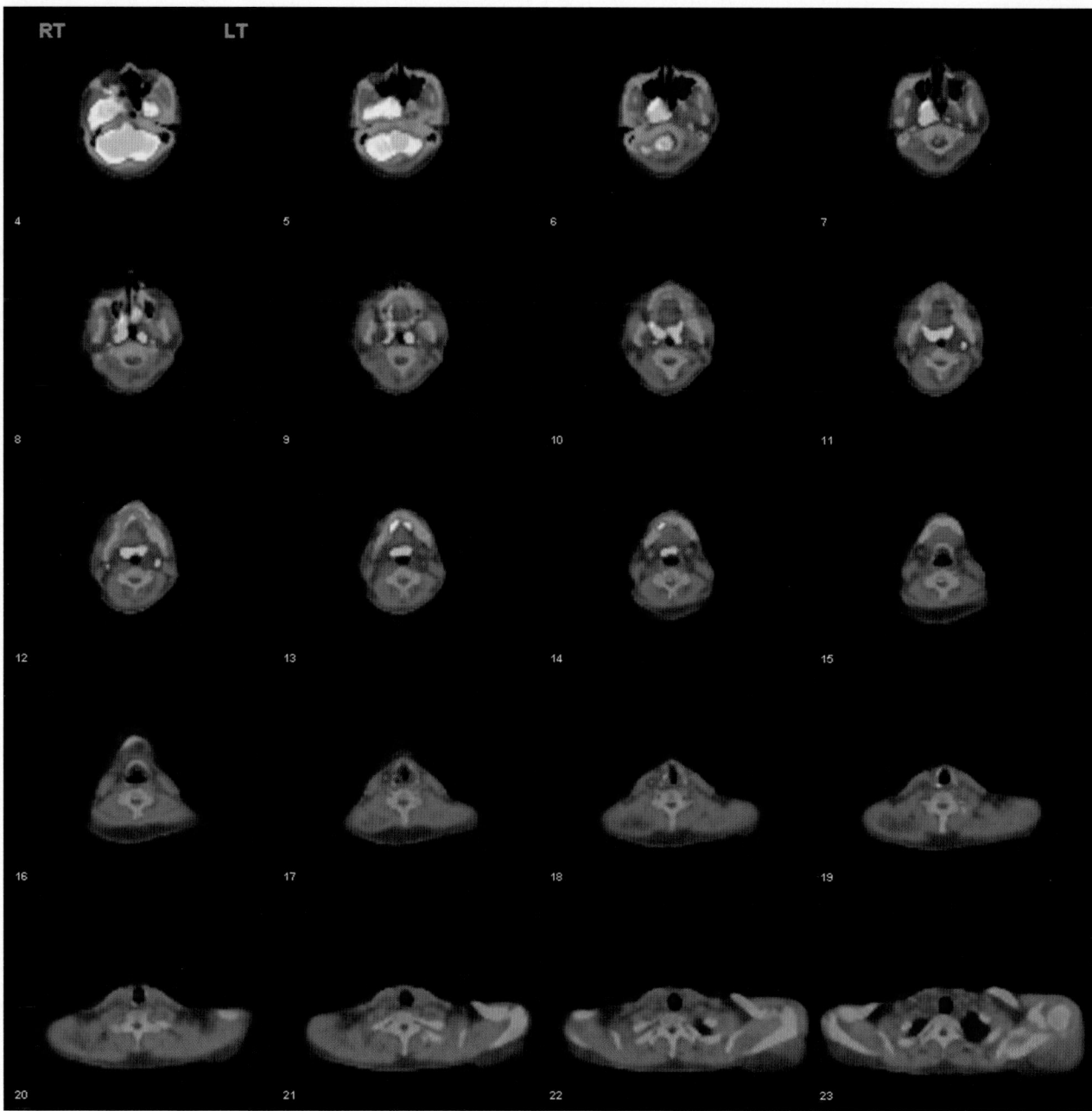

Figure 17–3. Initial PET scan images.

hearing loss had resolved after placement of the tympanostomy tube. Radiation therapy was recommended along with referral to medical oncology for a discussion of concomitant chemotherapy.

Medical Oncology Consultation

The patient was seen by medical oncology for initial consultation 2 days after his initial visit with radiation oncology. At that time, combined chemoradiation was recommended with the plan to administer Cisplatin (100 mg/m^2) on days 1, 22, and 43 during radiation therapy and upon completion of radiation, administration of Cisplatin plus 5-FU every 4 weeks for three cycles. Magnetic resonance imaging (MRI) of the head and neck, a bone scan, and a chest x-ray were recommended to determine any other sites of disease.

Further Imaging

A bone scan was completed 2 weeks following the medical oncology consultation and findings were normal, indicating no bone metastases. MRI of the head and neck showed the known right nasopharyngeal mass which extended into the right pterygopalatine fossa, the right sphenopalatine fossa, and the right nasal cavity with evidence for muscle denervation involving the right medial pterygoid muscle. There was subtle evidence for tumor invading along the right Vidian nerve with asymmetric prominence of the right geniculate ganglion. There was no significant extension to the right internal auditory canal noted. There was no evidence of intracranial metastatic disease and no definite invasion of the right orbit. A chest x-ray showed no active pulmonary pleural disease.

TREATMENT

Radiation therapy (external beam) was initiated 17 days following the medical oncology consultation with a combination of 6 and 10 MV photons utilizing intensity-modulated radiation therapy (IMRT) techniques designed to target a tumor and spare surrounding healthy tissue. For this case, IMRT would spare the adjacent critical structures, including the optic apparatus, brainstem, and contralateral parotid gland. Radiation Oncology prescribed Caphosol for xerostomia as well as PreviDent fluoride rinse. Concurrent chemotherapy was also initiated. Epistaxis was noted early in his treatment. Interventional radiology was consulted and completed tumor embolization 3 days after the onset of chemoradiation.

Following the embolization, the patient's course was complicated by decreased oral intake. Unfortunately, the patient had initially declined placement of a percutaneous endoscopic gastrostomy (PEG) tube and began losing weight with the onset of treatment. The patient experienced complications following his second cycle of chemotherapy and required hospitalization for profound mucositis, malnutrition, and dehydration 3 weeks into his treatment. A patient-controlled analgesia (PCA) pump was necessary during that time for pain control. PEG placement was ultimately completed during this hospitalization. All treatment (radiation therapy and chemotherapy) was put on hold during the 20-day hospitalization. The patient required re-fitting of his radiotherapy mask secondary to weight loss, and repeat radiotherapy simulation was completed 1 week following discharge from the hospital. The patient also experienced acute renal failure during his hospitalization (creatinine peaked at 6.78; normal level: 0.5–1.5 mg/dL), and medical oncology elected not to continue with chemotherapy during the completion of radiation therapy. The patient completed radiation therapy in mid-September. Treatment consisted of a total tumor dose of 7000 cGy in 35 treatment fractions.

INITIAL POST TREATMENT IMAGING

A post treatment CT scan of the neck and positron emission tomography (PET)/CT scan skull to thigh were completed (Figures 17–4 and 17–5) approximately 1 month following conclusion of treatment. Impressions of the CT scan of the neck included a 5-mm focus of mild mucosal enhancement on the left at the level of the nasopharynx. There was no correlating increased activity on the PET/CT. The remainder of the neck demonstrated no significant mass or adenopathy. The PET/CT revealed normal distribution of isotope throughout the head and neck. The hypermetabolic foci seen on the pretreatment scan were noted to be resolved. The paranasal sinuses were well aerated. Thorax/axilla, abdomen/pelvis, and axial skeleton were normal. Impressions were noted as follows: normal PET scan; excellent response to therapy.

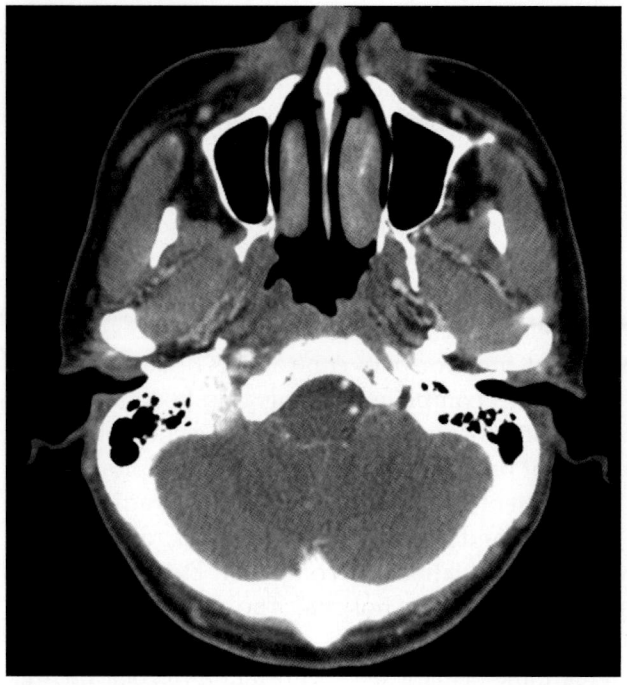 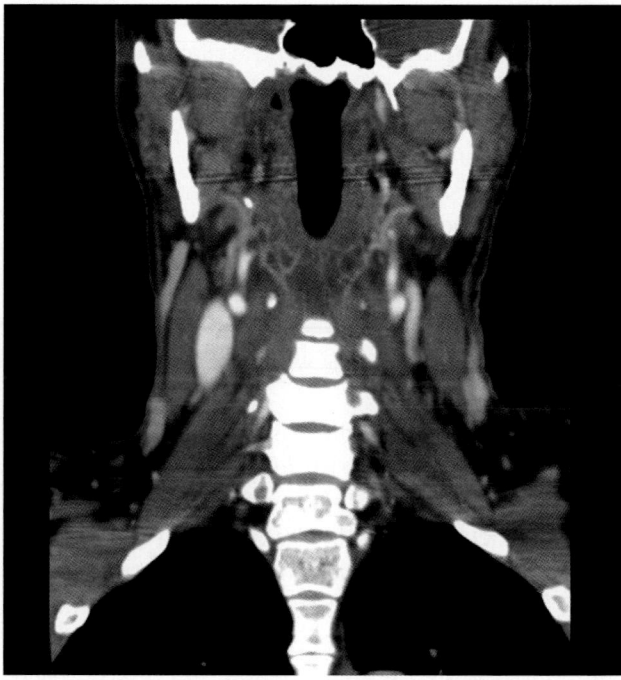

A   **B**

Figure 17–4. CT scan images 1 month following treatment.

SPEECH PATHOLOGY INTERVENTION

The patient was initially referred to Speech Pathology upon conclusion of chemoradiation. At that time, the patient was receiving his primary nutrition via the PEG tube (six to seven cans of Jevity 1.5). He was encouraged to initiate oral intake by radiation oncology and had initiated puree consistencies including pudding, yogurt, and water. The patient noted that he felt that he was swallowing small sips of water without difficulty. He reported that he was sensing puree foods sticking in the throat region after the swallow. He reported at that time that use of a liquid wash was of benefit in clearing the sensation of pharyngeal residue. A fiberoptic endoscopic evaluation of swallowing (FEES) was completed; the patient was presented with thin liquid, nectar-thick liquid, honey-thick liquid, puree, and mechanical soft consistencies. The patient exhibited mild oral dysphagia with premature spillage to the pharynx prior to the swallow on all consistencies and mild-moderate pharyngeal phase dysphagia. Decreased tongue base retraction and pharyngeal constriction were noted, and mild/mild-moderate pharyngeal residue (primarily in the valleculae) was evident after the swallow on increased viscosities, including puree and mechanical soft consistencies. Pharyngeal residue cleared with use of a liquid wash. There was no evidence of supraglottic penetration or aspiration during the initial FEES. Based on the examination findings, it was recommended that the patient increase his oral intake, primarily a pureed diet with thin liquids. Pharyngeal swallowing exercises were initiated.

POST TREATMENT COURSE

The patient was seen for follow-up by Otolaryngology approximately 2 months following completion of radiation therapy. At that visit, the patient reported some right-sided tinnitus but felt that hearing acuity had returned to normal. The patient's primary complaint was dysphagia and a burning

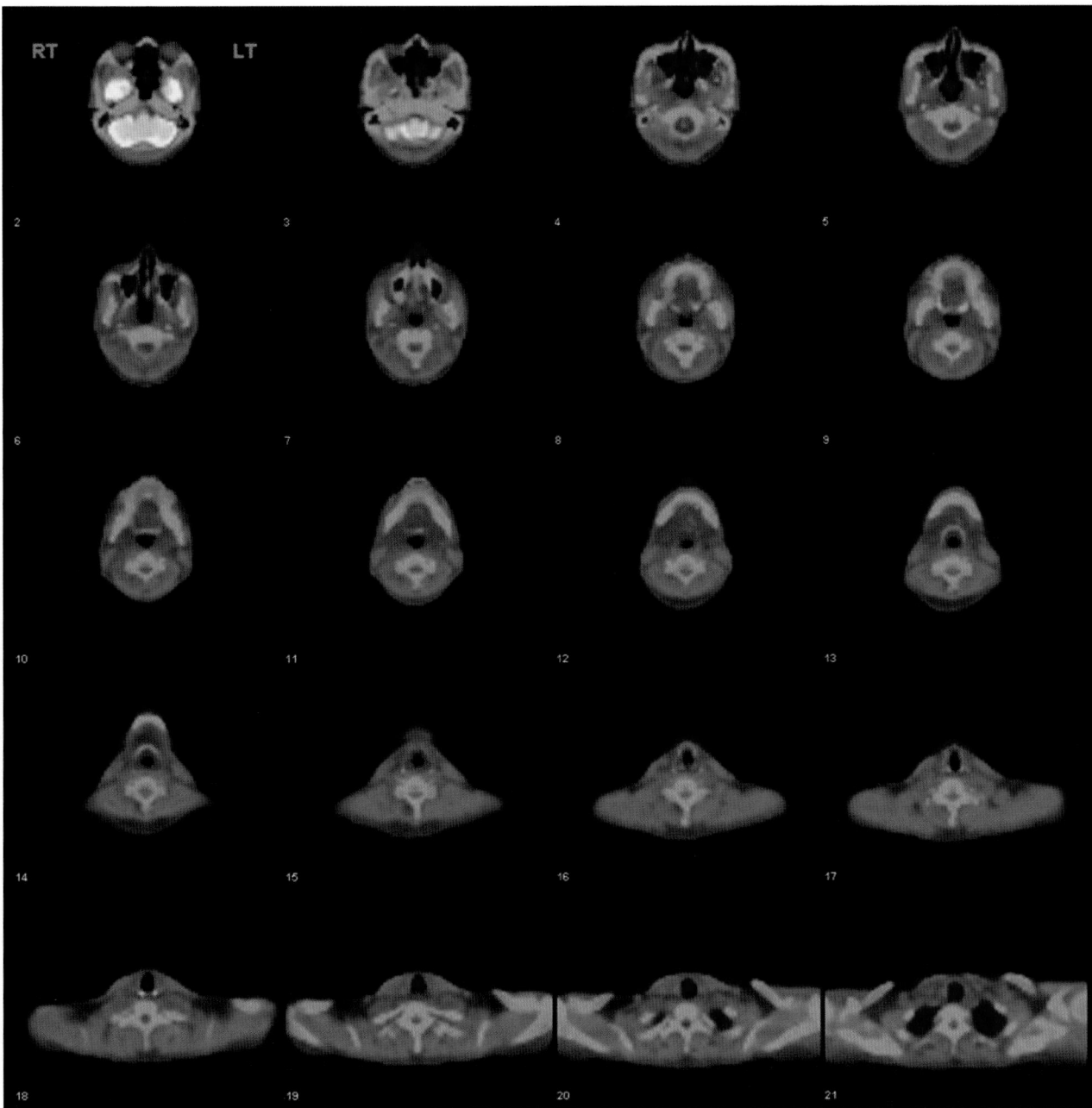

Figure 17–5. PET scan images 1 month following treatment.

sensation in his throat. Examination showed that the right tympanostomy tube was in place with no middle ear effusion or acute infection. The left tympanic membrane was noted to be clear and intact. Nasal endoscopy was completed and showed no evidence of the previously seen nasopharyngeal mass. The eustachian tube orifices were widely patent. Base of the tongue and the epiglottis were normal in appearance. Some edema of the aryepiglottic folds as well as some edema of the vocal folds was evident bilaterally. Mild pooling of secretions was evident in the pyriform sinuses, bilaterally. Follow-up with speech pathology for further dysphagia management was recommended. A proton pump inhibitor (PPI), Zegerid powder for oral suspension 40 mg q.d., was prescribed for reflux control. This was later switched to Prevacid Solutabs 30 mg daily for insurance reasons. Rotating monthly visits with Otolaryngology, Radiation Oncology, and Medical Oncology were set up for cancer surveillance.

Follow-up with otolaryngology was completed 2 months later. At that time, the patient was continuing to take all nutrition via the PEG tube. Further evaluation with videofluoroscopic swallowing study was recommended based on the patient's persisting dysphagia complaints and limited progress in increasing his oral intake. Nasal endoscopy completed by Otolaryngology again showed no evidence of nasopharyngeal mass recurrence. The eustachian tube orifices were widely patent. Some edema of the epiglottis and aryepiglottic folds was noted along with some mild edema of the true vocal cords and some mild pooling of secretions in the pyriform sinuses bilaterally. Some tissue changes in the posterior larynx consistent with possible laryngopharyngeal reflux were evident. The patient admitted to not being compliant with taking his PPI medication.

CONTINUED SPEECH PATHOLOGY INTERVENTION

The patient did not follow up with speech pathology following his initial FEES for swallowing intervention. He was seen for two repeat FEES examinations; the second FEES was completed 2 months following the initial exam, and the third was completed 1 month later. The examinations showed some slight improvement in swallowing function from the initial FEES. Tongue base retraction and pharyngeal constriction remained reduced. Mild-moderate pharyngeal residue was evident (in the valleculae and pyriform sinuses) after the swallow with mild pharyngeal residue after the swallow on puree and mild-moderate pharyngeal residue after the swallow on mechanical soft consistencies. On the second FEES examination, some white plaque-like formations were evident on the lingual surface, soft palate, and along the posterior pharyngeal wall. This appeared

to be consistent with *Candida* (thrush). Additionally, some interarytenoid tissue edema was noted that appeared to be somewhat more pronounced than on the initial FEES examination. Otolaryngology prescribed a 14-day course of Diflucan. The patient was encouraged to continue to increase his PO intake with thin liquids, puree, and high-calorie supplements/smoothies. It was recommended that the patient continue to complete pharyngeal swallowing exercises. On his visit for the third FEES, the patient complained of persistent pain with swallowing and subsequent pain involving the left oropharynx approximately 5 minutes following PO intake. He also noted that he was experiencing occasional regurgitation of tube feedings into his mouth. He continued to be poorly compliant with his antireflux medication. The patient exhibited a persistent slight delay in pharyngeal onset of the swallow, although it was noted that this delay may have actually been a hesitation due to discomfort. Mild pharyngeal residue was noted after the swallow on increased viscosities. The patient winced during each swallow and reported discomfort. As the patient's swallowing complaints appeared to be greater than the instrumental assessment findings, further evaluation of swallowing function was recommended to include assessment of upper esophageal function. The videofluoroscopic swallowing study (VFSS) ordered by Otolaryngology was completed on an outpatient basis at a nearby hospital 2 weeks following the third FEES examination (see Video 17–1). Radiologic findings revealed a functional oral phase of the swallow. Some oral hesitance and piecemeal deglutition that did not appear to be correlated with any oral weakness was noted. The pharyngeal swallow onset was timely. Mild stasis was evident in the valleculae after the swallow which cleared completely with a second swallow. The patient exhibited a hyperreactive response to the vallecular stasis; he coughed vigorously immediately after the swallow. A-P view showed symmetric bolus passage through the pharynx and brisk passage of the 12-mm barium tablet. There was no evidence of supraglottic penetration or aspiration. The patient exhibited postradiation sensitivity with a significant discrepancy between the degree of dysphagia evident on the instrumental examination compared to what was seen on clinical exam. It was unclear as to how much of this might be psychological in origin. At that time, swallowing rehabilitation was recommended to guide the patient through desensitization of the pharynx. Completion of a food diary was recommended to target weaning from the PEG tube.

Following the VFSS, the patient's compliance for swallowing therapy increased, and he attended treatment sessions on a more regular basis. Weaning from PEG tube feedings was prolonged. Dysgeusia, increased pharyngeal sensitivity for mild pharyngeal residue, and odynophagia were factors that limited the patient's progress to oral intake. Based on the patient's persisting issues, he was referred to Gastroenterology, and an EGD was completed 4 months following the VFSS. An esophageal ring was reported in the proximal esophagus which was subsequently dilated. Some fragments of degenerating food were noted in this region; biopsy was negative for malignancy. The remainder of the esophagus, stomach, and the first and second portions of the duodenum were found to be normal, otherwise. The patient gradually increased his oral intake from puree consistencies initially, to soft solids over the course of several months.

CANCER SURVEILLANCE IMAGING

A follow-up PET scan skull to thigh with CT was completed 5 months following treatment (Figures 17–6 and 17–7). Impressions included evidence of increased activity within a new ill-defined nodular density versus infiltrate within the left lower lobe. There was also evidence of increased uptake within a single mediastinal node and a single right axillary lymph node. These were noted to be resolved on a repeat PET scan skull to thigh with CT completed 3 months later and were not felt to indicate recurrence of a malignancy.

OTOLARYNGOLOGY FOLLOW-UP

By the 4-month post–cancer treatment follow-up visit with Otolaryngology, the patient was taking all nutrition by mouth. The patient, however, reported issues with xerostomia. Two and a half years following chemoradiation, the patient continued to have some right-sided eustachian tube dysfunction.

LONG-TERM POST TREATMENT PLAN

A repeat VFSS was completed 4 years following chemoradiation and showed normal oral and pharyngeal phases of the swallow. The patient has been followed for 5 years since the conclusion of his cancer treatment with no evidence of recurrence of neoplasm. He has remained on a regular consistency diet with continued complaints of xerostomia.

SUMMARY

This case outlines a challenging case of a patient with an extensive nasopharyngeal carcinoma with a favorable outcome. His clinical course during cancer treatment was complicated by the need for hospitalization for tumor embolization early in his chemoradiation. Other complications during treatment included profound mucositis, malnutrition, and dehydration. The latter was likely a result of the patient's initial refusal to consent to PEG tube placement. The patient's treatment was delayed by 20 days due to weight loss which required refitting of the radiotherapy mask and repeat radiotherapy simulation. The patient's progress during and following his treatment was limited at times due to financial and patient compliance issues. The patient's oral intake during treatment was nearly nil, and his return to oral intake following his treatment was prolonged, despite only mild oropharyngeal swallowing deficits noted on swallowing studies. Odynophagia, dysgeusia, and xerostomia persisted and were felt to negatively impact on the patient's return to full oral intake. Issues with xerostomia are very common during and following treatment for nasopharyngeal carcinoma; Patterson et al. (2014) reported that 83.3% of the patients surveyed in their study noted dry mouth and 61.1% reported dysgeusia as issues on a quality of life (QOL) scale 24 months following treatment. Additionally, Tong, Lee, Yuen, and Lo

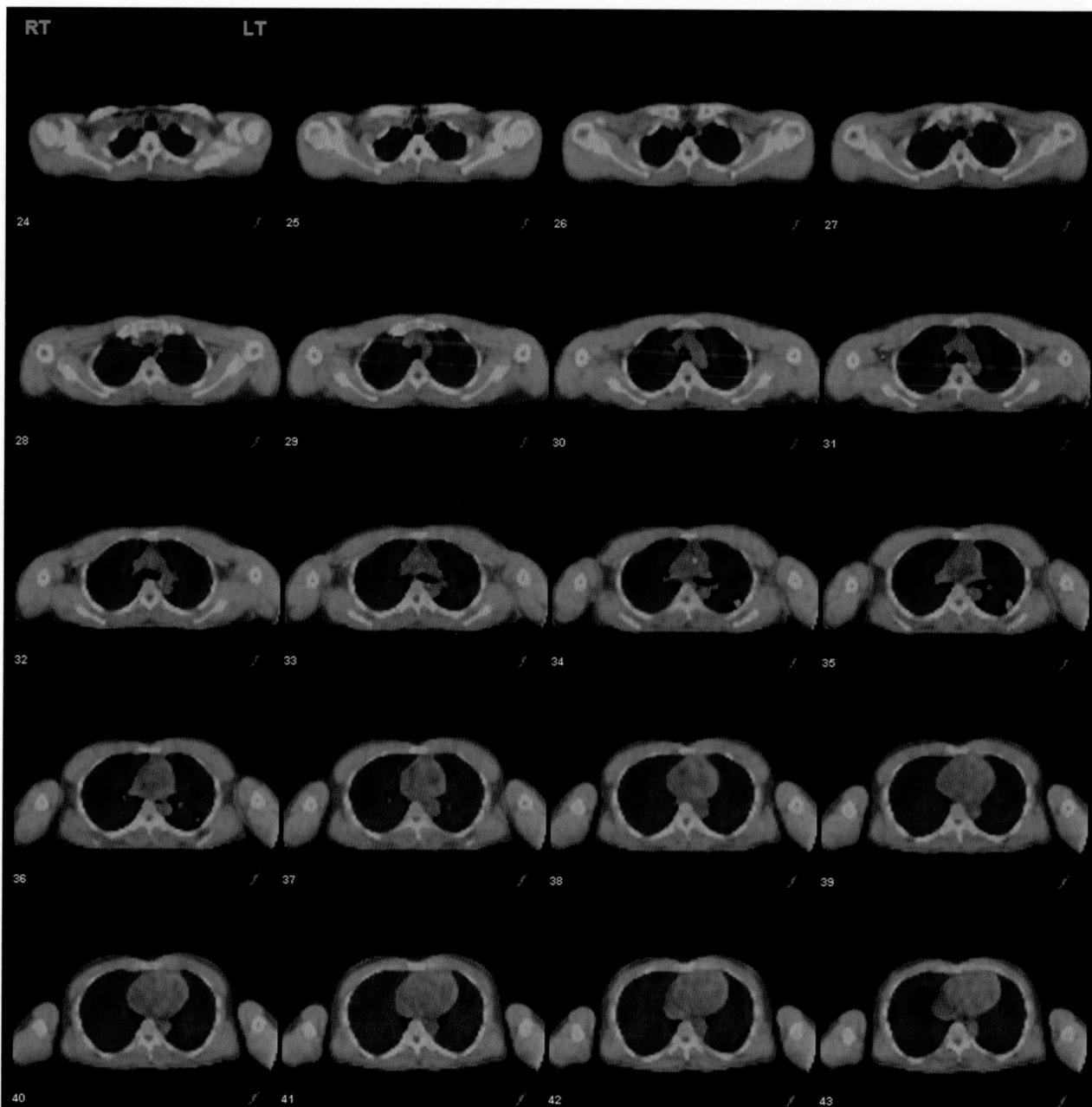

Figure 17–6. PET scan images 5 months after treatment.

(2010) reported that 97% of the nasopharyngeal cancer survivors they studied reported xerostomia. This patient's perception of swallowing difficulty following his treatment was greater than the deficits noted on instrumental examination. It is possible that there was a significant psychological component to his prolonged swallowing issues. This may be a consideration for assessment/research with this population

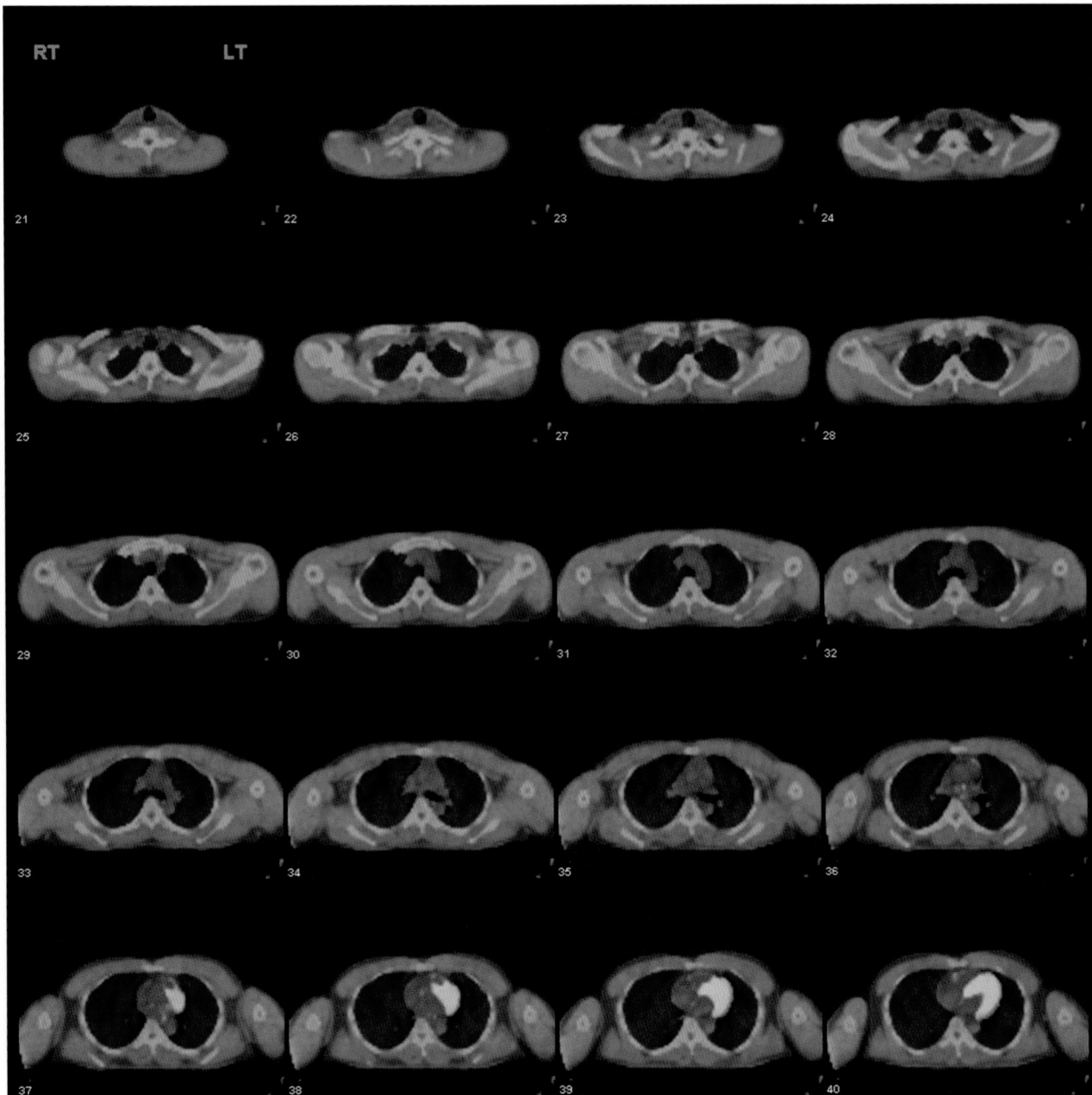

Figure 17–7. PET scan images 8 months after treatment.

when considering use of patient scales to determine degree of swallowing impairment. In long-term follow-up, this patient was found to have persisting issues with eustachian tube dysfunction. This is likely a result of damage caused by the nasopharyngeal tumor as well as a sequela of radiation therapy. Repeat VFSS several years post treatment showed normal oral and pharyngeal phases of the swallow.

REFLECTION AND ANALYSIS FOR FURTHER STUDY

1. How would you approach treatment with a patient whose perception of his or her swallow impairment was in conflict with objective measures obtained during dysphagia examination?
2. What are three distinct ways that the ability to take foods by mouth affects quality of life?
3. Many patients are resistant to initiation of tube feeds. Imagine that you had a patient who, in order to avoid malnutrition and maximize recovery, needed to initiate feeding by nonoral means. What would you say to this patient and to his or her caregivers in order to lessen fear and increase understanding of the benefits of nonoral feeding for patients at high risk for malnutrition and/or aspiration?

REFERENCES

Chang, E. T., & Adami, H. (2006). The enigmatic epidemiology of nasopharyngeal carcinoma. *Cancer Epidemiology Biomarkers and Prevention, 15*(10), 1765–1777.

Patterson, M., Brain, R., Chin, R., Veivers, D., Back, M., Wignall, A., & Eade, T. (2014). Functional swallowing outcomes in nasopharyngeal cancer treated with IMRT at 6 to 42 months post-radiotherapy. *Dysphagia, 29*(6), 663–670. doi:10.1007/s00455-014-9559-0

Tong, M. F., Lee, K. S., Yuen, M. Y., & Lo, P. Y. (2011). Perceptions and experiences of post-irradiation swallowing difficulties in nasopharyngeal cancer survivors. *European Journal of Cancer Care, 20*(2), 170–178. doi:10.1111/j.1365-2354.2010.01183.x

18

Case of Occult Primary Head and Neck SCCA Presented With Lymphadenopathy

Nikhil Rao, Vicki Lewis, Henry Ho, Aftab H. Patni, Erin P. Silverman, Lee Zehenbot, and Bari Hoffman Ruddy

INTRODUCTION AND HISTORY

This case report is of a 74-year-old male who presented to our practice in late October 2014 for evaluation of a right neck lymphadenopathy. The mass was first noticed 3 weeks prior during a routine dental appointment. The patient is a retired professor of engineering and mathematics. At the time of initial evaluation the patient denied any pain, dysphagia, or dyspnea. He did claim recent-onset hoarseness and xerostomia.

Past Medical History

Past medical history was significant for hypertension, hyperlipidemia, cataracts (status postcataract removal), dermatologic scalp lesions, and prostate cancer diagnosed in 2006. Surgical history included robotic prostatectomy for successful resolution of prostate cancer in 2006, penile implant, and detached retina repair.

Social and Family History

Social history was negative for use of tobacco products, although the patient reported that he did have a history of exposure to secondhand smoke. Alcohol consumption was noted to be two to four drinks per day and patient denied any health issues relating to alcohol consumption. Family history was significant for a female sibling with a history of cancer (unspecified), heart disease, and hypertension.

DIAGNOSTIC FOCUS AND ASSESSMENT

Prior to presenting to our practice, the patient underwent computed tomography (CT) of the neck which revealed a 3.7 × 2.6 × 3.3 cm rounded, well-defined mass, in Level II of the right neck. No other evidence of pathologic lymphadenopathy was noted. Additionally, the patient underwent fine-needle aspiration (FNA) of the mass, the results of which were positive for squamous cell carcinoma.

The patient was referred to otolaryngology, and a positron emission tomography (PET) scan (skull to thigh) was completed. This revealed a right Level II lymph node with a maximum SUV of 10.9 correlating with the 3.7-cm neck mass. Distribution within the remainder of the head and neck was normal and neither CT nor PET was able to identify a primary cancer site. Fine-needle aspiration of the lymph node was P16 positive, resulting in a diagnosis of HPV-positive squamous cell carcinoma of the right neck.

On initial physical examination by Otolaryngology, a right-sided Level II neck mass approximately 6 cm in diameter was identified. Flexible fiberoptic laryngoscopy was completed with topical (4% lidocaine) anesthesia and was unremarkable with the exception of prominent lingual tonsils. The true vocal folds were noted to be symmetrical with no visible lesions and normal mobility bilaterally.

At the conclusion of the initial Otolaryngology assessment, plans were made for a direct laryngoscopy, possible tonsillectomy, right selective neck dissection (Levels II, III, and IV), and a PET scan was ordered.

TIMELINE

October 2014

- Initial observation of right-sided neck mass by dentist
- FNA positive for SCAA
- Neck CT
- PET scan
- Fine-needle aspiration of right neck mass

November 2014

- FEES and oral intake assessment (preop)

December 2014

- Preoperative counseling
- Bilateral tonsillectomy and right selective neck dissection
- Postoperative clinic visit
- Radiation oncology intake and radiation therapy begin

January 2015

- Repeat FEES and oral intake assessment (postop)
- Radiation therapy continues
- Chemotherapy begins

February 2015

- Completion of radiation therapy
- Completion of chemotherapy

THERAPEUTIC FOCUS AND ASSESSMENT

Following initial evaluation, the patient returned to the Otolaryngology clinic for two preoperative visits. On the first visit a flexible fiberoptic endoscopic evaluation of swallowing (FEES) and oral intake assessment was conducted by a speech pathologist. At the second preoperative clinic visit, the patient was examined by Otolaryngology and underwent counseling regarding the planned surgery, peri- and postoperative course, and expectations. Preoperative prescriptions and orders were also finalized. At this visit, swallow function was again assessed, and the patient continued to deny dysphagia symptoms and oral intake assessment using the EAT-10 (Belafsky et al., 2008) was normal. Multiple oral consistencies, including thin liquid through solids were presented during FEES, which revealed normal oral and pharyngeal function without clinical signs of airway penetration or aspiration. The patient was advised to continue his current (regular) diet but was counseled on the potential for developing dysphagia symptoms postoperatively. Aspiration precautions and swallowing exercises including strategies to increase tongue base retraction, laryngeal elevation, and pharyngeal constriction were introduced and practiced in order to prepare patient for potential postoperative changes to swallow function. A postoperative FEES and oral intake assessment were scheduled.

SURGICAL OUTCOME

In mid-December 2014, the patient underwent direct laryngoscopy with biopsy, transoral laser microsurgical lingual tonsillectomy, and right selective neck dissection (Levels II, III, IV, and V) under general anesthesia. Following passage of the laryngoscope, all regions of the oro- and hypopharynx were examined, and no obvious mucosal source for the neoplasm was located. Mucosa and lymphoid tissue were excised from both the right and left tongue bases using a micromanipulator attached with a CO_2 laser. An additional sample was taken from the base of tongue at midline in a similar fashion. Bilateral tonsillectomy was completed using an Omniguide laser fiber with a short, curved tip hand piece. Care was taken to obtain a generous margin on both sides, removing both mucosa and constrictor musculature so as to remove both tonsils in their entirety along with a region of normal tissue. On the right tonsil, no obvious neoplasm was noted on initial inspection; however, there was a significant amount of cryptic debris with associated inflammation. Both right and left tonsils were immediately sent to pathology.

Following bilateral tonsillectomy, the patient underwent a right neck dissection. In order to remove the abnormal lymph node within Level II, a surgical specimen was developed from the sternocleidomastoid (laterally), omohyoid (anterior border), and digastric sling (inferior border). Encapsulated within this specimen was a very large (approximately 6 cm) lymph node with no visible spillage of contents or other impact to the normal surrounding tissues. This node was marked and immediately sent to pathology.

Final pathology findings revealed metastatic nonkeratinizing squamous cell carcinoma in one out of five Level II lymph nodes obtained during right selective neck dissection. All Level III, VI, and V lymph nodes were negative for metastasis. The right tonsil specimen was significant for invasive, nonkeratinizing squamous cell carcinoma with basaloid morphology, completely excised with free margins. The left, and remaining right tonsillar tissue, displayed reactive lymphoid hyperplasia and filamentous mycobacteria consistent with actinomyces. No malignancy was found within the left tonsil. Samples obtained from the piriform recesses bilaterally consisted of benign squamous mucosa and were negative for malignancy. Samples taken from the left, right, and midline tongue base displayed benign squamous mucosa with underlying lymphoid hyperplasia but were negative for malignancy.

POSTSURGICAL FOLLOW-UP

One week following surgery the patient returned to clinic for his initial postoperative visit. He denied any new complaints and reported minimal postsurgical pain. The patient was afebrile, and on physical examination the surgical site was noted to be heal-

ing well. Radiation and medical oncology follow-up was initiated.

Two weeks after surgery, the patient presented to radiation oncology for initiation of adjuvant radiation therapy. The risks, benefits, and side effects of treatment were discussed with the patient in detail, who opted to proceed. The primary site, right tonsil, and right neck were targeted. The clinical target volume at the highest risk for recurrence was planned to be treated to a dose of 60 at 2 Gy per fraction with intensity-modulated radiation therapy (IMRT). Elective regions of the right neck at lower risk for recurrence were planned to be treated to a dose of 54 at 1.8 Gy per fraction during this time. The patient was to be scheduled for 6 weeks of daily radiation Monday to Friday. With IMRT, planning allowed avoidance of critical organs including the uninvolved oropharynx, oral cavity, cochlea, parotid glands, submandibular glands, larynx, trachea, and spinal cord (Figure 18–1). In addition to IMRT, he was scheduled to receive six doses (once per week during radiation therapy) of Cisplatin as a radiation sensitizer. The patient underwent 30 fractions of radiation therapy from January 14 to February 25, 2015. He was advised to use baking soda and salt water rinses during radiation and also prescribed Neutrasal, a calcium phosphate rinse, to improve mucosal healing after surgery and during radiation. The patient underwent prophylactic PEG feeding tube placement prior to the initiation of chemoradiation.

POSTSURGICAL AND POSTRADIATION SPEECH-LANGUAGE PATHOLOGY FOLLOW-UP

At nearly 1 month postop, immediately prior to the onset of chemoradiation, the patient returned to clinic for repeat FEES examination and oral intake assessment with speech-language pathology. He reported some postoperative dysphagia, which had resolved; the patient had resumed a regular consistency diet with thin liquids and denied any symptoms of dysphagia. Repeat administration of the EAT-10 was normal, and repeat FEES revealed no pharyngeal phase swallowing deficits and no clinical signs of airway penetration or aspiration.

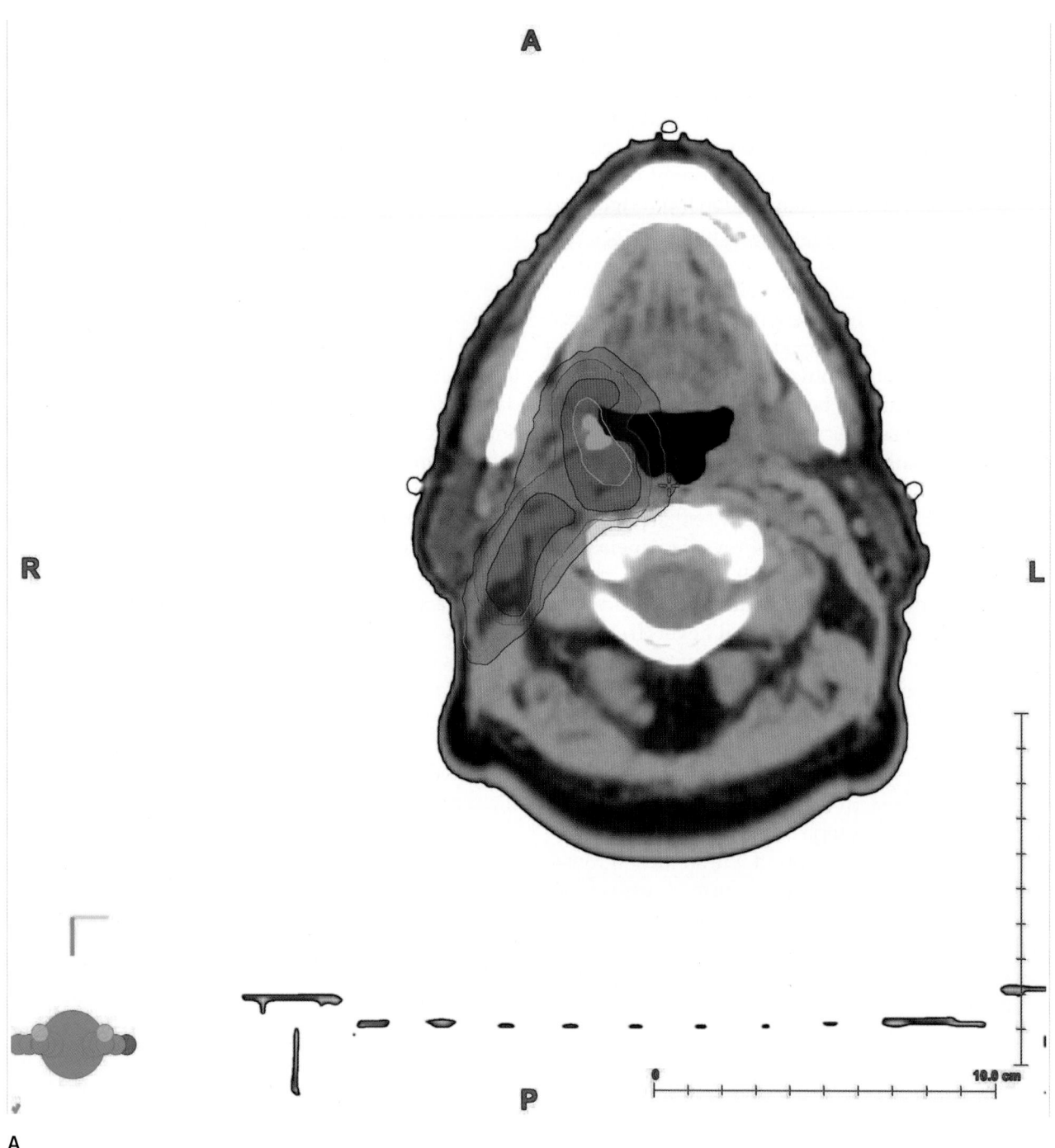

A

Figure 18–1. A. Radiation treatment volume. *continues*

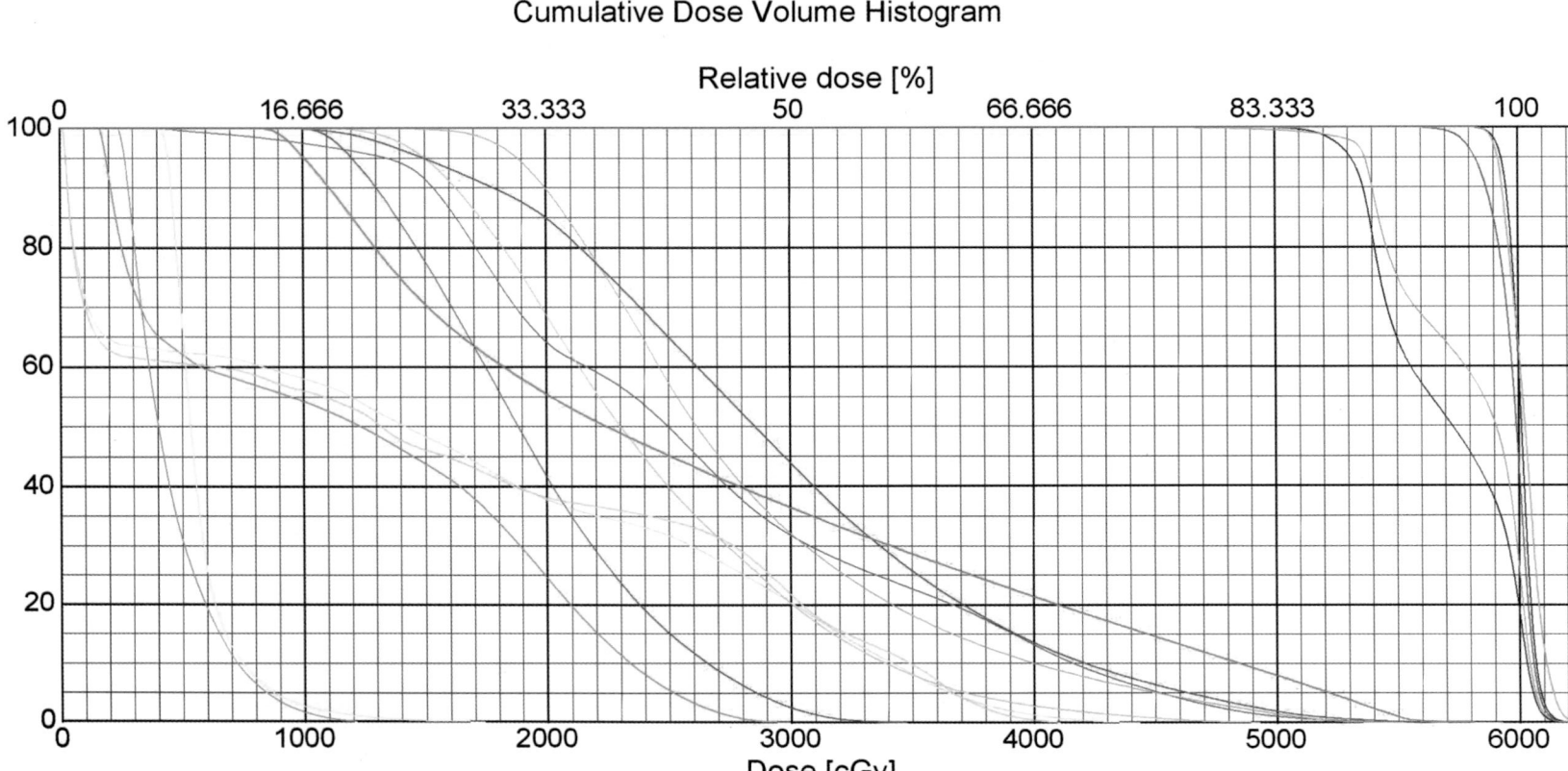

Figure 18–1. *continued* **B** and **C.** Dose volume histogram. *continues*

Structure	Structure Status	Coverage [%/%]	Volume	Min Dose	Max Dose	Mean Dose	Modal Dose	Median Dose	Std Dev
rcochlea	Approved	100.0 / 99.7	0.1 cm³	984.8 cGy	3474.1 cGy	1933.9 cGy	1736.3 cGy	1882.4 cGy	502.2 cGy
GTV	Approved	100.0 / 99.8	5.3 cm³	5802.4 cGy	6258.6 cGy	6024.6 cGy	6056.3 cGy	6026.8 cGy	67.2 cGy
lsmg	Approved	100.0 / 100.3	8.8 cm³	408.2 cGy	1740.5 cGy	574.5 cGy	487.9 cGy	533.7 cGy	146.5 cGy
trachea	Approved	100.0 / 99.9	19.8 cm³	1100.4 cGy	4931.2 cGy	2426.6 cGy	1963.0 cGy	2301.3 cGy	691.1 cGy
cord	Approved	100.0 / 100.1	19.9 cm³	6.3 cGy	4107.5 cGy	1517.0 cGy	24.7 cGy	1316.6 cGy	1381.5 cGy
r parotid	Approved	100.0 / 100.0	28.4 cm³	812.5 cGy	5931.4 cGy	2630.9 cGy	1136.1 cGy	2243.3 cGy	1388.0 cGy
brain stem	Approved	100.0 / 100.0	29.3 cm³	156.3 cGy	2996.8 cGy	1200.9 cGy	197.1 cGy	1230.5 cGy	860.2 cGy
l parotid	Approved	100.0 / 100.0	29.7 cm³	233.8 cGy	1213.4 cGy	456.3 cGy	303.1 cGy	401.0 cGy	182.1 cGy

Structure	Structure Status	Coverage [%/%]	Volume	Min Dose	Max Dose	Mean Dose	Modal Dose	Median Dose	Std Dev
larynx	Approved	100.0 / 100.0	41.6 cm³	1348.8 cGy	5534.1 cGy	2820.0 cGy	2441.5 cGy	2616.4 cGy	783.6 cGy
mandible	Approved	100.0 / 100.0	56.0 cm³	391.8 cGy	5562.0 cGy	2632.1 cGy	1803.1 cGy	2498.8 cGy	1023.5 cGy
cord+5mm	Approved	100.0 / 100.1	93.0 cm³	5.7 cGy	4435.2 cGy	1522.7 cGy	24.3 cGy	1414.6 cGy	1344.8 cGy
CTV60	Approved	100.0 / 100.0	108.0 cm³	5475.5 cGy	6258.6 cGy	6010.8 cGy	6012.2 cGy	6011.8 cGy	47.8 cGy
oroavoid	Approved	100.0 / 100.0	139.4 cm³	902.3 cGy	5705.7 cGy	2931.9 cGy	2661.4 cGy	2855.1 cGy	916.5 cGy
PTV60	Approved	100.0 / 100.0	188.0 cm³	5384.7 cGy	6258.6 cGy	5976.8 cGy	6012.2 cGy	5991.3 cGy	77.8 cGy
CTV54-1	Approved	100.0 / 100.0	303.7 cm³	4043.0 cGy	6258.6 cGy	5781.2 cGy	6012.2 cGy	5907.6 cGy	266.5 cGy
PTV54	Approved	100.0 / 100.0	435.5 cm³	4637.2 cGy	6258.6 cGy	5703.6 cGy	6012.2 cGy	5728.5 cGy	275.6 cGy

C

Figure 18–1. *continued*

As a precautionary measure, potential changes to swallow function that can occur during radiation therapy were reviewed with the patient. The speech pathologist also reviewed aspiration precautions and swallowing exercises including strategies to increase tongue base retraction, laryngeal elevation, and pharyngeal constriction. Additional strategies to minimize symptoms of xerostomia were reviewed, including the importance of oral hygiene and use of oral moisturizers prior to eating. The patient was provided with information on maximizing caloric intake including the preparation of high-calorie supplements. The patient was instructed to follow up with speech pathology 3 weeks into chemoradiation therapy to monitor swallowing function.

CONTINUED SPEECH-LANGUAGE PATHOLOGY AND OTHER FOLLOW-UP

Three weeks following the start of chemoradiation therapy the patient returned to speech pathology for follow-up. At that time he reported reduced appetite, nausea and constipation, and xerostomia which mildly adversely affected his swallow. A weight loss of 5 to 6 pounds was noted compared to his pretreatment weight baseline. The patient had opted to not use the feeding tube since beginning chemoradiation. He was prescribed antinausea medication by his medical oncologist and instructed to continue his regular-consistency diet with high-calorie supplements as tolerated. During this visit with speech pathology, the patient reported that he was experiencing decreased hearing acuity, bilaterally. The patient did report that he had some chronic baseline hearing loss; however, his hearing had noticeably worsened over the course of treatment. This was discussed with Otolaryngology, and the patient was referred to the Neurotology department. Out of concern for chemotherapy-related ototoxicity, chemotherapy was discontinued. At that time, the patient reported that his hearing loss continued to progress with new-onset intermittent bilateral tinnitus. Clinical examination revealed impacted cerumen bilaterally, which was removed. Repeat basic comprehensive audiometry threshold and discrimination testing was then completed and revealed a significant sensorineural hearing loss (Figure 18–2). The potential role of steroids to improve, but not guarantee, nerve recovery was discussed and a Prednisone 16-day burst with taper was prescribed. The option of adding a series of three bilateral intratympanic steroid (ITS) injections to possibly further increase the chance of recovery was also discussed, and the patient verbalized his desire to proceed. The patient was seen 1 week later by Neurotology for an initial ITS. At that time, he was taking the 16-day course of Prednisone. Appropriate expectations were discussed including the fact that the patient's prognosis for full recovery of hearing was poor. The injection was completed, and it was recommended that the patient continue taking the course of oral steroids. One week follow-up was recommended for a repeat audiogram and the second bilateral ITS injection. A hearing aid evaluation by audiology was also recommended. The patient followed up with Neurotology 9 days later. At that time, the patient continued to note bilateral hearing loss with sound distortion and tinnitus. Repeat hearing testing was completed by audiology, revealing persistent bilateral sensorineural hearing loss. A second bilateral ITS injection was completed 1 week later; at that time, follow-up was recommended in 1 week for repeat audiogram and the third ITS injection. A third ITS injection was completed 11 days later. At that time, the patient reported continued bilateral hearing loss with sound distortion and tinnitus; a repeat audiogram showed stable sensorineural hearing loss. Follow-up with audiology for hearing aids was recommended and Otolaryngology follow-up, including completion of a repeat audiogram, was recommended in 3 months.

OUTCOMES AND DISCUSSION

This case demonstrates the successful treatment of a patient who presented with squamous cell metastasis to the right neck with no obvious primary site. P16 positivity was very important in his case both as an important prognostic marker and to help guide therapy. The surgical approach chosen for this patient was both diagnostic and therapeutic. We were able to surgically excise bulky lymphadenopathy

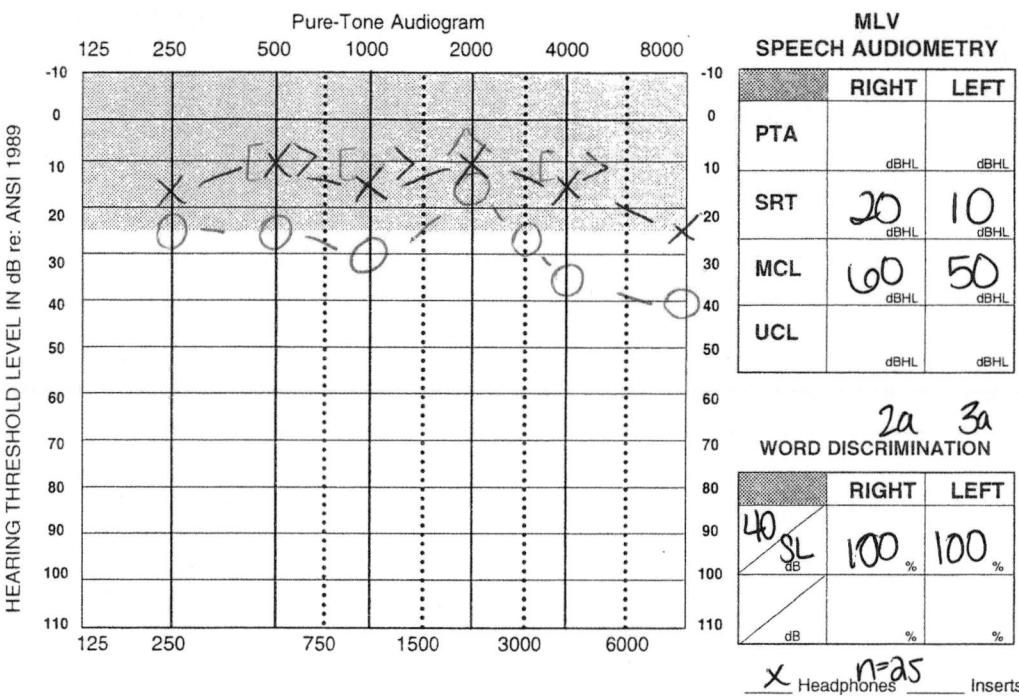

Figure 18–2. Audiogram depicting significant sensorineural hearing loss.

from the right neck and also localize the primary site to the right tonsil. After surgery, accurate staging information was obtained. This allowed for a further refinement with the delivery of concurrent chemoradiation in the adjuvant setting. Given the improvements in technology and technique with IMRT, patients are better able to tolerate chemoradiation. In this particular case, mucositis was localized and confined to the right tonsil and oropharynx. This allowed the patient to complete treatment and recovery without need of his intact feeding tube and without any significant weight loss. Remarkably, during treatment the patient lost less than 5% of his body weight and did not require narcotics, topical anesthetics, or medications for mucus control. At the conclusion of chemoradiation therapy, he still had not used the feeding tube and it was subsequently removed.

Regular and ongoing involvement of speech-language pathology, pre- to postoperatively, was a critical factor relating to the ability of this patient to maintain excellent swallow function both during and after treatment. Finally, regular use of baking soda salt water rinses and Neutrasal mouth rinses

appeared to be effective as supportive care measures during chemoradiation and highlight the importance of nonmedication supportive care measures in the treatment of patients with radiotherapy or chemoradiation. The patients is now 5 months post chemoradiation treatment; PET scan results (skull to thigh) were negative for recurrence.

He is consuming a regular-consistency diet and reports minimal symptoms of xerostomia. He has returned to the work schedule he was completing following his head and neck cancer diagnosis. Follow-up with Otolaryngology is planned in 6 months.

REFLECTION AND ANALYSIS FOR FURTHER STUDY

1. One of the aspects that is rarely discussed in the literature is the level of pain that the patient may be experiencing is a function of the surgical procedure and or radiation treatment. Because tolerance of pain and coping with pain is an

individual response, what might you use as a clinician to assess and recognize the level of pain in your patients

2. Patients who are diagnosed with HPV-related malignancies are shocked to learn that this is a causative factor. Provide evidence as to what our discipline has recently done to support education regarding this quiet contribution to head and neck cancer.

3. Imagine that you are referred a patient with HPV-related HNC who is 59 years old, single, and interested in dating. He is concerned about his HPV status given his medical history. As a clinician, how would you approach the dialogue with this patient?

REFERENCE

Belafsky, P. C., Mouadeb, D. A., Rees, C. J., Pryor, J. C., Postma, G. N., Allen, J., & Leonard, R. J. (2008). Validity and reliability of the Eating Assessment Tool (EAT-10). *Annals of Otology, Rhinology, and Laryngology, 117*(12), 919–924.

PART VII

Consideration of Communication Options and Patient-Centered Treatment

19

Consideration of Communication Options in Head and Neck Cancer: Augmentative and Alternative

Laura J. Ball, Jennifer Kent-Walsh, and Nancy A. Harrington

INTRODUCTION

Individuals who are treated for head and neck cancer in its various forms may discover significant unmet communication needs as a result of treatment, including surgical resection, radiation, and chemotherapy. In one study examining functional speech at 3 months post cancer treatment for 158 patients, only 63% of postsurgical patients and 55% of postsurgical plus radiation patients reported broadly functional speech (Perry & Shaw, 2000). Another 22% of postsurgical patients and 26% of postsurgical plus radiation patients reported at least moderate speech disabilities, defined as speech that was perceived by the patients themselves to be intelligible only when the context of the message was known to the communication partners (Perry & Shaw, 2000). These patients reported frequent need to repeat spoken messages and write to supplement their speech to convey intended meaning (Perry & Shaw, 2000). Likewise, 12% of postsurgical and 19% postsurgical plus radiation patients reported having poor speech, which was defined as having only occasional, or no, functional communication, and/or having speech that is at least 50% unintelligible (Perry & Shaw,

2000). These results are distressing given that other research indicates even 80% speech intelligibility scores correspond with significant difficulties in functional communication and highly problematic unmet communication needs in everyday contexts (Ball, Beukelman, & Pattee, 2004).

Unmet Communication Needs in Head and Neck Cancer Patients

The communication impairments observed among head and neck cancer patients can be mild to profound, and are frequently unmet. Such impairments have the potential to impact countless aspects of daily activity, from participation in medical decision making to socialization with friends and family (Hemsley & Balandin, 2014; Light & Mcnaughton, 2015). It is important to identify optimal levels of communicative support throughout the phases of cancer treatment and to consider variations in medical status and personal needs over time. In particular, individual interventions must be considered in the context of the cancer site (e.g., tongue, maxilla, larynx), phase of recovery (e.g., presurgical, acute postsurgical, speech restorative, medical instability), preexisting communication skills and demands, and ongoing communication needs (Sullivan, Gaebler, & Ball, 2007a).

For those with head and neck cancer, speech intelligibility decreases with increases in tumor size, increases in resected tissue volume, need for reconstructive surgery, and tumor site—with poorer intelligibility in cases involving the floor of the mouth or lower alveolar crest (Blythe et al., 2014; Borggreven et al., 2007). Such features have important implications for these individuals when considering functional communication interventions as a component of rehabilitation. Situational communication effectiveness of individuals using esophageal speech, electrolarynx, or both has been reported to range from 80% to 100% intelligibility (Sullivan, Beukelman, & Mathy-Laikko, 1993). Speakers have reported the necessity to increase the number of communication methods they implement based on communication complexity within their environment; for example, when needing to talk over background noise or intercoms, speakers note that they must add writing, gestures, and/or interpreters to supplement their spoken communication (Sullivan et al., 1993). Although writing supplementation of spoken communication may be useful in some situations, it can be restricted by limited literacy skills for some patients. One recent report indicated that 17.1% of individuals with head and neck cancer read at or below the eighth-grade level (Jesse et al., 2014). Because reduced speech intelligibility is associated with reduced quality of life, timely identification of patients experiencing reduced intelligibility is necessary to identify appropriate communication options to facilitate overall recovery (Borggreven et al., 2007).

On a related note, recent years have seen an increase in communication technologies for patients. Esophageal speech and electrolarynx use are no longer the only options available to head and neck cancer patients and, in many cases, have fallen out of favor with patients. The increase in availability and acceptability of mobile technologies and associated communication applications has changed the landscape of functional communication intervention (e.g., McNaughton & Light, 2013).

The significance of including functional communication as an aspect of treatment and recovery with head and neck cancer patients is an ongoing subject of interest within research literature. For example, one qualitative study examining interview responses to open-ended questions from caregivers of individuals with head and neck cancer identified communication impairment as a central topic of concern. Caregivers reported that strategies to identify problems and meet patient needs (e.g., "giving voice, being there, giving control, saving face, normalizing, relieving pain, and giving hope") were primarily self-taught and required intensive effort and creativity on their part. The study concluded that postsurgical patients and their caregivers are in critical need of assistance to meet communication needs (McGrory, 2011). Similarly, nurses have attributed nurse-patient communication breakdowns to lack of a readily manageable and interpretable communication systems (Happ, Roesch, & Kagan, 2004). Caregivers of adult patients with complex communication needs desire viable modes of communication to fulfill the following needs: (a) regulate the behavior of others for basic wants and needs (e.g., getting needs met, giving instructions/directions, providing clarifications); (b) stay connected with friends and family members (e.g., social closeness); and (c) discuss important issues (e.g., information transfer; Fried-Oken et al., 2006). These findings are alarming given that the overwhelming majority of individuals with severe speech impairments have limited or no access to augmentative or alternative communication modalities while in the hospital and therefore struggle to provide medical information and to have medical needs met. Additionally, these patients are at increased risk for poor health outcomes (Blackstone, Beukelman, & Yorkston, 2015; Hemsley & Balandin, 2014).

Individual survivors of head and neck cancer may encounter the need to communicate:

- changing social roles associated with the cancer diagnosis;
- specific and urgent messages related to dysphagia;
- information to medical personnel (e.g., symptoms, pain management information, anxiety);
- detailed messages with new communication partners who may not readily understand them;

- messages associated with confronting addictions (e.g., tobacco, alcohol);
- messages critical to counseling and support group interactions; and
- personal messages with family, friends, and social network (Sullivan et al., 2007a).

In order to ensure that patients with head and neck cancer are able to successfully meet these communication needs, augmentative and alternative communication (AAC) assessment and intervention procedures should be implemented routinely in conjunction with traditional speech restoration options to augment intelligibility, decrease communication breakdowns, facilitate repair when communication breakdowns occur, and provide alternate methods of communication when traditional methods result in ongoing unmet communication needs. AAC includes all forms of communication (other than oral speech) that are used to express thoughts, needs, wants, and ideas (ASHA, 2002). To inform the provider of potential options for increasing the standard of care for head and neck cancer patients experiencing significant communication challenges, the remainder of this chapter covers (a) key AAC system considerations for developing or identifying AAC options for individual patients, (b) key AAC options for patients with head and neck cancer, and (c) key AAC service-delivery intervals for patients with head and neck cancer to support presurgical care, acute care (immediately postsurgical care), initial outpatient care, and ongoing outpatient care AAC (e.g., in cases of treatment change or new disease states; Sullivan et al., 2007a).

KEY CONSIDERATIONS FOR DEVELOPING OR IDENTIFYING AAC OPTIONS FOR INDIVIDUAL PATIENTS

It is proposed that AAC options for individuals with head and neck cancer should meet the following basic guidelines drawn from the common needs and circumstances of this population combined with standard considerations in AAC service-delivery (Beukelman & Mirenda, 2013):

1. *Portability.* Given that most individuals with head and neck cancer remain independent and often drive themselves to medical appointments, lightweight portability is an essential feature of the selected AAC system. It should be noted that portability is less of a concern when the person uses a wheelchair for ambulation, in which case the system may be mounted to the chair for transport.

2. *Direct Access.* The majority of patients will have full functioning of their hands and the natural tendency to access a communication system using their hands to type directly on an onscreen keyboard or by selecting onscreen images from a visual array to communicate. It is noteworthy that the system must be large enough to provide a means of selecting individual items with few miss-hits (i.e., the ability to isolate individual letters for typing messages).

3. *High-Quality Display.* The system must have good visibility to accommodate for visual impairment; this might include adaptable font sizes and screen angles to remain visible in multiple lighting contexts.

4. *High-Quality Voice Output.* For those who will be communicating in adverse situations (e.g., noisy environments, traveling in vehicles), high-quality voice output with adjustable volume is essential because it can be highly problematic to be writing messages and handing them to communication partners in such contexts.

5. *Traditional Orthography.* For individuals with literacy skills sufficient to represent their utterances, the standard orthography of their native language(s) will prove to be the most effective symbol set for implementation. Some consideration may be made to identify the optimal keyboard layout (e.g., alphabetic order versus QWERTY layout—the standard English-language typewriter keyboard layout with the characters q, w, e, r, t, and y positioned in the top left row of alphabetic characters on the keyboard) for improved rate and message formulation efficiency.

6. *Message Formulation.* Because of the wide variety of messages that must be conveyed, the ability to formulate novel messages is a key feature of a communication system. Although message

banking may be helpful for recording some high-frequency messages, the array of messages necessary will extend beyond what can be pre-recorded. Text-to-speech voice output provides the ability to formulate unique messages based on the communicative interaction.

7. *Rate Acceleration.* The speaking rate of a typical message produced by an AAC system is considerably slower than a message produced via natural speech; therefore, any features that will increase the rate of communication are generally highly valued by patients. Some options for rate acceleration include word and phrase prediction.

8. *Ease of Use.* The majority of individuals with head and neck cancer will seek an established long-standing system for effective communication. Often, people prefer a system that is akin to a "point-and-shoot" camera for their communication. They do not typically wish to spend extended periods of time learning to use a new communication system, programming extensive messages, or learning new representational systems (e.g., icons, symbols); simplicity is frequently key with this patient population.

KEY AAC OPTIONS FOR HEAD AND NECK CANCER PATIENTS

As previously referenced, technology advancements continue to yield an increasing array of AAC options for individuals with complex communication needs. There are several common categories of AAC options that will be applicable to individuals with head and neck cancer, including mobile technologies, traditional speech-generating devices, and communication software.

Mobile Technologies

Recently developed communication applications for use with standard smartphone and computer tablet technologies have expanded available options for all individuals with significant communication impairments, including head and neck cancer patients. His-

torically, a great deal of stigma has been associated with speech disabilities, and there have been common misconceptions that intelligence is somehow correlated with speech clarity (DO-IT, 2012). As portable devices have become an intrinsic part of daily life for people from many cultures, languages, and traditions, they provide a readily accessible means of supporting communication without adding to visible disability (McNaughton & Light, 2013). Additionally, they reduce the need to purchase separate equipment focused solely on communication and provide an adaptable means of achieving communication goals.

Desired features of mobile technology communication systems include those mentioned previously (e.g., portability, high-quality display). Additionally, options to obtain extended battery life (e.g., communication during an 8-hr work shift), durability and protection (e.g., a case that increases durability of the system without compromising access) with screen protection, and voice output amplification are key considerations. If the person places high premium on small devices but may not be able to isolate individual items on the display because of hand/finger size or mobility, identifying a stylus that will provide access to the keyboard and a means of ensuring its location without loss (i.e., storage slot) also will become key.

There are many communication applications available for use on iOS and Android platforms, although the number of options is currently much greater on iOS platforms. Table 19–1 includes examples of currently available AAC applications and a summary of some of the relevant features for patients with head and neck cancer in the following categories: operating system platform options, voice output options, select rate enhancement options, and two notable additional options including multilingual functionality and accessibility features. Table 19–1 is not intended to provide an exhaustive list of all available applications; rather, it provides an overview the nature of available applications in the context of some of the most salient features that may have relevance for individual patients with head and neck cancer. The reader is encouraged to periodically consult the Apple App Store or Google Play for available applications.

Table 19–1. Sample Text-to-Speech Augmentative and Alternative Communication Applications

	Platform Options		Voice Output Options		Rate Enhancement Options				Additional Options	
Application	iOS	Android	Synthesized Speech Voices	Blended Personal Voices[a]	Word Prediction Intelligent[b]	Stored Phrases	Customizable Keyboard	Write-to-Text[c]	Multiple Languages	Accessibility Features
Abilipad	X		X		X[b]	X	X			
Assistive Express	X		X		X[b]	X		X		
EZ Speech Pro	X	X	X		X[b]	X				
Flip Writer AAC	X		X		X					
iMean	X		X		X		X			
Predictable	X	X	X	X	X[b]	X	X	X	X (iOS)	X
Proloquo4Text	X		X	X	X[b]	X	X		X	X
Rocket Keys	X		X		X[b]		X			
Speak It!	X		X			X			X	X
Touch Voice	X	X	X		X	X				
Type2Speak	X		X			X				
Verbally	X		X		X[b]	X	X			
VidaTalk	X		X			X			X	X

Note. [a]Intelligent word prediction is a feature that goes beyond standard word predication functionality by learning a person's patterns of use and, therefore, increasing the efficiency of message prediction. [b]Blended personal voices involve integration with voice and/or message banking software. [c]This incorporates handwriting recognition technology combined with text-to-speech voice output.

Traditional Speech-Generating Devices

Although mobile technologies and communication applications enhance AAC service-delivery as patient awareness and openness to technology increase (McNaughton & Light, 2013), they are not the only available AAC options. More traditional, dedicated, speech-generating devices (SGDs) have existed for decades. Because these technologies were specifically designed for communication purposes, traditional AAC systems may afford the most effective means of meeting daily communication needs through highly customizable and variable features (Beukelman & Mirenda, 2013; McNaughton & Light, 2013). For example, at present, most SGDs provide superior voice output quality and access options compared to AAC applications on mainstream smartphones and tablets. Other features of interest for patients with AAC needs relate to available language options and options for connectivity to other computer technologies. As evidenced in Table 19–1, AAC mobile technology options often do not provide options for such extended functionality. One example of an SGD with multilingual capabilities is the NOVA Chat 5, which supports communication on a small dedicated system (i.e., 5″ screen) with Canadian French, Dutch, English, Spanish, and German languages (Saltillo, 2015). The NOVA Chat 5 also offers a variety of software options that may be customized for individual purposes (e.g., word-based vocabulary, core words, phrase-based communication). Another popular SGD, The Lightwriter SL40 Connect, essentially works like a talking typewriter with a variety of rate-enhancing features, includes a SIM card to support texting, and can easily transfer notes to/from a computer (Tobii Dynavox, 2015). As with any type of technology, SGD technologies are constantly evolving, so emerging SGD technologies are expected to continue to provide even better options to assist individuals in meeting daily communication needs with increased efficiency and effectiveness.

Communication Software. Communication software programs designed for use on laptop or desktop computers also provide options for head and neck cancer patients to communicate directly or to design and print low-tech communication displays useful for communicating basic messages in a wide range of settings. Since such communication software options represent language using symbols other than traditional text (e.g., via pictures and line drawings), these options may be particularly helpful to individuals with literacy and/or cognitive limitations. One example is *DynaVox Compass*, a communication software program that can be installed on a SGD or tablet system (e.g., Dynavox T10, Apple iPad). It provides preprogrammed messages and formats, such as QuickPhrases. QuickPhrases are messages designed to provide rapid social commenting that may reduce or eliminate the need to create the same message repeatedly (e.g., "How are you?"; "What's going on?"; "Have a great day!") (Tobii Dynavox, 2015). *Pogo Boards* is another communication software program with multiple functionalities that is both Mac and PC compatible (Talk to Me Technologies, 2015). Pogo Boards also has preprogrammed message formats and has a sharing feature that enables sharing of created layouts. It can be implemented on a computer or tablet-based system and can be used to print communication boards.

OVERVIEW OF AAC ASSESSMENT AND INTERVENTION PROCEDURES FOR HEAD AND NECK CANCER PATIENTS

Given the range of AAC options that exist, it is necessary to consider how appropriate supports will be identified and implemented with individual patients. The proposed model for AAC assessment for patients with head and neck cancer differs from the typical lengthy AAC evaluation process that yields a communication system following an extended series of assessment sessions and trials. Instead, the focus is on supporting communication in a rapid, just-in-time manner (i.e., not waiting for emergency-intense communication needs to arise, but methodically targeting communicative supports as needed). With this population, communication systems frequently undergo multiple transformations to meet changing communication needs. Many approaches are simple, and clinicians may not see a need for direct instruction, although many patients require explicit instruction, even with simple or "low-tech" strategies, to adapt to and implement

AAC (Sullivan, Gaebler, & Ball, 2007b). Another contributing factor is that most medical professionals (e.g., nurses, physicians) do not receive instruction to know how to interact with their patients who are not able to communication effectively via natural speech (Hemsley & Balandin, 2014). Therefore, some form of instruction and therapeutic support for both patients *and* providers is likely to improve patient-provider communication, which can in turn influence treatment satisfaction and outcomes (Downey & Happ, 2013; Hemsley & Balandin, 2014).

PRESURGICAL ASSESSMENT

Individuals with head and neck cancer may lose their voice as a result of cancer treatment; therefore, assessment should begin prior to, or in concert with, medical treatments (e.g., chemotherapy or radiation). As with traditional means of speech restoration, individuals facing surgical treatment for head and neck cancer will benefit from presurgical AAC assessments. The goal of presurgical AAC assessments is to identify communication needs, determine communication options for implementation immediately after surgery, and evaluate potential usefulness of various AAC options. At this stage, the clinician completes a communication needs assessment and determines individual patterns of communication (e.g., does the person communicate intensively in her/his profession . . . teacher, lawyer, coach?), establishes the level of communication interest (e.g., does the patient wish to communicate via phone with family/friends at a distance?), and identifies potential supports and needs following surgery (e.g., which family members, friends, or caregivers can provide support?). Although it is difficult to anticipate the extent of postsurgical communication challenges, consideration should be made regarding the size of tumor, location, and type of surgery planned. Having this knowledge will inform the potential speech outcome (i.e., individuals who have large tumors, a large volume of tissue resected, and floor of mouth or lower alveolar crest tumors typically have poorer speech outcomes). This is particularly relevant to considering a speech-generating device option and the potential

need to identify important messages for digital storage (i.e., voice banking) and future implementation in advance of surgery.

A communication needs assessment involves collection of personal information and prospective communication topics that form the individual's typical communicative interactions on a day-to-day basis. This information is used to determine context-specific impairment (e.g., noise, poor lighting), identify potential for situational communication breakdowns (e.g., speaking with preliterate children or a frequent need to communicate in noisy environments), and suggest possible AAC solutions. Examples of information obtained include birthdate/age; family names and relationships; significant other names, locations, and relationships; recent family changes or events; language spoken by family members; home and community features (e.g., leisure interests, hobbies, home responsibilities, pets); community activities (e.g., faith-based activities, clubs, volunteer), mobility (e.g., drive, walk, wheelchair, bicycle); neighborhood people (e.g., neighbors, friends, grocer, dog walker); noisy environments frequented (e.g., restaurants, casino, sports, concerts); employment (e.g., location, FT/PT, duties); and telephone use (e.g., amount, familiarity of person called/calling). It is also helpful to obtain information on cooccurring conditions that may impact communication effectiveness and treatment options, such as hearing, vision, or cognitive impairment, so that they may be optimized or accommodated during treatment. The next component of evaluation includes examining the person's general effectiveness, efficiency, and overall satisfaction with a variety of communication strategies that include natural gestures, message supplementation, written messages, communication boards, communication applications for use with mobile technologies, and speech-generating devices.

The assessment will involve identifying a few natural gestures the person easily uses and assigning them meaning, perhaps creating a "gesture dictionary" as a resource for caregivers (i.e., when I do X gesture, it means Y or Z). For example, the person can associate certain gestures with messages (e.g., click tongue, snap fingers, or clap hands to get another person's attention). Combining gestures with mouthed words may provide sufficient context to produce intelligible utterances at least in the immediate short term after surgery (e.g., mouthing "talk with wife" with a hand gesture for talking on the telephone).

"Mouthing" words and entire messages without voicing immediately after surgery may be effective, particularly for familiar listeners and basic, frequently used messages. If the individual is literate, *alphabet* supplementation is a simple strategy using a small paper with the alphabet typed on it (lamination increases durability and stability). The person points to the first letter of each word as he or she simultaneously "mouths" it. This system has been shown to help communication partners by slowing speaking rate, providing linguistic context for the word, and identifying word boundaries (Hanson, Beukelman, Fager, & Ullman, 2004). A *topic* supplementation board may provide additional contextual information by first establishing the topic of conversation. After establishing the topic, the person uses alphabet supplementation for the remainder of the message. By using personally relevant photographs that are contextually rich, *picture* supplementation may augment natural speech productions (Hanson et al., 2004). Supplementation has been found to be more acceptable to individuals when speech output is less intelligible, becoming less acceptable as intelligibility improves (Hanson et al., 2004). For message supplementation options, it is important to evaluate the layout for efficiency of locating alphabet, topics, and photos; determine optimal font or image size for easy and rapid visualization, and consider finger size (i.e., a male with large fingers may have difficulty isolating small, narrowly spaced letters/images). Typically, select a layout that is large enough to identify letters rapidly and isolate each with the fingertip but keep the size small enough for portability in a pocket or purse.

A small, portable white board and dry erase markers also may prove to be useful to write temporary, short messages (i.e., written and then erased). A notebook and pen may be used to write more detailed messages and can also serve as a memory aid and may be useful in writing questions that the person wants to remember to ask various medical personnel or caregivers. In addition, messages written on paper can be retrieved for communication multiple times if necessary (e.g., flip through pages to locate a written message from previous days). This system may not be efficient if the person writes multiple messages and then must comb through multiple notes for several minutes to locate an earlier item, but may serve as an effective repository for a few messages that are communicated multiple times. For written language options, it is important to evaluate handwriting legibility and literacy skills prior to implementation; if using for retrieval, it also will be necessary to examine the person's ability to locate a message on multiple pages.

Picture communication boards with a series of basic messages may be used and displayed in text (if the patient is literate) or with symbols or photographs (if the patient has limited literacy skills and/or intellectual disabilities). In this case, it will be necessary to evaluate and prioritize anticipated message needs with the person, determine the optimal size and location for various messages, and to group messages systematically so it is most intuitive for that individual (e.g., by topic, urgency). Additionally, it may be necessary for the person to learn a new symbol "language" in order to be efficient with communication; therefore, the assessment should incorporate time to learn a new message representation in order to afford efficient selection of symbols/photographs.

Picture communication boards may be paired with digital voice output speech-generating devices (SGDs) to provide voicing along with each message. Speech-generating devices may produce either digitized (i.e., recorded) or synthesized (i.e., computerized) voice output and may display text or picture symbols. Digitized SGDs with preformulated/recorded messages have proved to be successfully implemented in acute care following surgery for head and neck cancer (Happ, Kagan, & Roesch, 2001). Voice assessment for AAC purposes prior to surgery involves (a) determining intelligibility of spoken utterances and (b) asking the person to indicate whether he or she finds that recordings of his or her voice are representative of their personality. Assumptions should not be made by clinicians about the viability of voice recordings, because in some cases, cancer has resulted in changes to vocal productions that render the voice as unnatural or foreign to the owner and therefore the individual prefers not to use recordings, even for "trademark" (Costello, 2012) utterances.

PRESURGICAL TREATMENT

It is vital to emphasize to patients that they will be able to communicate following surgery while providing educational materials/information regarding some of the different ways they will communicate in both the short and long term. The earliest possible intervention can enable patients to capture their own voices using either voice banking or message banking. Voice banking and message banking provide two viable avenues for presurgical treatment which may be of interest to patients. *Voice banking* involves recording speech that is then used to create a personalized synthetic (i.e., computerized) voice. One example, ModelTalker (Bunnell et al., 2015), requires recording of approximately 1,600 sentences (i.e., 4–6 hr over 3–4 days) and as such, must be initiated well prior to surgery. The resulting synthetic voice may not meet individual expectations for naturalness, and any changes to voice that have occurred as a result of the cancer will also be captured; therefore, it is suggested that the person listen to several examples to get a realistic idea of the output prior to making a decision as to the whether or not the long-term use benefit will outweigh the time and effort necessary to pursue this type of treatment. Patients must consider if lower-quality personalized voices are more acceptable to them than higher-quality non-personalized synthesized voices available within standard AAC application for mobile technologies or SGDs (Bode, 2015).

Message banking involves digitally recording phrases, messages, and vocabulary for the purpose of incorporating them into an SGD. These digital recordings will retain the naturalness and vocal qualities of the original voice (also reflecting changes due to cancer). An example of a banked message is the digital recording used for voicemail or an answering machine. The banked recordings are labeled and categorized for storage and can easily be imported into an SGD as needed at a later time (Bode, 2015). This strategy is often particularly effective for "trademark"(Costello, 2012) messages (e.g., "Bless your heart!"; "Not!") that patients would prefer to have in their own voices due to personal or sentimental reasons (e.g., "love you more") and for frequently relayed or repeated messages (e.g.,

"Good night my love"). One questionnaire created to elicit potential messages for message banking asks the patient to report how they ask or answer questions (e.g., when you first wake from surgery, what do you think will be important to say?) (Costello, 2012). These messages do not enable novel message generation but also can be "spoken" using an SGD.

ACUTE-CARE AAC

Because poor patient-provider communication is associated with negative health outcomes, the 2010 Joint Commission Standards established guidelines to ensure effective care of individuals with communication vulnerability (e.g., inability to produce speech that is intelligible, no voice, altered mental status, inability to speak/understand the language of the medical team, literacy limitations) (Bartlett, Blais, & Tamblyn, 2008; Hurtig, Czerniejewski, Bohnenkamp, & Na, 2013; Joint Commission, 2009, 2010). The goal of acute-care AAC assessment is to evaluate effectiveness of selected short-term AAC techniques identified for acute-care communication and to continue to evaluate additional AAC options for longer-term implementation. As is apparent immediately following surgery, patients will be considered communication vulnerable and likely require alternate modes to express basic care messages (e.g., discomfort, emotions, positioning), to ask questions about their surgery and health status, to communicate reassuring messages to family and friends, and to request items or actions. Based on the assessment and planned intervention completed during presurgical assessment, it is important to evaluate the effectiveness of the strategies implemented during medical staff interactions and with family and friends.

OUTPATIENT AAC INTERVENTION

The goal of outpatient AAC assessment is to identify daily communication needs that are not being met by the speech restorative procedures. As the speech restorative procedures are implemented, ongoing monitoring of communication breakdowns is conducted. Some considerations for assessment include examining intelligibility and comprehensibility. In addition, communication efficiency (intelligible words per minute) is monitored. A communication effectiveness scale was adapted for use by individuals with head and neck cancer that may be useful in identifying ongoing areas of communication impairment in functional situations (e.g., talking at home, on the telephone, in the car, when excited, in noise) (Sullivan et al., 1993).

ONGOING AAC INTERVENTION

The goal of ongoing AAC intervention is to evaluate newly identified communication needs, specify additional sources of communication breakdown, and identify AAC solutions. When a communication system that meets all of the individual's daily communication needs is established, the person may require no additional assessment. However, cancer recurrence or development of a new medical condition may require additional medical treatments that subsequently impact the effectiveness of the communication system. Additionally, if SGD options are in use, there is also the possibility of technology failure or advancement that must be addressed. In such instances, it may be useful to readminister the communication effectiveness scale to identify contextual communication breakdowns (Sullivan et al., 1993). Situations where communication breakdowns occur are identified at this phase, and methods for repair of these interactions are attempted, trialed, and practiced.

CONCLUSIONS

Although many patients with head and neck cancer become effective communicators with traditional speech restoration interventions, the large number of patients for whom postsurgical treatment remains ineffective for meeting all of their daily needs requires serious consideration. It is of vital importance that these individuals be provided with effective alternative modes to communicate with all of their communication partners in all of their required and desired environments. Contemporary AAC technologies and service-delivery options provide a myriad of options for supporting the functional communication of all patients with head and neck cancer.

REFLECTION AND ANALYSIS FOR FURTHER STUDY

1. How might a head and neck cancer patient's needs change relative to treatment stage: presurgical, acute recovery, subacute recovery, outpatient and ongoing (lifelong) recovery?
2. Give three examples of simple, "low-tech" AAC approaches and three examples of more sophisticated technologies, and provide a description of a hypothetical patient for which each example might be most appropriate.
3. Why might patients opt for the work of programming a system to use his or her own voice rather than going with a more readily deployable approach?
4. What would be the most important skills to entrain with the caregiver of an individual using AAC technology?

REFERENCES

American Speech-Language-Hearing Association. (2002). *Augmentative and alternative communication: Knowledge and skills for service delivery* [Knowledge and skills]. Retrieved from http://www.asha.org/policy

Ball, L. J., Beukelman, D. R., & Pattee, G. L. (2004). Communication effectiveness of individuals with amyotrophic lateral sclerosis. *Journal of Communication Disorders, 37*(3), 197–215. http://doi.org/10.1016/j.jcomdis.2003.09.002

Bartlett, G. R., Blais, R., & Tamblyn, R. (2008). Impact of patient communication problems on the risk of preventable adverse events in the acute care setting. *Canadian Medical Association Journal, 178*, 1555–1562.

Beukelman, D., & Mirenda, P. (2013). *Augmentative and alternative communication: Supporting children and adults with complex communication needs* (4th ed.). Baltimore, MD: Paul H. Brookes.

Blackstone, S. W., Beukelman, D. R., & Yorkston, K. M. (2015). *Patient-provider communication roles for speech-language pathologists and other health care professionals*. San Diego, CA: Plural.

Blythe, K. M., McCabe, P., Heard, R., Clark, J., Madill, C., & Ballard, K. J. (2014). Cancers of the tongue and floor of mouth: Five-year file audit within the acute phase. *American Journal of Speech-Language Pathology, 23*(November), 668–678. http://doi.org/10.1044/2014

Bode, T. (2015, January 14). *Road testing ModelTalker* [Web log comment]. Retrieved from http://www.zyteq.com.au/blog/

Borggreven, P. a, Verdonck-de Leeuw, I. M., Muller, M. J., Heiligers, M. L. C. H., de Bree, R., Aaronson, N. K., & Leemans, C. R. (2007). Quality of life and functional status in patients with cancer of the oral cavity and oropharynx: Pretreatment values of a prospective study. *European Archives of Oto-Rhino-Laryngology, 264*(6), 651–657. http://doi.org/10.1007/s00405-007-0249-5

Bunnell, H. T., Chandlee, J., Lilley, J., Gray, J., Moyers, B., & Warren, B. (2015). *ModelTalker*. Wilmington, DE.

Costello, J. M. (2012, August). *Preserving legacy: A guide to message banking*. Presentation handout from ISAAC Biennial Conference, Pittsburgh, PA.

DO-IT. (2012). *Effective communication: Faculty and students with disabilities*. Seattle, WA: University of Washington.

Downey, D., & Happ, M. B. (2013). The need for nurse training to promote improved patient-provider communication for patients with complex communication needs. *Perspectives on Augmentative and Alternative Communication, 22*(2), 112. http://doi.org/10.1044/aac22.2.112

Fried-Oken, M., Fox, L., Rau, M. T., Tullman, J., Baker, G., Hindal, M., . . . Lou, J.-S. (2006). Purposes of AAC device use for persons with ALS as reported by caregivers. *Augmentative and Alternative Communication, 22*(3), 209–221. http://doi.org/10.1080/07434610600650276

Hanson, E. K., Beukelman, D. R., Fager, S., & Ullman, C. (2004). Listener attitudes toward speech supplementation strategies used by speakers with dysarthria. *Journal of Medical Speech-Language Pathology, 12*, 161–166.

Happ, M. B., Kagan, S. H., & Roesch, T. (2001). Using a complementary design to test augmentative communication device for head and neck cancer patients. In *6th National Conference on Cancer Nursing Research*. Pointe Verde Beach, FL.

Happ, M. B., Roesch, T., & Kagan, S. H. (2004). Communication needs, methods, and perceived voice quality following head and neck surgery. *Cancer Nursing, 27*(1), 1–9. http://doi.org/10.1097/00002820-200401000-00001

Hemsley, B., & Balandin, S. (2014). A metasynthesis of patient-provider communication in hospital for patients with severe communication disabilities: Informing new translational research. *Augmentative and Alternative Communication, 30*(4), 329–343. http://doi.org/10.3109/07434618.2014.955614

Hurtig, R., Czerniejewski, E., Bohnenkamp, L., & Na, J. (2013). Meeting the needs of limited English proficiency patients. *Perspectives on Augmentative and Alternative Communication, 22*(2), 91. http://doi.org/10.1044/aac22.2.91

Jesse, M., Fei, N., Goldstein, E., Rakitin, I., Shama, L., Hall, F., & Ghanem, T. (2014). Head and neck cancer screenings and human papillomavirus knowledge across diverse suburban and urban populations. *American Journal of Otolaryngology, 36*, 223–229. doi:http://doi.org/10.1016

Light, J., & Mcnaughton, D. (2015). Designing AAC research and intervention to improve outcomes for individuals with complex communication needs. *Augmentative and Alternative Communication, 31*(2), 85–96. http://doi.org/10.3109/07434618.2015.1036458

McGrory, A. (2011). Communicating with head and neck cancer patients. *ORL Head and Neck Nursing, 29*(3), 7–11.

McNaughton, D., & Light, J. (2013). The iPad and mobile technology revolution: Benefits and challenges for individuals who require augmentative and alternative communication. *Augmentative and Alternative Communication, 29*(2), 107–116. http://doi.org/10.3109/07434618.2013.784930

Perry, A. R., & Shaw, M. A. (2000). Evaluation of functional outcomes (speech, swallowing and voice) in patients attending speech pathology after head and neck cancer treatment(s): Development of a multi-centre database. *Journal of Laryngology and Otology, 114*(March), 605–615.

Saltillo. (2015). *NOVA chat 5*. Millersburg, OH: Author.

Sullivan, M., Beukelman, D. R., & Mathy-Laikko, P. (1993). Situational communication effectiveness of rehabilitated individuals with total laryngectomies. *Journal of Medical Speech-Language Pathology, 1*, 73–80.

Sullivan, M., Gaebler, C., & Ball, L. J. (2007a). AAC for people with head and neck cancer. In D. R. Beukelman, K. L. Garrett, & K. M. Yorkston (Eds.), *Augmentative communication strategies for adults with acute or chronic medical conditions* (pp. 347–367). Baltimore, MD: Paul H. Brookes.

Sullivan, M., Gaebler, C., & Ball, L. J. (2007b). Supporting persons with chronic communication limitations: Head and neck cancer. In *ASHA Convention* (pp. 1–6). Boston, MA.

Talk to Me Technologies. (2015). Pogo Boards, Cedar Falls, IA.

The Joint Commission. (2009). *Hospitals, language, and culture: A snapshot of the nation*. Oakbrook Terrace, IL: Author.

The Joint Commission. (2010). *Advancing effective communication, cultural competence, and patient- and family-centered care: A roadmap for hospitals*. Oakbrook Terrace, IL: Author.

Tobii Dynavox. (2009). *QuickFires. Quickfires: Big impact with little words*. Retrieved from http://uk.dynavoxtech.com/tips/series5/details.aspx?id=119

Tobii Dynavox. (2015). *Lightwriter SL40 Connect*. Pittsburgh, PA: Author.

20

Rehabilitation of the Laryngectomized Individual: Alaryngeal Communication Options

Bari Hoffman Ruddy, Vicki Lewis, and Christine Sapienza

TOTAL LARYNGECTOMY INTRODUCTION

With a total laryngectomy, communication is dependent on alaryngeal speech modes. A *total laryngectomy* refers to removal of the entire larynx. The hyoid bone is cut from the suprahyoid musculature, and the thyroid and cricoid cartilages are removed from the pharyngeal muscles and trachea. Figure 20–1 depicts the normal anatomic orientations prior to a total laryngectomy. Figure 20–2 depicts a total laryngectomy. As a result of this procedure, the trachea is redirected to form an opening in the front of the neck, known as a *stoma*. A total laryngectomy is performed when the extent of the laryngeal carcinoma is not amenable to conservation surgical or nonsurgical procedures. Other times, total laryngectomy is completed as a second-order approach, after the first choice treatment of radiation therapy has failed to resolve the cancer, and when the patient is no longer a candidate for additional radiation.

Prior to laryngectomy, the normal anatomy of the upper respiratory tract filters air through the nose hairs where it is warmed and humidified by the mucous membranes of the nasal and pharyngeal cavities. After total laryngectomy, normal head and neck anatomy is altered, resulting in inhaled air flowing through the neck stoma, directly into the trachea without filtration, warming, or humidification. These changes often result in irritation, inflammation, and possibly infection as bacteria multiply within lower airway structures. In addition, loss of heat and humidity to inhaled air contributes to increasing thickness or *viscosity* of mucus throughout the respiratory tract. Because inspired air no longer passes through the nasal, oral, and pharyngeal cavities, airflow resistance decreases, resulting in reduced oxygenation of upper airway tissues, decreased olfaction (loss of smell), increased production of mucus secretions, and decreased ability to mobilize or remove these secretions.

THE ROLE OF THE SPEECH-LANGUAGE PATHOLOGIST PRIOR TO LARYNGECTOMY

Similar to counseling techniques used with patients undergoing organ preservation treatment for head and neck cancer (HNC), the speech-language pathologist plays a key role counseling patients prior to surgery. During the counseling session, a

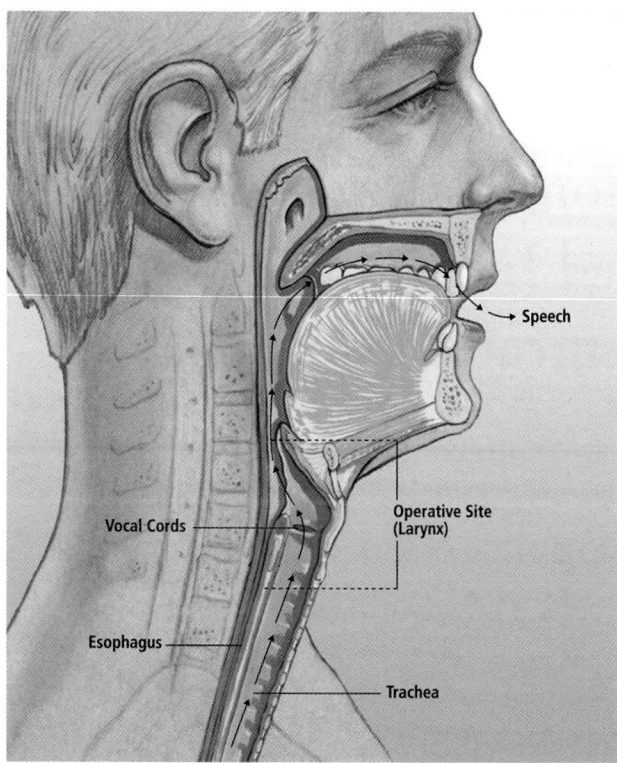

Figure 20–1. Head and neck anatomy prior to laryngectomy. (Courtesy of InHealth Technologies, http://www.inhealth.com)

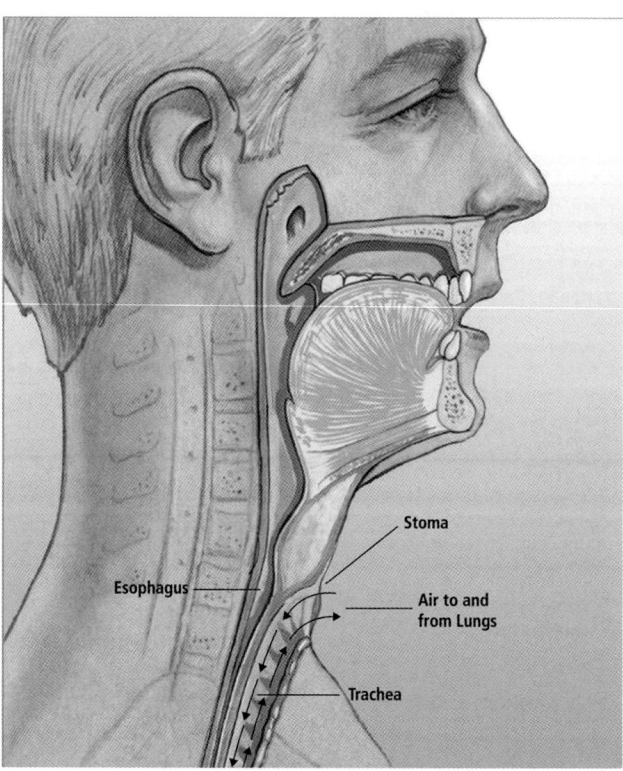

Figure 20–2. Head and neck anatomy after laryngectomy. (Courtesy of InHealth Technologies, http://www.inhealth.com)

wide range of psychosocial issues are addressed. The unique needs, preferences, coping strategies, support systems, and financial resources available to each patient must be taken into careful consideration. The speech-language pathologist will explain anticipated postsurgical changes to anatomy as well as the impact of these changes on swallowing, voice, and speech.

Augmentative and alternative means of communication may be introduced and practiced in advance of surgery. Use of an electrolarynx may be introduced, and the patient can initiate use of the device (without use of voicing) to begin to learn techniques to communicate effectively, including overarticulation, proper phrasing, and proper placement of the device on the neck. Additionally, presurgical measures of quality of life, voice, and swallow are obtained. Instrumental assessments such as videofluoroscopy or endoscopy allow for quantification of presurgical laryngeal and pharyngeal function.

THE ROLE OF THE SPEECH-LANGUAGE PATHOLOGIST FOLLOWING LARYNGECTOMY

In many settings, education pertaining to post-laryngectomy changes is provided by the speech-language pathologist. Key topics for discussion include filtration of inspired air through a stoma cover or similar device as well as stoma-related safety concerns. Additionally, the speech-language pathologist is central to the provision of postsurgical counseling and entraining new means of communication, including alaryngeal speech.

Filtration After Laryngectomy

Cloth stoma covers serve to protect the lower airways and can be homemade or purchased by the patient. Disposable foam stoma covers are also available (Figures 20–3 and 20–4). Air inspired through the stoma can also be warmed and filtered through use of a heat and moisture exchange (HME) system. Multiple HME products are commercially available. These feature a disposable filter cassette that attaches to the stoma with an adhesive baseplate, laryngectomy button, or laryngectomy tube (Figures 20–5 through 20–9).

The HME device works on the principle that, during exhalation, heat and moisture are absorbed by the filtration mechanism prior to being transferred back into the inspired air (Hilgers, Aaronson, Ackerstaff, Schouwenburg, & VanZanwijk, 1991).

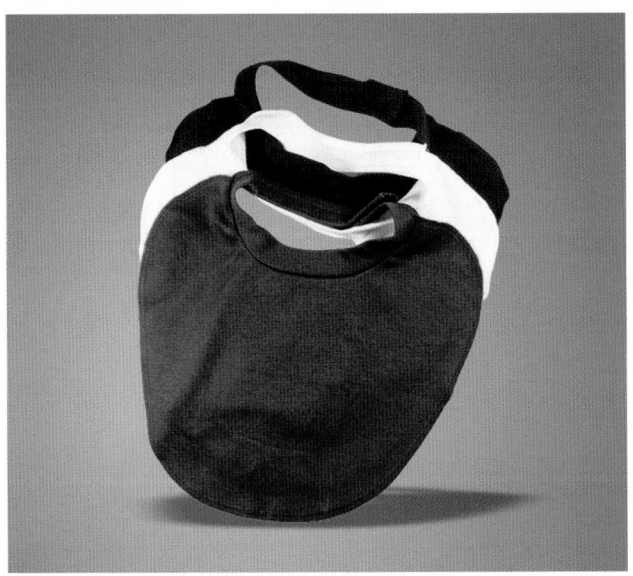

Figure 20–3. Cloth stoma covers.

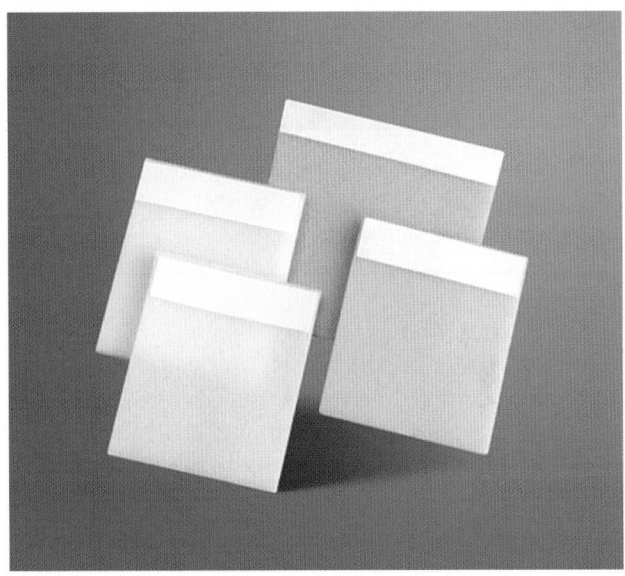

Figure 20–4. Disposable foam stoma covers.

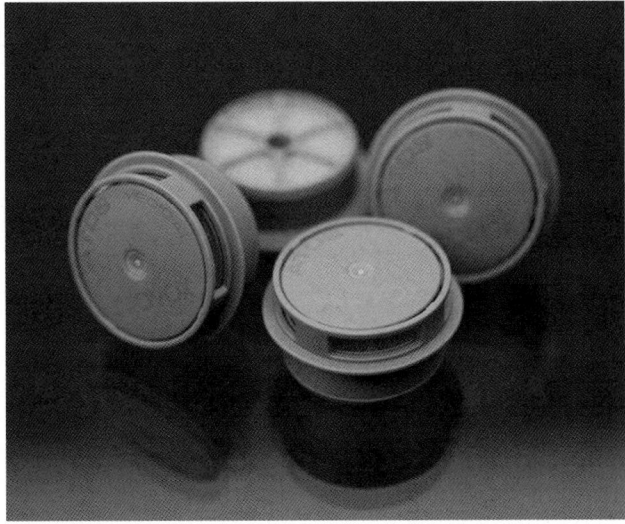

Figure 20–5. HME cassette. (Courtesy of Atos Medical, http://www.atosmedical.com)

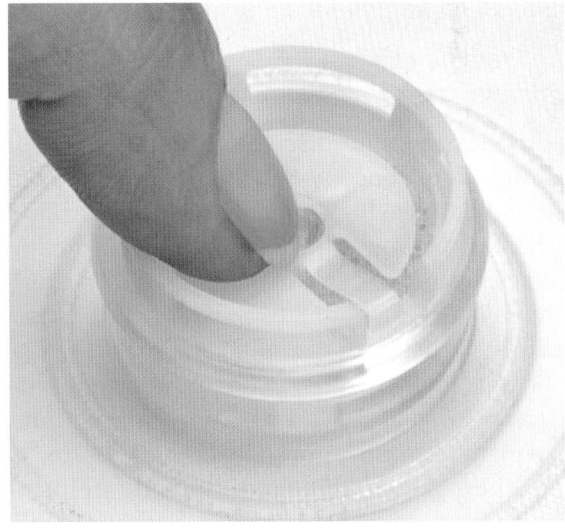

Figure 20–6. HME Easy Touch Speech Button. (Courtesy of InHealth Technologies, http://www.inhealth.com)

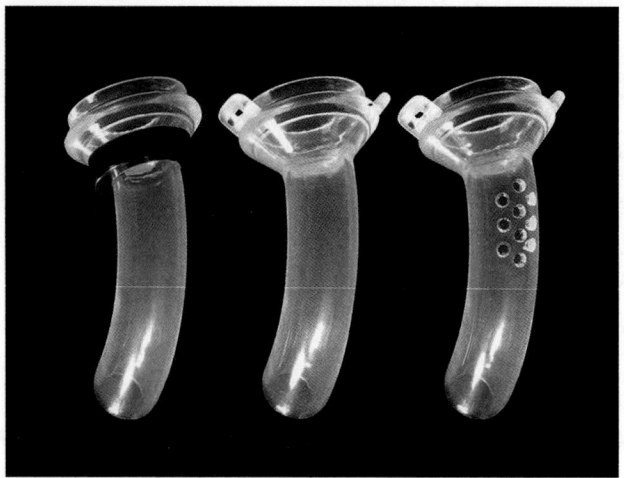

Figure 20–7. Provox LaryTubes, which can be used for stomal attachment of an HME cassette. (Courtesy of Atos Medical, http://www.atosmedical.com)

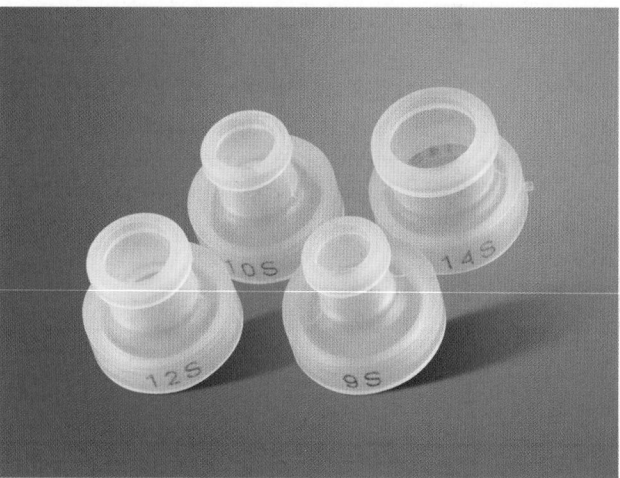

Figure 20–8. Barton-Mayo buttons, which can be used for stomal attachment of an HME cassette. These buttons are custom sized for individual patients by the speech pathologist. (Courtesy of InHealth Technologies, http://www.inhealth.com)

Although these products vary in design, resistance to airflow, and efficiency of use, in general, HMEs increase the air temperature and the humidity of inspired air, thereby promoting normal function of cilia in the lungs. Return of ciliary action improves pulmonary hygiene through improvements in *pulmonary toilet*, the ability to clear (cough or expectorate) secretions from the airway. This in turn decreases the overall volume of mucus within the lower airway, lessening the risk of mucus accumulation.

Safety Concerns Relating to Stomas

Additional topics for discussion after laryngectomy include safety concerns relating to the presence of a stoma. Because the stoma opens directly into the trachea, providing unhindered access to the lower airways, water barriers are necessary during certain activities such as bathing or showering. After laryngectomy the patient is classified as a "neck breather." A shower shield or collar made of waterproof material can be used to provide a barrier while permitting the patient to breathe normally (Figure 20–10).

Other safety principles include refraining from swimming and awareness of changes to the procedure for administering or receiving cardio-

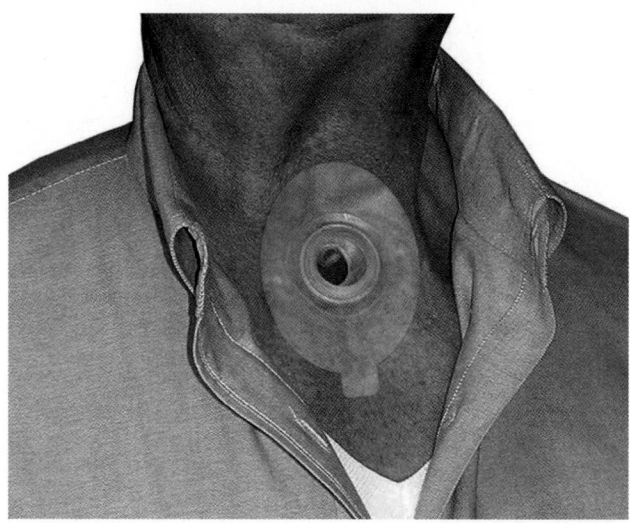

Figure 20–9. View of a stoma with a disposable adhesive baseplate holding an HME device in place. (Courtesy of InHealth Technologies, http://www.inhealth.com)

pulmonary resuscitation (CPR) including explicit instruction for caregivers on mouth-to-stoma resuscitation. Special considerations and safeguards are necessary particularly in an emergency situation. Typically, when someone stops breathing, a rescuer may blow air into the individual's mouth. Mouth-to-

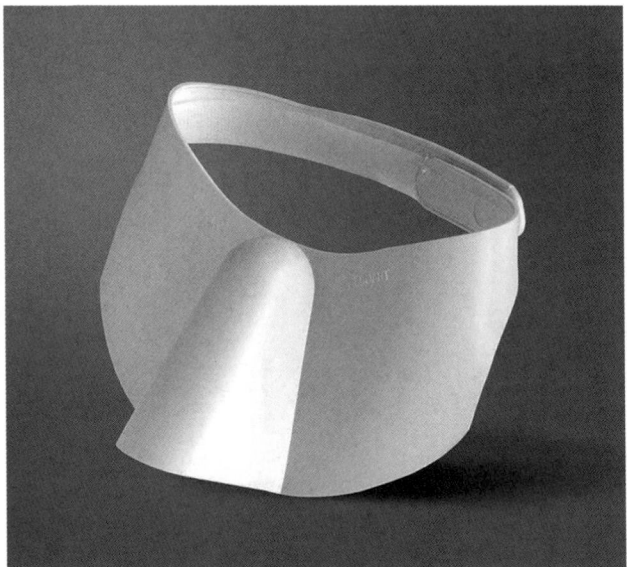

Figure 20–10. Rubber shower collar. (Courtesy of InHealth Technologies, http://www.inhealth.com)

mouth rescue breathing is a quick and effective way to provide oxygen to an individual. This technique will no longer work if the person is a neck breather, because the only way the individual will get oxygen into the lungs is if it is provided through the neck opening and not through the mouth or nose. It is critical that the rescuer is knowledgeable about this distinction as a lack of understanding can present a life-threatening situation. Individuals with a total laryngectomy may decide to obtain a brightly colored emergency card to carry with them on their person or to keep in their vehicle or on their vehicle window or choose to wear a special "medic alert" bracelet or necklace in order to identify themselves as someone with a total laryngectomy and provide vital medical information in an emergency situation. Clinicians should also advocate that their patients contact their local emergency medical service (EMS) following total laryngectomy to alert the local responders of their address and register that they are a neck breather. Last, patients and their families should be educated about purchasing an Ambu bag at a local medical supply store. Should the individual with a total laryngectomy require CPR by a family member, the Ambu bag can be utilized with

a pediatric mask that can be placed on the stoma for CPR administration. If the individual with the total laryngectomy is the one administering CPR to another, he or she can pair the Ambu bag with a regular-sized CPR mask.

Postsurgical Counseling and Management

Postsurgical counseling and management focuses on readdressing psychosocial issues, talking about patient and family support systems, available community resources, lifestyle changes, and nutritional changes that will need to occur as a result of the surgery. Patients are encouraged to participate in support groups to aid in coping with the postsurgical outcomes, facilitate socialization, and assist in the emotional recovery. Management should focus on practicing with voice, speech, and swallowing strategies as necessary. The speech pathologist maintains close collaboration with the physician, nurse, dietitian, social worker, physical therapist, psychiatric professional, and other team members to ensure comprehensive care of the patient (Stemple, Glaze, & Klaben, 2000).

The rehabilitation goal for the individual with a total laryngectomy is to learn to communicate through a wide array of means in addition to knowing how to use a backup method. The next section provides an overview of the modes of communication for patients following total laryngectomy.

COMMUNICATION FOLLOWING TOTAL LARYNGECTOMY

There are several rehabilitation options available following a total laryngectomy, including artificial/ electromechanical, esophageal, or prosthetic. The "best" technique for the patient to use as an alternative mode of communication depends on a number of factors including age, cognitive status, motor coordination, and cultural and personal preferences. The goal of rehabilitation is to learn to communicate with whatever option is best to improve functional communication and quality of life (Table 20–1).

Table 20–1. Description of Primary Alaryngeal Modes of Communication

Type	Production	Disadvantages	Advantages	Troubleshooting for SLPs	Outcome Studies
Artificial larynx	An electrical-powered vibration that functions as a sound source Types: *Transcervical:* vibratory device is placed against the neck *Transoral:* vibration/sound is delivered directly to the mouth via tube *Intraoral:* remote-controlled operated device that is custom built into the upper denture or orthodontic retainer	• A monopitch sound with metallic quality that may sound unusual and distracting • Requires clear articulation skills • Handheld device • Difficult to use with the telephone	• Fast and easy way to communicate after surgery (portable) • Can be used as a backup to another means of communicating • Battery operated • Volume and pitch control features	• Find the right placement • Work on eliminating distracters, such as on/off timing, body movement, and stance • Increase intelligibility by teaching appropriate articulation, rate, phrasing, pitch, loudness, and stress	• Adaptive filtering and subtractive-type algorithms will reduce the noise level associated with electrolarynx and improve the speech quality and intelligibility (Liu & Ng, 2007) • Breathiness during speech has a higher acceptability rating than during quick breathing and exhalation. The results showed that newer electrolarynxes can control pitch by expiration pressure (Liu, Wan, Wang, & Niu, 2004)
Esophageal speech	Air is trapped into the mouth and then forced back up, causing the walls of the esophagus and pharynx to vibrate. The sound is then shaped into speech using the remaining articulators.	• Low-pitch sound, derived from a controlled belch or burp • Difficult to learn how to do • Articulation must be clear • Reduced length of utterance	• No devices are needed to produce speech • It is possible to produce a "normal" sounding voice (may improve quality of life)	Build skill level of patient: • Voice: increase length of utterance and develop appropriate stress patterns • Develop consistency and duration of speech • Eliminate distracters: stoma noise, lip smacking, intruding consonants	• Most preferred by laryngectomee patients, however, least intelligible during 5 and 10 dB message-to-competition ratios (Clark & Stemple, 1982)

Type	Production	Disadvantages	Advantages	Troubleshooting for SLPs	Outcome Studies
Tracheoesophageal speech (TEP)	A small surgical passage is created inside the stoma, from the back wall of the trachea into the esophageal wall. A small-valved tube (voice prosthesis) is placed into this passage to enable tracheoesophageal speech. Voice is produced by blocking the stoma.	• Requires a good seal around the perimeter of the stoma • Requires ability to maintain prosthesis • Costly: some equipment needs to be replaced daily	• More natural speech • Improved intelligibility • Greater sound duration	Monitor for: • Leakage of liquids through or around the TEP • *Candida* • Poor cleaning: brushing and flushing device • Wrong-size prosthesis • Muscle tension of overall body	• Research shows that there is a normal airstream source in speech production using a TEP device, which contributes to speech timing and intelligibility of alaryngeal speakers

Electromechanical Speech

An electromechanical device (also referred to as an artificial larynx or *electrolarynx*) is a useful treatment option in the early postoperative phase when the patient cannot use other alternative voicing techniques. It can also be used as a means of long-term communication. One advantage to introducing a device such as an electrolarynx early in the postoperative course is providing the patient with a useful means of communication, potentially limiting frustration and facilitating continued participation in the plan of care. The speech-language pathologist (along with the patient) selects the most appropriate device and teaches basic use/care of device in acute care. Immediately following surgery, the patient will need to use an intraoral adaptor because placement of the device on the neck tissues is contraindicated while the surgical site heals. Training in variable communication settings including one-on-one, communication in a noisy environment, and over the telephone can be addressed prior to discharge from the hospital.

Electromechanical speech is achieved through use of an "on the neck" (*transcervical*) or intraoral device. Most of the artificial larynges available today are able to be used for either transcervical or intraoral placement. These devices feature a vibrating head that can be used for on the neck (transcervical) placement; additionally, a cap can be placed on the vibrating head, attached to an intraoral tube that transmits sound for intraoral use. All of these devices rely on the principle of introducing an electromechanical vibration, heard as a tone or buzz. Most devices available are rechargeable and have loudness and pitch control.

Transcervical placement involves placing the device against the neck (in an area of soft tissue, not in contact with bone). The device vibration is transmitted as a tone/buzz through the tissue of the neck to the oral cavity where it is then acoustically "shaped" into recognizable speech sounds by movements of the speech articulators (Figures 20–11, 20–12, and 20–13). Intraoral placement introduces the tone/buzz directly into the oral cavity through a tube. From here the sound is shaped into recognizable speech in a manner identical to transcervical methods.

A major advantage of the electrolarynx is the ability for immediate production of basic speech.

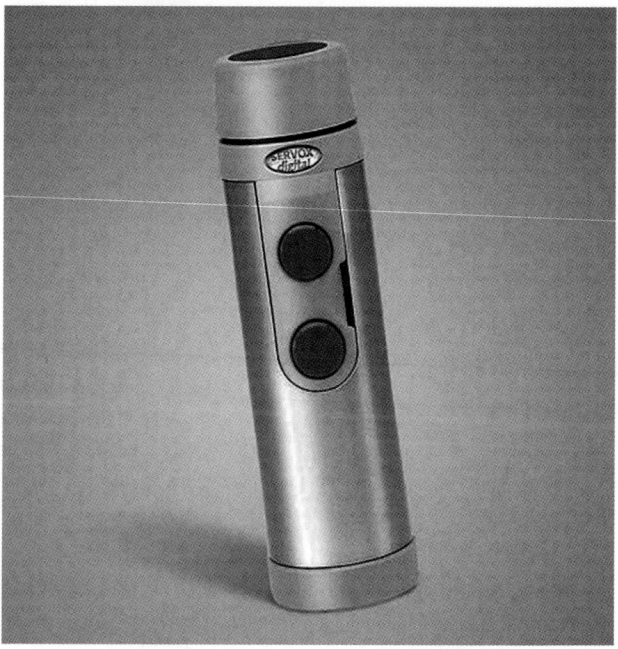

Figure 20–11. Servox electrolarynx. (Courtesy of InHealth Technologies, http://www.inhealth.com)

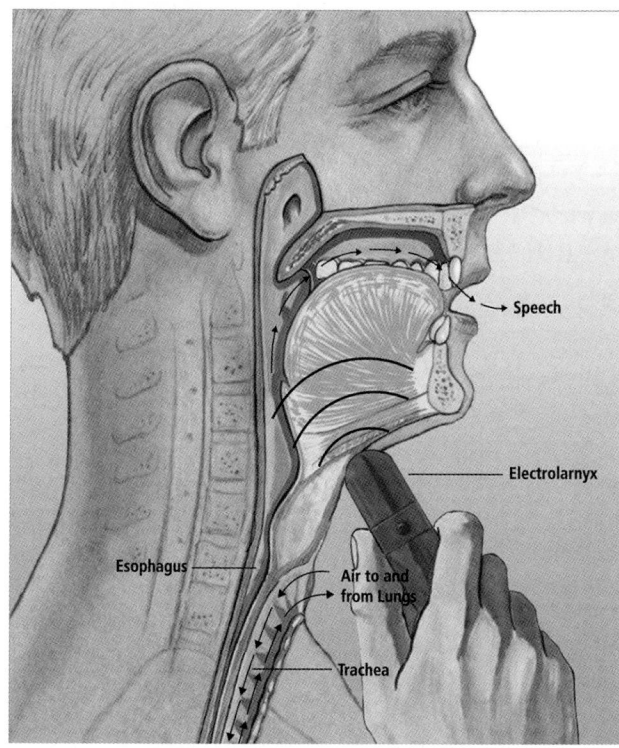

Figure 20–12. Optimal transcervical placement of electrolarynx. (Courtesy of InHealth Technologies, http://www.inhealth.com)

This approach is commonly used early in the post-surgical period and will not interfere or delay progress mastering other forms of alaryngeal speech. The devices can also help facilitate other forms of alaryngeal speech.

There exist certain contraindications to use of an electrolarynx. Patients who have undergone extensive surgery and radiation therapy many demonstrate fibrosis of neck tissues that may otherwise impede the transmission of the tone/buzz toward the oral cavity. Limited dexterity and reduced cognitive function may also preclude successful use of these devices. The major disadvantage associated with the electrolarynx is the artificial, "robotic" sound quality produced by the devices. This sound quality is sometimes embarrassing to patients and can be distracting to listeners. In spite of these known disadvantages, Hillman, Walsh, and Heaton (2005) reported that artificial larynx use was the predominant mode of alaryngeal communication at follow-up. Eighty-five percent of patients in their study used an artificial larynx at 1-month postop and 55% still used it as their primary means of communication 24 months postoperatively. Other investigations have revealed similar results with more than half of the individuals undergoing total laryngectomy continuing to use an electrolarynx postoperatively (Carr, Schmidbauer, Majaess, & Smith, 2000).

Esophageal Speech

Esophageal speech (Figure 20–14) is another option for alaryngeal communication following laryngectomy. During some surgical procedures, when the larynx is removed, the upper portion of the trachea

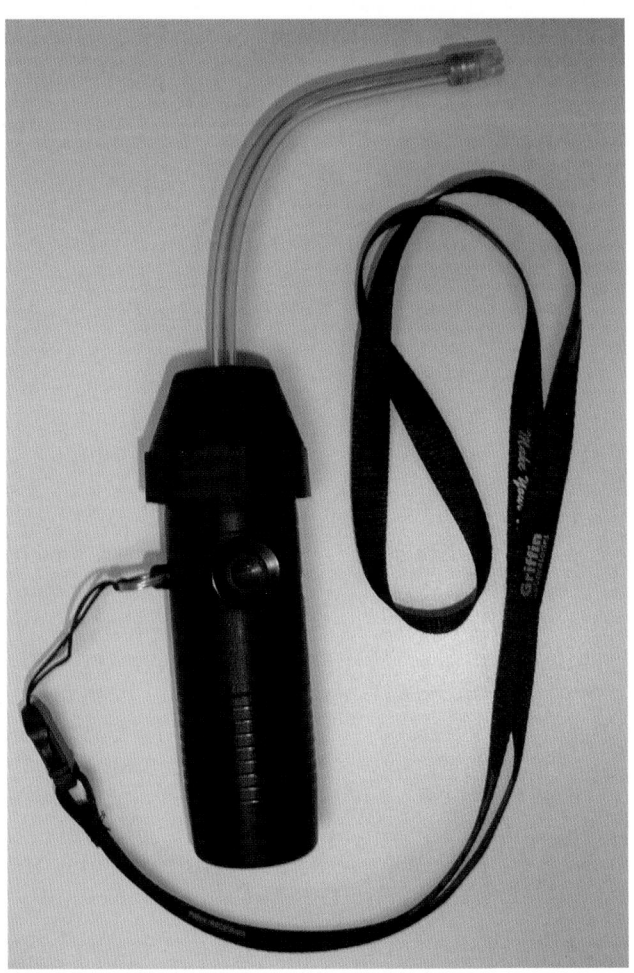

Figure 20–13. Electrolarynx with intraoral adapter in place.

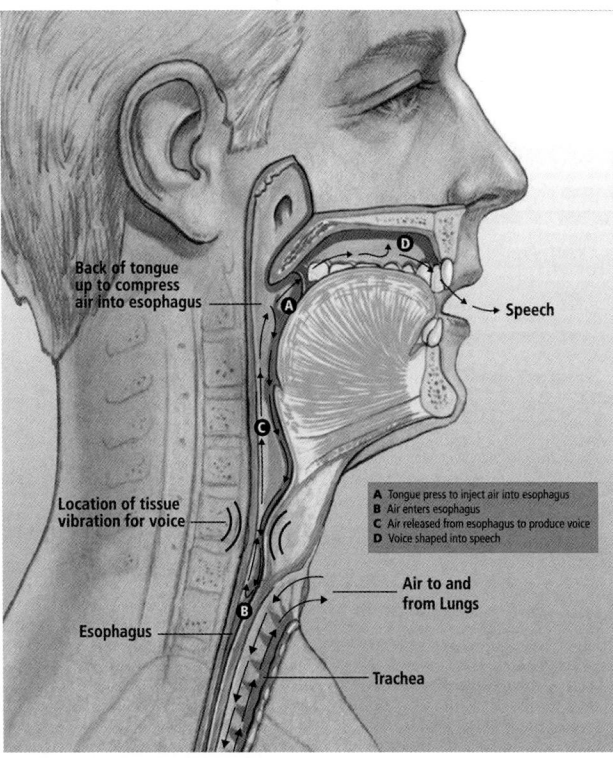

Figure 20–14. Esophageal speech production. (Courtesy of InHealth Technologies, http://www.inhealth.com)

is pulled forward and attached superiorly to the sternum, and the reconstructed pharynx is joined directly to the esophageal opening. The junction at which the hypopharynx joins the esophagus is called the *pharyngoesophageal (PE) segment*. The PE segment is composed of striated muscle: the cricopharyngeeus muscle, the lower strands of the inferior pharyngeal constrictor, and the superior esophageal sphincter (Zemlin, 1998). During esophogeal speech, sound is produced by the vibration of the pharyngoesophageal (PE) segment (Zemlin, 1998).

Esophageal speech can be produced when the individual transports a small amount (75 mL) of air from the oral and pharyngeal cavity into the esophagus. The air is redirected back through the PE segment to create vibration of the tissue. Repeating this process over and over rapidly can ultimately produce intelligible esophageal speech. The process is similar to a controlled belch or burp that is then formed into words through movements of the tongue, lips, teeth, and palate (Salmon, 1986). Advantages for esophageal speech are that it does not require expensive electromechanical devices or prostheses and is a hands-free speech technique. The main disadvantage is that most patients are unable to master the technique sufficiently for useful voice production, which is reported to be only as high as 20% to 25% (Gates, Ryan, Cooper, et al., 1982) and in recent studies as low as 7% to 10% (Hillman et al., 2005). Furthermore, esophageal speech results in low-pitched (50–80 Hz) and low-intensity speech that can be difficult to understand.

Factors associated with successful acquisition of esophageal speech include type and extent of surgery, positive attitude, psychosocial adjustment, frequency of therapy, and positive family support. Failures in developing esophageal speech have been associated with poor attitude, lack of patient motivation, limited physical strength, postoperative radiation effects, dysphagia, and limited therapy (Gates, Ryan, Cantu, & Hearne, 1982; Graham, 2005). Patients who master esophageal speech should also be provided with training on a backup method of communication, typically an electrolarynx. If a patient becomes ill or is feeling fatigued, ability to produce esophageal speech may deteriorate, and having a backup method of communication can become necessary.

There are two primary techniques that can be used to transport air from the oral cavity to the esophagus to produce esophageal speech: injection (a positive-pressure approach) and inhalation (a negative-pressure approach). These variations of esophageal speech are based on how the PE segment opens to allow air intake (Salmon, 2005).

Injection Method

The injection method requires the use of the tongue to force air back into the pharynx and esophagus. Here, the lip and tongue movements increase the already positive air pressure in the oral cavity, forcing air through the closed PE segment and into the upper portion of the esophagus (Duguay, 1999; Graham, 2005). The tightening of the thoracic and abdominal muscles prevents the air from moving farther down the esophagus. The trapped air moves upward through the PE segment, setting the surrounding musculature (pharyngeal-esophageal) into vibration, thereby producing sound (Graham, 2005). As the patient articulates, the vibrations are then further shaped by the resonant capacities of the nasal and oropharyngeal cavities (Edels, 1983). There are two techniques used to inject air into the esophagus: the consonant press injection method and the glossopharyngeal press (Graham, 2005).

The consonant press injection method (also referred to as injection method for obstruents or consonant injection) uses the natural intraoral air pressures created by plosive and fricative sounds to inject air into the esophagus. When a patient produces sounds such as /t/, /p/, or /k/, or words such as "poach," "toad," or "kick," the strength of contact in the lips and tongue musculature builds and compresses intraoral air pressure sufficient enough to overcome the resistance of the closed PE segment (Edels, 1983; Graham, 2005). Sound is produced as the air is redirected to vibrate the PE segment.

The tongue pump or glossopharyngeal press method creates a seal using the lips and tongue to increase intraoral air pressure to move the air toward the PE segment. The tongue creates a pumping action that reduces the size of the oral cavity, compressing the air, which, in turn, increases intraoral air pressure causing the PE segment to open and vibrate.

Inhalation Method

The inhalation method uses a rapid expansion of the thoracic cavity during inspiration to draw air into the esophagus. The patient is instructed to take a quick, short breath through the stoma. As the diaphragm moves downward, there is an increase in the negative pressure within the thoracic cavity (where the esophagus is located). A vacuum effect is created in the esophagus as the negative air pressure begins to increase. This allows air from the oral and pharyngeal cavities to be drawn passively into the esophagus. Once the air has entered the upper esophagus, the PE sphincter closes, thereby trapping the air in the esophagus. The procedure for returning the air to the oropharynx parallels that of the consonant press injection method (Graham, 2005).

Tracheoesophageal Puncture (TEP)

Transesophageal puncture was first introduced by Singer and Blom (1980) and, since that time, has gained popularity as a technique for restoring voice and speech production in patients following laryngectomy (Webster & Duguay, 1990). Similar to esophageal speech, patients who utilize a TEP should also be provided with training on a backup method of communication. If the prosthesis malfunctions, an alternate means of communication may become necessary.

The tracheoesophageal puncture (TEP) is performed either at the time of the laryngectomy surgery (referred to as a primary TEP), or later once sufficient healing has occurred (referred to as a secondary TEP). The secondary TEP typically takes place approximately 6 weeks or more following laryngectomy or radiation therapy. The tracheoesophageal puncture creates a surgical opening (fistula) between the posterior wall of the trachea and the anterior wall of the esophagus for insertion of a voice prosthesis. Once the puncture is created, a balloon catheter is directed downward through the fistula into the esophagus (Gress & Singer, 2005) or an indwelling prosthesis can be placed by the surgeon at the time of the procedure. When a primary TEP is performed and a balloon catheter is placed in the TE tract, the catheter serves as a feeding tube that is ultimately replaced by the voice prosthesis after

sufficient healing has occurred. In cases where a surgeon places an indwelling prosthesis during a primary TEP, another means of nonoral nutrition such as a nasogastric tube or percutaneous gastrostomy tube will be necessary until the patient has healed sufficiently to initiate oral intake.

In patients who do not have a prosthesis placed during the TEP surgery, eventually the catheter is removed, and a small one-way valve (prosthesis) is inserted into the puncture in order to prevent its spontaneous closure and prevent the aspiration of pharyngoesophageal contents into the trachea (Figures 20–15 and 20–16). Once in place,

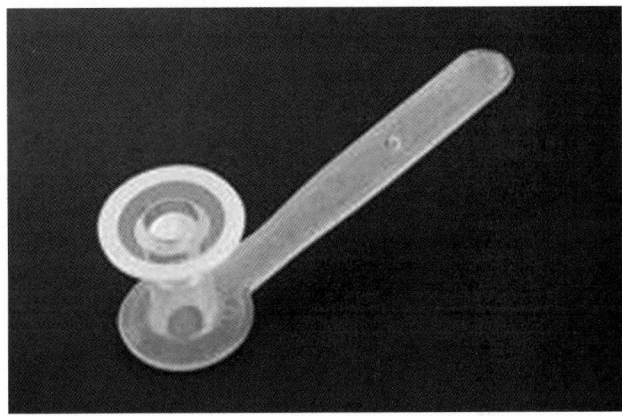

Figure 20–15. InHealth voice prosthesis. (Courtesy of InHealth Technologies, http://www.inhealth.com)

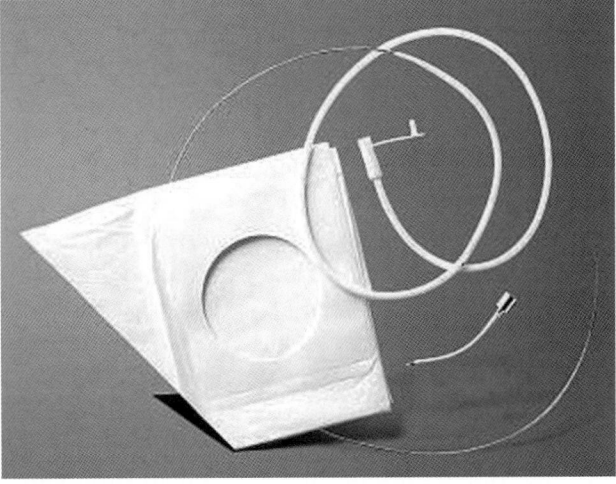

Figure 20–16. Tracheoesophageal puncture set. (Courtesy of InHealth Technologies, http://www.inhealth.com)

the voice prosthesis allows for a one-way flow of air from the trachea into the region below the PE segment. The puncture permits diversion of pulmonary air to drive pharyngoesophageal vibration for the production of tracheoesophageal speech (also referred to as TE voice and speech) (Gress & Singer, 2005).

Tracheoesophageal (TE) Sound Generation

To produce the TE sound, the patient inhales, then exhales while occluding (typically with a finger) the tracheostoma. Patients need to be able to coordinate finger occlusion of the tracheostoma and the associated release with inhalation and exhalation for speech. Stoma occlusion can also be achieved through the use of a tracheostoma valve to allow for hands-free speech production. This valve opens under positive pressure as the air enters the esophagus and closes by elastic recoil. Therefore, when pulmonary air enters the prosthesis, it opens the one-way prosthesis valve, directing air into the pharyngoesophagus, setting these tissues into vibration for sound generation. As the sound enters the oral and nasopharyngeal cavities, articulation and resonance shape the sounds for speech (Gress & Singer, 2005). Figure 20–16 depicts TE speech production.

Types of Prostheses for TEP Voice

The voice prosthesis is a cylindrical-shaped tube, usually made from medical-grade silicone. Two categories of devices are available: the indwelling prosthesis (placed by the clinician) and the non-indwelling prosthesis (placed by the patient). The neck strap on the indwelling prosthesis is usually cut following insertion and, thus, taping to the neck is not necessary. For both types of prostheses, at the distal end, a slit, hinged, or ball valve is placed through the front wall of the esophagus. The tracheal flange of the prosthesis is flush with the back wall of the stoma/trachea. During voice production, exhaled air flows through the opening at the tracheal flange of the prosthesis, when the stoma is occluded. Air enters into the esophagus through the prosthesis and then flows through the PE segment producing audible vibration (voice).

Cleaning of the prosthesis can be completed via the opening of the device at the back wall of the stoma; tools for cleaning the prosthesis are provided by the prosthesis manufacturer. Keeping the prosthesis free of debris is very important as food debris that collects at the level of the esophageal flange of the prosthesis can lead to yeast (*Candida*) growth. When this occurs, the *Candida* will invade the surface of the prosthesis valve and will result in malfunction of the valve. This causes leakage, initially of fluids, through the prosthesis when the patient drinks. Once this occurs, the prosthesis must be replaced due to aspiration risk.

Non-Indwelling Prostheses

- *Duckbill Style:* This is the original prosthesis designed by Singer and Blom (1980) with use of a slit-type valve (Figure 20–17).
- *Low Pressure/Low Resistance:* This is a hinged valve with a lower opening pressure. This design requires less respiratory effort for sound generation to occur as compared with the duckbill devices (Gress & Singer, 2005; Pauloski, 1998) (Figure 20–18).

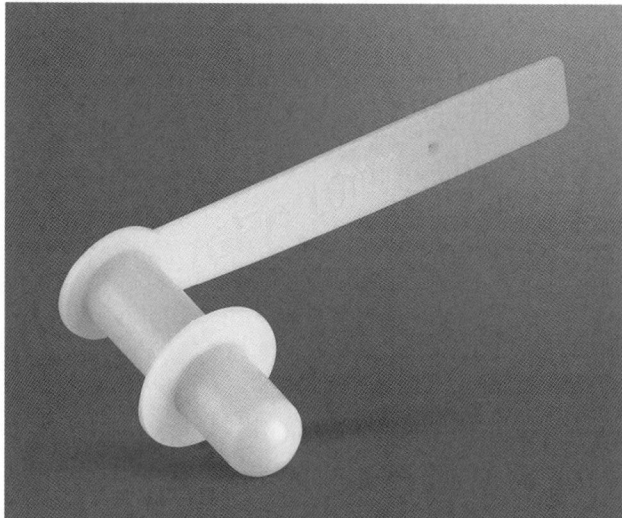

Figure 20–17. The duckbill style of non-indwelling devices, with use of a slit-type valve. (Courtesy of InHealth Technologies, http://www.inhealth.com)

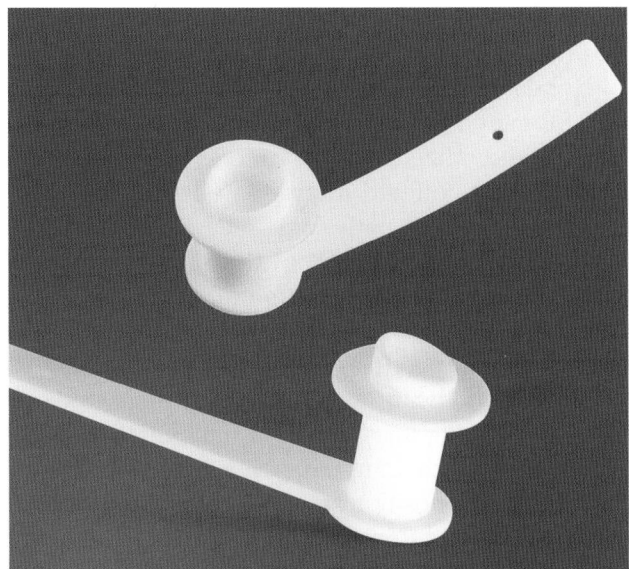

Figure 20–18. The low-pressure/low-resistance style of non-indwelling devices, with a hinged valve with a lower opening pressure. (Courtesy of InHealth Technologies, http://www.inhealth.com)

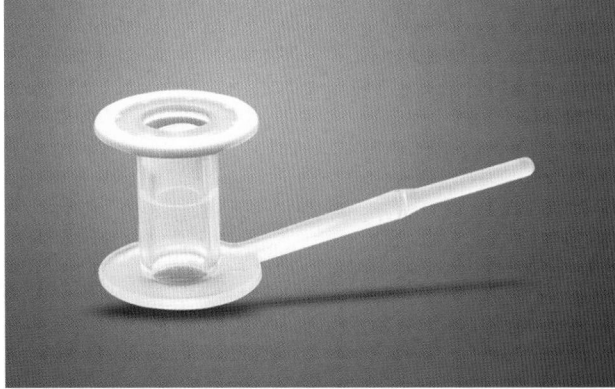

Figure 20–19. Classic indwelling device. (Courtesy of InHealth Technologies, http://www.inhealth.com)

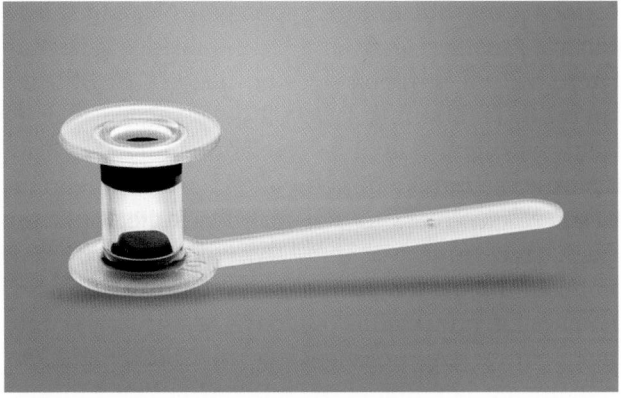

Figure 20–20. Blom Singer dual-valve prosthesis. (Courtesy of InHealth Technologies, http://www.inhealth.com)

Indwelling Prosthesis. An indwelling prosthesis is an extended-wear clinician-inserted prosthesis that requires minimized maintenance (Gress & Singer, 2005) (Figures 20–19, 20–20, and 20–21).

Prosthesis length and methods for sizing vary by each manufacturer. Prosthesis product literature should be consulted to determine proper sizing tools, protocol, and other specifications of the selected prosthesis. Voice prostheses lengths range in size from 4 to 28 mm; prosthesis diameters range from 16 French to 22.5 French. There are several manufacturers of voice prostheses. Note: French is a unit of measure in medicine for the outer diameter of a tube (1 Fr = 0.33 mm).

The main advantages of the TEP method of voice production include a relatively good voice quality when compared to the other alaryngeal methods. Although similar in quality to voice produced with esophageal speech, the duration of TEP voice production on one breath is often greater than with production of esophageal speech. Disadvantages of TEP can include postoperative complications, the daily maintenance of the prosthesis by the patient, recurrent

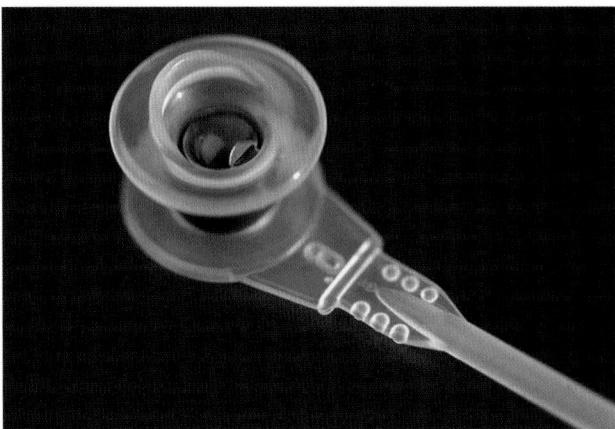

Figure 20–21. Provox 2 voice prosthesis. (Courtesy of Atos Medical, http://www.atosmedical.com)

leakage of the prosthesis after a period of time requiring replacement by the clinician, the cost, and the need to use a finger to occlude the tracheostoma.

Some of the more current voice prostheses tend to be more reliable and safe to use, have a front-loading insertion technique, indwelling fixation, and low resistance to airflow. Overall, satisfaction with speech quality, fluency of speech, overall intelligibility, ease of phone use, satisfaction with social interactions, and quality of life tend to be high with the TEP method in comparison to artificial and esophageal methods (Clements, Rassekh Seikaly, Hokanson, & Calhoun, 1997; Hillman, Walsh, & Heaton, 2005).

Prosthesis Placement

Various prosthetic products are available, and selection of a prosthesis type and style is a patient-specific process. If the surgeon does not place a prosthesis during the TEP surgical procedure, prosthesis placement can occur as soon as the tissue in the TEP site has healed. This can be completed by the surgeon or the speech-language pathologist. The catheter placed during the surgery is removed, and the TEP tract diameter can be dilated as necessary. Dilation occurs by insertion of catheters of increasing diameter until the puncture is approximately a size 2 French greater in diameter than that of the selected TEP prosthesis. This gradual process helps to decrease tissue trauma when the prosthesis is inserted.

Accurate measurement is critical for determining the proper length for the prosthesis. If a prosthesis that is placed is too short in length, it may not be fully in place in the esophageal wall. If this occurs, the back wall of the tract will close, and the TEP tract will be lost. If a prosthesis that is placed is too long, a pistoning (back and forth) movement of the prosthesis can occur with use, and this can result in inadvertent dilation of the tract diameter and tissue irritation. As a result, the patient may leak fluids around the outer surface of the prosthesis while drinking. The prosthesis is typically inserted from the tracheal side using a standard insertion tool supplied by the manufacturer (Gress & Singer, 2005). The clinician needs to orient himself or herself to the position of TE tract, "line it up," and firmly insert the prosthesis until it is positioned flush with the back wall of the trachea. The methods for insertion

will vary based on the type and manufacturer of the prosthesis (Gress & Singer, 2005).

Evaluation and treatment of patients utilizing the TEP method of alaryngeal speech require training and specialized clinical practice beyond what is traditionally offered in graduate-level programs in speech-language pathology. There are a number of voice institutes throughout the country offering courses in laryngectomy rehabilitation; for example, the International Association of Laryngectomees Voice Rehabilitation Institute offers a yearly training conference; another option would be to apprentice at a facility offering laryngectomy rehabilitation. The American Speech Language-Hearing Association has published a position statement of practice policy entitled *Roles and Responsibilities of Speech-Language Pathologists With Respect to Evaluation and Treatment for Tracheoesophageal Puncture and Prosthesis* (ASHA, 2004). In some facilities the speech pathologist aids the surgeon in evaluation of a patient's suitability to use a voice prosthesis, assists in sizing and fitting, determines prosthesis placement, trains the patient how to fit and care for their prosthesis, and implements therapy to maximize the patient's ability to communicate while using the voice prosthesis (Stemple, Glaze, & Klaben, 2000).

REFLECTION AND ANALYSIS FOR FURTHER STUDY

1. Identify a facility near you that offers training in the placement of voice prostheses.
2. What prototypical patient is ideally suited for each of the types of alaryngeal speech? In other words, for each type of alaryngeal speech generate a "best for" and "not suited for" list.
3. What would you say to a patient who initially rejects alaryngeal speech out of fear of sounding different?

REFERENCES

American Speech-Language-Hearing Association. (1992, March). Position statement and guidelines for evaluation and treatment for tracheoesophageal fistulization/puncture. *American Speech and Hearing Association, 34*(Suppl. 7), 17–21.

Carr, M. M., Schmidbauer, J. A., Majaess, L., & Smith, R. L. (2000). Communication after laryngectomy: An assessment of quality of life. *Otolaryngology-Head and Neck Surgery, 122*(1), 39–43.

Clark, J., & Stemple, J. (1982). Assessment of three modes of alaryngeal speech with a synthetic sentence identification (SSI) task in varying message-to-competition ratios. *Journal of Speech and Hearing Research, 25*(3), 333–338.

Clements, K. S., Rassekh, C. H., Seikaly, H., Hokanson, J. A., & Calhoun, K. H. (1997). Communication after laryngectomy. An assessment of patient satisfaction. *Archives of Otolaryngology-Head and Neck Surgery, 123*(5), 493–496.

Duguay, M. J. (1999). Esophageal speech training: The initial phase. In S. J. Salmon (Ed.), *Alaryngeal speech rehabilitation: For clinicians by clinicians* (2nd ed., pp. 155–201). Austin, TX: Pro-Ed.

Edels, Y. (1983). Pseudo voice theory and practice. In Y. Edels (Ed.), *Laryngectomy: Diagnosis rehabilitation* (pp. 107–141). London, UK: Croom Helm.

Gates, G., Ryan, W., Cantu, E., & Hearne, E. (1982). Current status of laryngectomee rehabilitation: II. Causes of failure. *American Journal of Otolaryngology, 3*(1), 8–14.

Gates, G., Ryan, W., Cooper, J., Lawliss, G., Cantu, E., Hayashi, T., . . . Hearne, E. (1982). Current status of laryngectomee rehabilitation: I. Results of therapy. *American Journal of Otolaryngology, 3*, 1–7.

Graham, M. (2005). Esophageal speech: Taking it to the limits. In P. Doyle & R. Keith (Eds.), *Contemporary considerations in the treatment and rehabilitation of head and neck cancer voice speech and swallowing* (pp. 379–430). Austin, TX: Pro-Ed.

Gress, C., & Singer, M. (2005). Tracheoesophageal voice restoration. In P. Doyle & R. Keith (Eds.), *Contemporary considerations in the treatment and rehabilitation of head and neck cancer voice speech and swallowing* (pp. 431–452). Austin, TX: Pro-Ed.

Hilgers, F., Aaronson, N., Ackerstaff, A., Schouwenburg, P., & VanZanwijk, N. (1991). The influence of a heat and mois- ture exchanger (HME) on the respiratory symptoms after total laryngectomy. *Clinical Otolaryngology, 16*, 152–156.

Hillman, R., Walsh, M., & Heaton, J. (2005). Laryngectomy speech rehabilitation. In P. Doyle & R. Keith (Eds.), *Contemporary considerations in the treatment and rehabilitation of head and neck cancer voice speech and swallowing* (pp. 75–90). Austin, TX: Pro-Ed.

Lui, H., & Ng, M. (2007). Electrolarynx in voice rehabilitation. *Auris Nasus Larynx, 34*(3), 327–332.

Liu, H., Wan, M., Wang, S., & Niu, H. (2007). Aerodynamic characteristics of laryngectomees breathing quietly and speaking with the electrolarynx. *Journal of Voice, 18*(4), 567–577.

Mohr, R. M., Quenelle, D. J., & Shumrick, D. A. (1983). Verticofrontolateral laryngectomy (hemilaryngectomy). Indications, technique, and results. *Archives of Otolaryngology-Head and Neck Surgery, 109*(6), 384–395.

Pauloski, B. (1998). Acoustic and aerodynamic characteristics of tracheoesophageal voice. In E. D. Blom, M. I. Singer, & R. C. Hamaker (Eds.), *Tracheoesophageal voice restoration following total laryngectomy* (pp. 123–141). San Diego, CA: Singular.

Salmon, S. J. (1986). Adjusting to laryngectomy. *Seminars in Speech and Language, 7*, 67–94.

Salmon, S. J. (2005). Commonalities among alaryngeal speech methods. In P. Doyle & R. Keith (Eds.), *Contemporary considerations in the treatment and rehabilitation of head and neck cancer voice speech and swallowing* (pp. 59–74). Austin, TX: Pro-Ed.

Singer, M., & Blom, E. (1980). An endoscopic technique for restoration of voice after laryngectomy. *Annals of Otology, Rhinology, and Laryngology, 89*, 529–533.

Stemple, J. C., Glaze, L. E., & Klaben, B. G. (2000). *Clinical voice pathology: Theory and management* (3rd ed.). San Diego, CA: Singular.

Webster, P., & Duguay, M. (1990). Surgeons reported attitudes and practices regarding alaryngeal speech. *Annals of Otology, Rhinology, and Laryngology, 99*(3, Pt. 1), 1727–1736.

Zemlin, W. R. (1998). *Speech and hearing science* (4th ed.). Boston, MA: Allyn & Bacon.

21

Patient Life Experiences Essential for Humanistic and Quality Care

Kathleen Ann Kavanagh

HUMANISTIC RESPONSE TO MEDICAL CRISIS

American society and the health care industry face many crises that affect the provision of humanistic and quality care. Some of these crises include high unemployment, fewer people having medical insurance, financial instability within the health care industry, increased longevity of the American people, ethical issues about end-of-life decisions, and the poor quality of health care. The Center for Disease Control and Prevention National Vital Statistics System (NVSS) 2013, reports the average life expectancy of a person born in the United States as 78.8 years. As the U.S. population ages, many of the people develop comorbidities that disrupt the quality of life.

The diagnosis of head and neck cancer is a life-changing event. Imagine yourself sitting in a medical office waiting for the results of a magnetic resonance image (MRI), computed technology (CT) scan, biopsy, and laboratory results. It has been agonizing to wait for the results, and you have been on pins and needles with family members over the past 2 weeks. You reflect back on how exhausting the past couple of weeks have been going to specialist appointments, obtaining diagnostic tests, and seeing loved ones express concern over you. The room is quiet and chilly. It feels so isolating. Nobody can

understand what you are feeling and thinking. Your mind continues to wander back to when you were a child and moves quickly to young adult years of marriage, children, grandchildren, and now the uncertain future.

After what feels like many hours (but in reality is only 15 min), the health care professional walks into the room. At the same time you begin to ask yourself if there is a difference in the professional's demeanor, eye contact, or body language during the initial greeting. The health care professional sits down next to you and discusses the diagnostic test results that indicate a diagnosis of head and neck cancer. You feel the floor collapse under you, and the health care professional's words begin to sound morphed and distant. Your mind begins speaking to itself in circles. What will I do now? How will this affect my family? Will I be able to continue working as I receive treatment? What is my prognosis? I want to live to see my grandchildren graduate college, and I have many more unfinished dreams that I want to experience.

Following a diagnosis of head and neck cancer, oftentimes diagnostic tests, procedures, and treatments become the focus of care. In this technologically advanced and driven society, we expect expedited and accurate diagnoses with quick cures for illnesses. The health care system reimbursement system does not provide financial incentives for extended discussions with patients in order to determine what is the best individualized plan of care. This plan of care requires the medical team to take into account the patient's past, current, and future life, within the context of this new diagnosis. It is time consuming to have lengthy discussions with the patient about their preferences for care, and quite often patients defer to the bias of their physician on a course of treatment that may or may not be focused upon the medical condition, and not the total life experience of the patient. Ideally, these life experiences, perspectives about life, and personal goals should drive the course of treatment to ensure humanistic quality care that includes their entire life-span experiences into the plan of care.

INCORPORATION OF NARRATIVE THEORY

Incorporation of narrative theory and a humanistic approach to the provision of care for cancer patients inform the health care professional as to the patients' values and goals. Just as any patient, patients with head and neck cancer want kind, humane, honest, and trustworthy relationships with the health care professionals who care for them. Many patients and their families assume that only ethical, humanistic, empathetic, and compassionate care will be provided over the course of their loved one's illness, treatment, and recovery.

How can this be achieved? What is the solution? How can confidence and trust in the patient–health care professional relationship be nurtured? Advancing technology that is meant to increase proficiency and the provision of quality care actually places greater time constraints on the health care professionals' ability to provide quality and humanistic care. Patients want their life narratives to be heard. They want their individual needs to be met. There needs to be a balance between science, technology, and the art of medicine to provide care that truly is individualized to the patient's experience during the time of illness.

A patient's sense of dignity is at risk when he or she receives a diagnosis of head and neck cancer or is suffering. Thoughts of being a burden to family members, experiencing invasion of privacy when receiv-

ing care from health care professionals, altered body appearance, and humiliation over requiring assistance during illness can result in a loss of dignity.

Health care professionals are expected to learn and follow the patient's wishes for care to prevent loss of dignity. The health care professionals working in this field need to ask themselves if the patient is receiving humanistic care, which includes high-quality, dignified, and ethical care. Again privacy and autonomy are often affected when receiving care in hospitals or rehabilitation centers. Patients with head and neck cancer have humanistic needs, which are often forgotten and replaced by a focus on the disease process and requisite regimented medical care. Having meaningful conversations and the inclusion of humanistic needs into the provision of care is often perceived as lower priority in comparison to medical needs. Patient rights, autonomy, and self-determination can be lost when receiving in-patient care at a health care facility.

From the moment we are born, every human being is immersed into a life of listening to and communicating with other human beings through storytelling. Health care professionals (physicians, nurses, respiratory therapists, nursing assistants, ancillary staff, etc.) gather objective and subjective data from patients as a means of determining how to diagnose and provide the best care to achieve patient wellness. Communication between human beings requires at least two people: a sender (person telling a narrative) and a receiver (person engaged in listening to the narrative). Communication between two people also consists of objective data in the form of nonverbal information, such as body language and facial expression. Objective data that are congruent with storytellers' verbal statements, known as subjective data, provide validity about the narrative.

Katherine Montgomery Hunter, professor of Medical Humanities and Bioethics, Northwestern University, states, "Medicine is fundamentally narrative—especially the scientific medicine practiced in a tertiary-care teaching hospital—and its daily practice is filled with stories" (Hunter, 1991). Each individual in this world has different life events that occur during our existence on earth. Interpretation and reaction to life events is very personal and unique to each human being. The patients' culture, spirituality, personal preferences, family influence, societal, and socioeconomic factors often play a large part in a person's decisions and actions toward life events. The only way to understand and include meaningful self-experience of a patient in the delivery of individualized care is to incorporate narrative. A patient with head and neck cancer may not be able to communicate their narrative verbally. To facilitate consistent alternative methods of communication, health care professionals could obtain the patient narrative by use of tablets, alphabet boards, lip reading, electrolarynx (artificial larynx), or a tracheoesophageal puncture valve (Passy-Muir valve). Life does not end for a patient diagnosed with head and neck cancer. Life gains greater meaning in the patient narrative including the patients' life experience prior to the illness, the life path that has been redirected to include the patients' illness, and the patients' future plans and goals.

For example, a 60-year-old female patient received a diagnosis of Stage II head and neck cancer that changed the future course of life by changing her formerly active lifestyle to one of radiation, surgery, chemotherapy, speech and language rehabilitation, follow-up diagnostic tests, medical appointments, and recovery. Depending on the course of treatment and rehabilitation results, multiple aspects of the patient's usual lifestyle could be affected: communication, and ability to eat and swallow food, degree of appetite, breathing and speaking abilities, personal relationships, employment, and psychosocial function.

Looking at the big picture, the head and neck cancer diagnosis changes the course of future events for a patient, but past events remain the same. Each of these events has meaning for individuals and is part of a bigger narrative about his or her life. The patient's past positive and negative life experiences remain important to the patient and are a factor in the patients' decision-making process about his or her care.

Health care professionals all too often impose their own values and care models on the patient, not taking into account the effects of the patient's past life experiences. The provision of health care needs to be collaboratively developed based on the patients' preferences and previous life experiences. Patient-centered, realistic, and measurable goals should be mutually decided on by the patient and health care professional, based on the patients' narration. Health care professionals should respond to and provide care with the intent of assisting the patient in achieving the best outcome possible. Relationships between patients and health care professionals must be based on an open and honest exchange of information. There must be mutual respect and trust between the patient seeking care and the attending health care professional. The ethical principles of autonomy, beneficence, nonmaleficence, and justice must, at all times, guide the intent and provision of care provided to patients with head and neck cancer.

In conclusion, patients must trust and openly confide accurate personal information in order for health care professionals to understand and collaboratively determine the best treatment plan for the patient. Greater patient compliance to a health care professional's advice or medical treatments occurs when the patient trusts the health care professional's good intent and resultant decisions. Once the patient develops a trusting and honest relationship with the health care professional, the patient will begin his or her narrative, and healing can begin for the head and neck cancer patient.

REFLECTION AND ANALYSIS FOR FURTHER STUDY

1. What are three specific actions that you could take when evaluating a patient for the first time, to foster a humanistic approach to care?
2. What is more important, professional expertise or humanistic manner when dealing with patients? Why?
3. Why do you think medicine moved away from a humanistic focus? What should be done to move it back?

REFERENCE

Montgomery Hunter, K. (1991). *Doctors' stories: The narrative structure of medical knowledge.* Princeton, NJ: Princeton University Press.

BIBLIOGRAPHY

Centers for Disease Control and Prevention. (2015). *National Vital Statistics System (NVSS)* 2013. Retrieved from http://www.cdc.gov/nchs/deaths.htm

Charon, R. (2001). Narrative medicine: A model for empathy, reflection, profession, and trust. *JAMA, 286*(15), 1897–1902. Retrieved from http://jama.jamanetwork.com/article.aspx?articleid=194300

Kavanagh, K. (2015). *Long-term care (ltc) residents' perceptions of care after humanistic patient narrative theory in-service training to ltc healthcare professionals.* Ann Arbor, MI: Proquest.

Pellegrino, E., & Thomasma, D. (1988). *For the patient's good: Restoration of beneficence in health care.* New York, NY: Oxford University Press.

Pellegrino, E., & Thomasma. D. (1996). *The Christian virtues in medical practice.* Washington, DC: Georgetown University Press.

Polkinghorne, D. (1991). Narrative and self-concept. *Journal of Narrative and Life History, 1*(2&3), 135–136. Retrieved from http://www.pasadena.edu/library/reserves/tfkeeler/engl1c/polkinghornenarrativeselfconcept.pdf

22

Health Literacy Implications for Head and Neck Cancer Patients

Kristie Hadden, Richard I. Zraick, and Samuel R. Atcherson

INTRODUCTION

Head and neck cancer information is often misunderstood by patients; even terms that seem basic to health professionals, like *tumor, malignant*, and *benign* are difficult for many patients to understand (Davis et al., 2001; Davis, Williams, Marin, Parker, & Glass, 2002; List, Lacey, Hopkins, & Burton, 1994). Health literacy can be a significant barrier to understanding for patients, and can affect interactions with health professionals, health decisions, self-care, and treatment outcomes. According to the Institute of Medicine (IOM), health literacy is defined as "the degree to which individuals have the capacity to obtain, process, and understand basic health information and services needed to make appropriate health decisions (Nielson-Bohlman, Panzer, & Kindig, 2004). According to the American Medical Association (AMA), health literacy is a stronger predictor of health status than age, income, employment status, education level, or racial and ethnic group (American Medical Association, 1999). Researchers have demonstrated that low patient health literacy is associated with many negative health consequences. Patients with lower health literacy are more likely to misuse health services (Bennett, Chen, Soroui, & White, 2009; Scott, Gazmararian, Williams, & Baker, 2002), have less knowledge about medical conditions and treatment (Arnold et al., 2001; Kalichman,

Catz, & Ramachandran, 1999; Schillinger et al., 2002; Williams, Baker, Parker, & Nurss, 1998), have higher rates of hospitalization (Baker et al., 2002; Baker, Parker, Williams, & Clark, 1998; Baker, Parker, Williams, Clark, & Nurss, 1997), have poorer health status (Baker et al., 2002), have higher health care costs (Baker et al., 2002; Baker et al., 1998; Howard, Gazmararian, & Parker, 2005; Scott et al., 2002), and have worse psychological effects than patients with higher health literacy (Parikh, Parker, Nurss, Baker, & Williams, 1996). Patients with lower health literacy also experience more serious medication errors (Schillinger, Machtinger, Wang, Rodriguez, & Bindman, 2005), overutilization of emergency departments (Baker et al., 2002), underutilization of preventive care, and increased mortality (Bostock & Steptoe, 2012; Sudore et al., 2009) compared to patients with adequate health literacy.

Unfortunately, low health literacy is common in the United States. The most recent results of the National Assessment of Adult Literacy (NAAL) illustrated that more than 36% of American adults scored at basic or below basic levels. This suggests that nearly 77 million Americans lack the health literacy skills needed to manage and prevent disease and to promote healthy communities (Baur, 2010). Research has revealed disease status, education, and race/ethnicity influence individuals' health literacy. Those at highest risk for low health literacy are older adults, adults with chronic diseases, those who have not attended any college, and those who self-identify as members of a racial minority group (Kutner, Greenberg, Jin, Paulsen, & White, 2006).

Although it is known that individual health literacy poses challenges to patients as well as the health systems that exist to provide them care, the problem and solution do not rest exclusively with the patient. Recent national and international commentary and research agendas in health literacy highlight the two sides of health literacy: the individual skills side, as well as the provider/health demands side. This literature identifies the problem with health literacy as being a mismatch between these two sides—that is, when the demands of health systems and/or providers outweigh the skills of the individual patient (Berkman et al., 2004; Davis et al., 1998; Davis, Michielutte, Askov, Williams, & Weiss, 1998).

The AMA describes patient health literacy as a complex "constellation of skills." These skills were divided into the following domains by the IOM expert panel on Health Literacy: (a) cultural and conceptual knowledge; (b) oral literacy, including speaking and listening skills; (c) print literacy, including writing and reading skills; and (d) numeracy (Baker, 2006). Language and communication are key elements of these skills and are required for patients to access health services, describe and discuss symptoms, answer questions, understand medical instructions, and ask relevant health care questions (Hester & Stevens-Ratchford, 2009). The "demand" side of health literacy includes the complexity of any health information and the effectiveness in which it is communicated. In this context, health information includes the information patients need to navigate their care, as well as understand their disease, the risks and benefits of treatments, implications of informed consent, and any other information that could affect patients' health. Individuals with communication disorders, including head and neck cancer patients, are at increased risk for health literacy challenges because of the high health information demands associated with cancer, as well as many predisposing factors that may be present that affect patient skills.

Because health literacy challenges are common, and because patients may feel ashamed or embar-

rassed to acknowledge when information is difficult to understand, health professionals may not be able to predict which patients have these challenges, or when these challenges may occur; in studies, physicians consistently overestimate patient health literacy level (Bass, III, Wilson, Griffith, & Barnett, 2002; Davis et al., 1998; Davis, Crouch, Wills, Miller, & Abdehou, 1990; Doak, Root, & Doak, 1996; Kelly & Haidet, 2007; Roter, 2005). Although there are known contributors to health literacy like age, race, and educational status, not all patients who are at risk for low health literacy struggle all of the time, and not all patients who are not at risk understand health information in all situations. Health literacy can therefore be considered a "hidden" problem (Rutherford et al., 2006). In order to ensure that all head and neck cancer patients understand the complicated information associated with combined modality management, treatment for cancer effects and side effects, complex care plans, multiple medication regimens, discharge plans, and survivorship information, a "universal precautions" approach to addressing health literacy is recommended (Dewalt et al., 2010). Just as with hidden blood-borne infections, health literacy universal precautions promote safe practices to ensure that all patients are protected, because you do not know who may be affected. These health literacy practices address spoken and written information, patient self-management, and supportive resources (Dewalt et al., 2010). By using a universal precautions approach to improve communication with patients, health professionals lessen the health literacy demands on the patient, communicating health information in ways that are easy to understand.

CHALLENGES TO UNDERSTANDING WRITTEN AND SPOKEN INFORMATION IN THE HEAD AND NECK CANCER CLINIC

The patient with head and neck cancer is faced with many challenges when receiving care within a comprehensive head and neck clinic. From the preoperative stage to the early postoperative stage to the postdischarge stage, patients and their caregivers are required to process an abundance of written and spoken health information. An early challenge, present upon the first visit to a new provider, is the multitude of medical case history forms that need to be filled out. Such forms are oftentimes filled with medical jargon and complex medical terms that can be difficult for patients to comprehend. Patients may rely upon a spouse or other caregiver to help them fill out the forms, yet that caregiver may also struggle with lower health literacy. Oftentimes, patients feel pressured to complete the forms in a timely manner, or in a busy waiting room environment, and such pressures may impact the patient's ability to provide accurate and complete information. Patients may be coming into the clinic with a constellation of fears and concerns related to their cancer diagnosis, and may not be in the ideal mindset to work through the more challenging questions presented on the case history forms.

Challenges for the patient may continue as they begin seeing nurses, physicians, therapists, and others involved in their care. Each specialist may have his or her own set of medical jargon and terminology, and idiosyncratic professional communication style, and may not be adept at gauging whether the patient truly understands the information that is being presented. Oftentimes, written information such as preoperative instructions, postoperative instructions, and general self-care guidelines are shared with patients in an effort to make the clinical interaction more expedient and supply material for the patient to refer to for future reference. One has to wonder how often a patient leaves the clinic believing he understands the procedure/surgery he has consented to, what is expected of him, or what is to come, only to get home and discover that he does not fully understand what he is about to experience. In an effort to better understand, he may turn to written supplemental instructions, only to find that he cannot fully comprehend what is written.

Postoperatively, patients are faced with many changes in the physical, psychological, social, and communication domains. Across these domains, it is incumbent upon clinicians to provide information at a level that can be understood by the patient and his or her caregiver. This is perhaps no more evident than in the management of self-care practices. Patients'

concerns include management of tracheostomy tubes, voice prostheses, speaking valves, and vents, bathing and personal hygiene, stoma care, clothing and stoma covers, adjustments in eating, treatment of minor respiratory ailments, activities and social involvement, communication difficulties, and awareness of potential problems and follow-up care (Roberts, 1994). Even the patient with adequate health literacy can easily become overwhelmed with the many changes he or she is facing. In the face of these challenges, the patient with lower health literacy is at increased risk of poorer postoperative outcomes.

Numeracy

In addition to struggling to understand cancer terms, instructions, and concepts, many patients lack adequate numeracy skills to comprehend and make informed decisions based on risks and probabilities (Davis et al., 1996; Lipkus, Samsa, & Rimer, 2001; Schwartz & Woloshin, 1997; Woloshin, Schwartz, Black, & Welch, 1999; Woloshin, Schwartz, Moncur, Gabriel, & Tosteson, 2001). Numeracy refers to a patient's quantitative skills and comfort with numerical expressions. As with health literacy, low numeracy is common in the United States; only 9% of Americans scored in the highest level of numeracy proficiency in a recent national survey (Centers for Disease Control and Prevention, 2014a). Head and neck cancer patients with low health literacy may have difficulty understanding risks associated with a particular medication or procedure, medication dosing, lab results, and even time schedules for appointments. The universal precautions approach to health literacy best practices supports simplifying numerical information for all patients, without assuming that some patients will understand and others will not. Numbers are important for decision making for all patients, and patients can struggle with numbers at any time. There are guidelines which can make numerical information that health professionals present to head and neck patients clearer and easier to understand, which can maximize the likelihood that appropriate health decisions are made (Centers for Disease Control and Prevention, 2014a; 2014b).

REDUCING HEALTH LITERACY DEMANDS FOR HEAD AND NECK CANCER PATIENTS

In order to reduce health literacy demands for head and neck cancer patients, health providers must consider the manner in which information is delivered to their patients. Health information is most often shared in two primary forms: spoken and written language. Spoken language is further understood to include both speaking (oral literacy) and listening (aural literacy) skills (Baker, 2006; Nouri & Rudd, 2015). For most patients, these two forms of information sharing are reasonable approaches provided that they can understand what they hear and what they read. For the average patient, health literacy demands can be reduced by using plain language (U.S. Department of Health and Human Services, n.d.) described as follows: Plain language is a strategy to meet patients where they are by speaking "plainly" (i.e., oral literacy on the part of the health provider) and providing health materials that are written "plainly." However, the concept of using plain language does not mean to oversimplify or "dumb down" information. Rather, plain language is about effective communication with a goal toward comprehension, compliance, and positive outcomes. The discussion and clarification of technical and medical terms is appropriate when using everyday examples, while also reducing or avoiding medical jargon as much as possible. The teach-back method described later in this chapter is a highly effective plain language strategy (Nouri & Rudd, 2015; Schillinger et al., 2003). For written materials, the NAAL revealed an estimated seventh- or eighth-grade average reading comprehension level for English-speaking adults in the United States (Kutner et al., 2006). To facilitate increased reading comprehension, however, it is recommended that health-related materials targeted to adults be written at the fifth- to sixth-grade reading level (Doak et al., 1996; Safeer & Keenan, 2005; Weiss & Coyne, 1997). The health literacy demand of written materials can be further reduced by ensuring that the information is suitable and user friendly, particularly in the manner in which it is displayed and organized (Doak et al., 1996; Meade & Smith, 1991). It is important to understand that everyone, regardless of education or expertise, may have difficulty understanding health information at one point or another. This is particularly true, for example, when head and neck cancer terminology is unfamiliar or when the diagnosis or prognosis of head and neck cancer is shared with the patient. Having a social support system and time to process information may be helpful in the long run.

For some patients the use of plain language will not be enough. Specifically, the plain-language strategies described previously may not be adequate when patients have (a) limited English proficiency, (b) cultural differences relative to the provider or providers, (c) lack of knowledge and experience, and/or (d) communication or other developmental disorders (Hester & Stevens-Ratchford, 2009; McKee & Paasche-Orlow, 2012; U.S. Department of Health and Human Services, n.d.). Health care providers who serve head and neck cancer patients can make a concerted effort to improve patient-provider communication by having a general fund of knowledge regarding speech-language-hearing disorders and cultural competency issues, and the ability to locate or access resources (e.g., qualified interpreters or materials in languages other than English) to address any of these areas.

Making Written Information More Understandable

Written information about head and neck cancer and treatment and management options can come in many forms including brochures, fact sheets, and electronic media. During office consultations, any of these resources can be provided, and it is the responsibility of the health provider to ensure that the information is readable, suitable, and user friendly. Evaluation of readability, suitability, and user-friendliness of written materials is already evident in a wide variety of health care disciplines and subspecialties including head and neck cancer (Greywoode, Bluman, Spiegel, & Boon, 2009; Hansberry et al., 2014; Kasabwala, Agarwal, Hansberry, Baredes, & Eloy, 2012; Svider et al., 2013) and communication disorders (Atcherson et al., 2014; Caposecco, Hickson, & Meyer, 2011; Zraick & Atcherson, 2012; Zraick, Atcherson, & Ham, 2012).

Many studies focused on the readability of health materials suggest that the reading grade level is incongruent with the health literacy skills of the average patient (i.e., the reading grade level demand is too high). However, when suitability and user-friendliness is considered, comprehension can be maximized. Readability formulas are mathematical computations and, with over 200 different readability formulas that have been put forth, they will each differ in what variables are included (Dubay, 2004). There is no agreed-upon standard for which readability formula to choose (Breese & Burman, 2005); however, two of the most common formulas used include Flesch Reading Ease (FRE) (FLESCH, 1948) and Flesch-Kincaid (F-K) (Kincaid, Fishburne, Rogers, & Chissom, 1975). Both of these formulas are easily available by activating a function in Microsoft Word following a "Spelling & Grammar" check. Alternatively, there are websites that will permit cutting and pasting portions of text for readability analysis as well. In general, the FRE and F-K formulas take into account sentence length and the number of syllables. The F-K formula provides an estimated reading grade level required to comprehend the information, while the FRE formula provides a score from 0 to 100 with 100 being the most readable. Readability forms should not be used in a vacuum, and careful thought and consideration should be taken to ensure that revisions toward improved readability will not alter the intended content of the material. In the case of validated questionnaires, modification should be avoided unless the questionnaire is reevaluated for validity and reliability (Zraick & Atcherson, 2012; Zraick et al., 2012). Hill-Briggs, Schumann, and Dike (2012) offer a five-step method for the evaluation and adaptation of printed patient health materials. Interested readers are encouraged to consult this paper to improve the readability of health materials they design and disseminate.

One of the major limitations of readability formulas is that they do not take into account human and nonhuman factors (Doak et al., 1996; Meade & Smith, 1991). For example, the organization or design of the material can help to ease its readability by use of an abundance of white space, use of bulleted lists, tables, graphics, "chunking" strategies, images, and larger font sizes. Health materials can be made easier to read by ensuring (a) that the content is accurate (Boyer, Selby, & Appel, 1998; Charnock, Shepperd, Needham, & Gann, 1999); (b) that the text size and font optimize legibility (Bernard, Liao, & Mills, 2001; Boyarski, Neuwirth, Forlizzi, & Regli, 1998); and (c) that there is an easy-to-follow layout of patient information and action items (Jacobs, Li, Schrier, Bargeron, & Salesin, 2004; Smith, Hetzel, Dalrymple, & Keselman, 2011). When approached together, improved readability coupled with suitable and user-friendly materials can help to improve dialogue by encouraging questions and seeking clarity on potentially confusing terms, procedures, treatment options, and follow-up care.

Confirming Understanding With Patients

Patients with low health literacy prefer communication about risks and benefits in verbal form over written form (American Medical Association, 1999; Tarn et al., 2006). Although these patients want spoken information from health professionals, they are also less likely to ask questions (Dewalt et al., 2010), making spoken communication an important but challenging communication channel in clinic and inpatient encounters. Compounding the issue, emotional responses in discussions about cancer diagnosis and treatment can also interfere with patients' understanding of verbal health information that is critical to their decision making, future self-care, and treatment outcomes (Berkman et al., 2004; Wicke, Lorge, Coppin, & Jones, 1994).

Patients have the right to understand all health information that is necessary to safely care for themselves, and health professionals have a duty to provide this information in simple, clear, and plain language so that it is understood (U.S.Department of Health and Human Services, 2005). Asking patients, "Do you have any questions?" is not an effective way to assess understanding, because patients are often ashamed and embarrassed to admit that they do not understand even complex information. Head and neck cancer patients are faced with heavy demands of multiple prescription medications, hygiene regimens, stoma care, prosthesis management, and many other issues related to their diagnosis and self-care. Health literacy best practices for verbal patient-provider communication should be used to lessen demands on patients and promote patient understanding of critical information. Confirming understanding with patients is not only a way to assess comprehension on the part of the patient, but it is also a way of taking responsibility for the message to determine how well it was communicated. Because health literacy can be a barrier to effective patient-provider communication, it is recommended that both sides of health literacy be considered, as well as using a universal precautions approach to confirming understanding.

Because patients recall or comprehend as little as half of what physicians convey during an outpatient encounter (Schillinger et al., 2003), it is essential that health professionals use best practices for effective spoken communication. Teach-back is a shame-free way of assessing patient understanding, and when paired with a feedback cycle, provides health professionals the opportunity to clarify information that was not understood. This technique involves first asking the patient to repeat or teach back the information in his or her own words. By taking responsibility for the message in its framing, health professionals can ensure that the patient does not feel like he or she is being tested. Phrases like, "I want to be sure that I explained your stoma care clearly. Can you show me what you will do when you get home?" can reduce the likelihood of shame and embarrassment when patients do not understand, because they focus on the health care professional's communication instead of the patient's skill level.

After the health professional assesses understanding in the teach-back cycle, the patient restates the information in his or her own words. Missing or misunderstood information is then clarified by the health professional and the assessment phrase is restated. This feedback loop continues until the patient recalls and restates all of the essential information conveyed. When understanding is confirmed, the teach-back cycle with feedback loop is complete. This cycle of assess, clarify, and confirm can be practiced and improved as can any communication skill.

Asking that patients recall and restate what they have been told is one of 11 top patient safety practices backed by scientific evidence (Shojania, Duncan, McDonald, Wachter, & Markowitz, 2001). Effective spoken communication techniques like teach-back have been associated with increased patient satisfaction (Ahrens & Wirges, 2013), improved knowledge, medication adherence and diet (Negarandeh, Mahmoodi, Noktehdan, Heshmat, & Shakibazadeh, 2013), more information retention, and lower hospital readmission rates (Healthcare Benchmarks and Quality Improvement, 2011; White, Garbez, Carroll, Brinker, & Howie-Esquivel, 2013). When conducted correctly, using a universal precautions approach, teach-back can improve head and neck cancer patient understanding of information in clinical encounters and lead to improved self-care.

HEALTH LITERACY RESOURCES

Always Use Teach-Back
http://www.teachbacktraining.org/

Teach-Back Method Extra Resources
http://www.nchealthliteracy.org/toolkit/Rheum/tool6xt.pdf

Teach-Back Method Tool 5
http://www.nchealthliteracy.org/toolkit/tool5.pdf

What does your patient really understand?
http://healthliteracymn.org/sites/default/files/images/files/Teach-Back_program_guide_updated_011212.pdf

Teach Back Basics
http://www.ihconline.org/aspx/general/page.aspx?pid=107#Educational_Materials

Centers for Disease Control and Prevention (CDC) Health Literacy Resources
http://www.cdc.gov/healthliteracy/learn/resources.html

Quick Guide to Health Literacy
http://www.health.gov/communication/literacy/quickguide/resources.htm

AHRQ Health Literacy Universal Precautions Toolkit
http://www.ahrq.gov/professionals/quality-patient-safety/quality-resources/tools/literacy-toolkit/

Plain Language Guidelines/Resources
http://www.plainlanguage.gov/

Health Literacy for Public Health Professionals
http://www.cdc.gov/healthliteracy/training/index.html

Effective Communication Tools for Healthcare Professionals
http://www.hrsa.gov/publichealth/healthliteracy/

Culture and Health Literacy Modules
http://cpheo1.sph.umn.edu/healthlit/#a

National Center for the Study of Adult Learning and Literacy
http://www.ncsall.net/index.html@id=25.html

Plain Language Association InterNational
http://www.plainlanguagenetwork.org/Resources/index.html

Health Literacy Special Collection
http://healthliteracy.worlded.org/funding.htm

U.S. National Library of Medicine
http://www.nlm.nih.gov/ep/healthlit.html

A Physician's Practical Guide to Culturally Competent Care
https://cccm.thinkculturalhealth.hhs.gov/

REFLECTION AND ANALYSIS FOR FURTHER STUDY

1. Aside from teach-back methods, what other means of improving health care literacy might be particularly applicable for use with head and neck cancer patients?

2. There is considerable literature discussing the deleterious effects of poor patient-provider communication. Given the reality that patients come from diverse backgrounds and cultures, how might you modify your treatment approach for a patient living in a large metropolitan city versus a patient who lives in a rural community with limited access to high-level medical facilities?

3. A fine line exists between successfully reducing health literacy burdens for patients and

conveying the impression that material is being "dumbed down." Generate specific strategies you would use to convey respect for the patient while still minimizing health literacy burden.

REFERENCES

Ahrens, S. L., & Wirges, A. M. (2013). Using evidence to improve satisfaction with medication side-effects education on a neuro-medical surgical unit. *Journal of Neuroscience Nursing, 45*(5), 281. doi:10.1097/JNN.0b013e31829d8ca5

American Medical Association. (1999). Health literacy: Report of the Council on Scientific Affairs. Ad Hoc Committee on Health Literacy for the Council on Scientific Affairs, American Medical Association. *Journal of the American Medical Association, 281*(6), 552–557.

Arnold, C. L., Davis, T. C., Berkel, H. J., Jackson, R. H., Nandy, I., & London, S. (2001). Smoking status, reading level, and knowledge of tobacco effects among low-income pregnant women. *Preventive Medicine, 32*(4), 313–320. doi:10.1006/pmed.2000.0815

Atcherson, S. R., DeLaune, A. E., Hadden, K., Zraick, R. I., Kelly-Campbell, R. J., & Minaya, C. P. (2014). A computer-based readability analysis of consumer materials on the American Speech-Language-Hearing Association website. *Contemporary Issues in Communication Sciences and Disorders, 41*, 12–23.

Baker, D. W. (2006). The meaning and the measure of health literacy. *Journal of General Internal Medicine, 21*(8), 878–883. doi:10.1111/j.1525-1497.2006.00540.x

Baker, D. W., Gazmararian, J. A., Williams, M. V., Scott, T., Parker, R. M., Green, D., . . . Peel, J. (2002). Functional health literacy and the risk of hospital admission among Medicare managed care enrollees. *American Journal of Public Health, 92*(8), 1278–1283. doi:10.2105/AJPH.92.8.1278

Baker, D. W., Parker, R. M., Williams, M. V., & Clark, W. S. (1998). Health literacy and the risk of hospital admission. *Journal of General Internal Medicine, 13*(12), 791–798. doi:10.1046/j.1525-1497.1998.00242.x

Baker, D. W., Parker, R. M., Williams, M. V., Clark, W. S., & Nurss, J. (1997). The relationship of patient reading ability to self-reported health and use of health services. *American Journal of Public Health, 87*(6), 1027–1030. doi:10.2105/AJPH.87.6.1027

Bass, P. F., III, Wilson, J. F., Griffith, C. H., & Barnett, D. R. (2002). Residents' ability to identify patients with poor literacy skills. *Academic Medicine, 77*(10), 1039–1041.

Baur, C. (2010). New directions in research on public health and health literacy. *Journal of Health Communication, 15*, 42–50. doi:10.1080/10810730.2010.499989

Bennett, I. M., Chen, J., Soroui, J. S., & White, S. (2009). The contribution of health literacy to disparities in self-rated health status and preventive health behaviors in older adults. *Annals of Family Medicine, 7*(3), 204–211. doi:10.1370/afm.940

Berkman, N. D., Dewalt, D. A., Pignone, M. P., Sheridan, S. L., Lohr, K. N., Lux, L., . . . Bonito, A. J. (2004). Literacy and health outcomes. *Evidence Report/Technology Assessment (Summary)*, (87), 1–8.

Bernard, M., Liao, C. H., & Mills, M. (2001). The effects of front type and size on the legibility and reading time of online text by older adults. *CHO '01 Extended Abstracts,* 175–176.

Bostock, S., & Steptoe, A. (2012). Association between low functional health literacy and mortality in older adults: Longitudinal cohort study. *British Medical Journal, 344,* e1602. doi:10.1136/bmj.e1602

Boyarski, D., Neuwirth, C., Forlizzi, J., & Regli, S. H. (1998). A study of fonts designed for screen display. *Proceedings of CHI '98,* 87–94.

Boyer, C., Selby, M., & Appel, R. D. (1998). The Health On the Net Code of Conduct for medical and health web sites. *Student Health Technology Informatics Journal, 52*(Pt. 2), 1163–1166.

Breese, P., & Burman, W. (2005). Readability of notice of privacy forms used by major health care institutions. *Journal of the American Medical Association, 293*(13), 1593–1594. doi:10.1001/jama.293.13.1593

Caposecco, A., Hickson, L., & Meyer, C. (2011). Assembly and insertion of a self-fitting hearing aid: Design of effective instruction materials. *Trends in Amplification, 15*(4), 184–195. doi:10.1177/1084713811430837

Centers for Disease Control and Prevention. (2014a). Understanding literacy and numeracy. *Program for the International Assessment of Adult Competencies, National Center for Education Statistics, U.S. Department of Education.* Retrieved from http://www.cdc.gov/healthliteracy/learn/understandingliteracy.html

Centers for Disease Control and Prevention. (2014b). *Using numbers and explaining risk.* U.S. Department of Health and Human Services. Retrieved from http://www.cdc.gov/healthliteracy/numeracy-course/index.html

Charnock, D., Shepperd, S., Needham, G., & Gann, R. (1999). DISCERN: An instrument for judging the quality of written consumer health information on treatment choices. *Journal of Epidemiology and Community Health, 53,* 105–111.

Davis, T. C., Arnold, C., Berkel, H. J., Nandy, I., Jackson, R. H., & Glass, J. (1996). Knowledge and attitude on screening mammography among low-literate, low-income women. *Cancer, 78*(9), 1912–1920.

Davis, T. C., Berkel, H. J., Arnold, C. L., Nandy, I., Jackson, R. H., & Murphy, P. W. (1998). Intervention to increase mammography utilization in a public hospital. *Journal of General Internal Medicine, 13*(4), 230–233.

Davis, T. C., Crouch, M. A., Wills, G., Miller, S., & Abdehou, D. M. (1990). The gap between patient reading comprehension and the readability of patient education materials. *Journal of Family Practice, 31*(5), 533–538.

Davis, T. C., Dolan, N. C., Ferreira, M. R., Tomori, C., Green, K. W., Sipler, A. M., & Bennett, C. L. (2001). The role of inadequate health literacy skills in colorectal cancer screening. *Cancer Investigation, 19*(2), 193–200.

Davis, T. C., Michielutte, R., Askov, E. N., Williams, M. V., & Weiss, B. D. (1998). Practical assessment of adult literacy in health care. *Health Education and Behavior, 25*(5), 613–624.

Davis, T. C., Williams, M. V., Marin, E., Parker, R. M., & Glass, J. (2002). Health literacy and cancer communication. *CA: A Cancer Journal for Clinicians, 52*(3), 134–153.

Dewalt, D. A., Callahan, L. F., Hawk, V. H., Broucksou, K. A., Hink, A., Rudd, R., & Brach, C. (2010). *Health Literacy Universal Precautions Toolkit* (AHRQ Publication No. 10-0046-EF). Rockville, MD: Agency for Healthcare Research and Quality.

Doak, C. C., Root, J. H., & Doak, L. G. (1996). *Teaching patients with low literacy skills* (2nd ed.). Philadelphia, PA: J.B. Lippincott.

Dubay, W. H. (2004). *The principles of readability.* Costa Mesa, CA: Impact Information.

Flesch, R. (1948). A new readability yardstick. *Journal of Applied Psychology, 32*(3), 221–233.

Greywoode, J., Bluman, E., Spiegel, J., & Boon, M. (2009). Readability analysis of patient information on the American Academy of Otolaryngology-Head and Neck Surgery website. *Otolaryngology-Head and Neck Surgery, 141*(5), 555–558. doi:10.1016/j.otohns.2009.08.004

Hansberry, D. R., Agarwal, N., Shah, R., Schmitt, P. J., Baredes, S., Setzen, M., . . . Eloy, J. A. (2014). Analysis of the readability of patient education materials from surgical subspecialties. *Laryngoscope, 124*(2), 405–412. doi:10.1002/lary.24261

Healthcare Benchmarks and Quality Improvement. (2011). Teach-back program reduces readmissions. *Healthcare Benchmarks and Quality Improvement, 18*(11), 123–125.

Hester, E. J., & Stevens-Ratchford, R. (2009). Health literacy and the role of the speech-language pathologist. *American Journal of Speech-Language Pathology, 18*(2), 180–191.

Hill-Briggs, F., Schumann, K. P., & Dike, O. (2012). Five-step methodology for evaluation and adaptation of print patient health information to meet the <5th grade readability criterion. *Medical Care, 50*(4), 294–301. doi:10.1097/MLR.0b013e318249d6c8

Howard, D. H., Gazmararian, J., & Parker, R. M. (2005). The impact of low health literacy on the medical costs of Medicare managed care enrollees. *American Journal of Medicine, 118*(4), 371–377.

Jacobs, C., Li, W., Schrier, E., Bargeron, B., & Salesin, D. (2004). Adaptive document layout. *Communications of the ACM, 47*(60), 66.

Kalichman, S. C., Catz, S., & Ramachandran, B. (1999). Barriers to HIV/AIDS treatment and treatment adherence among African-American adults with disadvantaged education. *Journal of the National Medical Association, 91*(8), 439–446.

Kasabwala, K., Agarwal, N., Hansberry, D. R., Baredes, S., & Eloy, J. A. (2012). Readability assessment of patient education materials from the American Academy of Otolaryngology-Head and Neck Surgery Foundation.

Otolaryngology-Head and Neck Surgery, 147(3), 466–471. doi:10.1177/0194599812442783

Kelly, P. A., & Haidet, P. (2007). Physician overestimation of patient literacy: A potential source of health care disparities. *Patient Education and Counseling, 66*(1), 119–122. doi:10.1016/j.pec.2006.10.007

Kincaid, J. P., Fishburne, R. P., Rogers, R. L., & Chissom, B. S. (1975). *Derivation of new readability formula for Navy enlisted personnel.* Millington, TN: Navy Research Branch.

Kutner, M., Greenberg, E., Jin, Y., Paulsen, C., & White, S. (2006). *Health literacy of America's adults: Results from the 2003 National Assessment of Adult Literacy.* National Center for Educational Statistics. Retrieved from https://nces.ed.gov/pubs2006/2006483.pdf

Lipkus, I. M., Samsa, G., & Rimer, B. K. (2001). General performance on a numeracy scale among highly educated samples. *Medical Decision Making, 21*(1), 37–44.

List, M. A., Lacey, L., Hopkins, E., & Burton, D. (1994). The involvement of low literate elderly women in the development and distribution of cancer screening materials. *Family and Community Health, 17*(1), 42–55.

McKee, M. M., & Paasche-Orlow, M. K. (2012). Health literacy and the disenfranchised: The importance of collaboration between limited English proficiency and health literacy researchers. *Journal of Health Communication, 17*(Suppl. 3), 7–12. doi:10.1080/10810730.2012.712627

Meade, C. D., & Smith, C. F. (1991). Readability formulas: Cautions and criteria. *Patient Education and Counseling, 17,* 153–158.

Negarandeh, R., Mahmoodi, H., Noktehdan, H., Heshmat, R., & Shakibazadeh, E. (2013). Teach back and pictorial image educational strategies on knowledge about diabetes and medication/dietary adherence among low health literate patients with type 2 diabetes. *Primary Care Diabetes, 7*(2), 111–118. doi:10.1016/j.pcd.2012.11.001

Nielson-Bohlman, L., Panzer, A. M., & Kindig, D. A. (2004). *Health literacy: A prescription to end confusion.* Washington, DC: Institute of Medicine National Academies Press.

Nouri, S. S., & Rudd, R. E. (2015). Health literacy in the "oral exchange": An important element of patient-provider communication. *Patient Education and Counseling, 98*(5), 565–571. doi:10.1016/j.pec.2014.12.002

Parikh, N. S., Parker, R. M., Nurss, J. R., Baker, D. W., & Williams, M. V. (1996). Shame and health literacy: The unspoken connection. *Patient Education and Counseling, 27*(1), 33–39.

Roberts, N. K. (1994). Nursing intervention for the laryngectomee: Management of change in self-care practices following hospitalization. In R.L. Keith & F. L. Darley (Eds.), *Laryngectomee rehabilitation* (3rd ed., pp. 119–132). London, UK: College-Hill Press.

Roter, D. L. (2005). Health literacy and the patient-provider relationship. In J. G. Schwartzberg, J. B. VanGeest, & C. C. Wang (Eds.), *Understanding health literacy: Implications for medicine and public health* (pp. 87–100). Chicago, IL: American Medical Association Press.

Rutherford, J., Holman, R., MacDonald, J., Taylor, A., Jarrett, D., & Bigrigg, A. (2006). Low literacy: A hidden problem in family planning clinics. *Journal of Family Planning and Reproductive Health Care, 32*(4), 235–240. doi:10.1783/14711 8906778586778

Safeer, R. S., & Keenan, J. (2005). Health literacy: The gap between physicians and patients. *American Family Physician, 72*(3), 463–468.

Schillinger, D., Grumbach, K., Piette, J., Wang, F., Osmond, D., Daher, C., . . . Bindman, A. B. (2002). Association of health literacy with diabetes outcomes. *JAMA, 288*(4), 475–482. doi:10.1001/jama.288.4.475

Schillinger, D., Machtinger, E., Wang, F., Rodriguez, M., & Bindman, A. (2005). Preventing medication errors in ambulatory care: The importance of establishing regimen concordance. In K. Henriksen, J. B. Battles, E. S. Marks, & D. Lewin (Eds.), *Advances in patient safety: From research to implementation (Volume 1: Research findings).* Rockville, MD: Agency for Healthcare Research and Quality.

Schillinger, D., Piette, J., Grumbach, K., Wang, F., Wilson, C., Daher, C., . . . Bindman, A. B. (2003). Closing the loop—Physician communication with diabetic patients who have low health literacy. *Archives of Internal Medicine, 163*(1), 83–90. doi:10.1001/archinte.163.1.83

Schwartz, L. M., & Woloshin, S. (1997). The role of numeracy in understanding the benefit of screening mammography. *Annals of Internal Medicine, 127*(11), 966.

Scott, T. L., Gazmararian, J. A., Williams, M. V., & Baker, D. W. (2002). Health literacy and preventive health care use among Medicare enrollees in a managed care organization. *Medical Care, 40*(5), 395–404.

Shojania, K. G., Duncan, B. W., McDonald, K. M., Wachter, R. M., & Markowitz, A. J. (2001). Making health care safer: A critical analysis of patient safety practices. *Evidence Report/Technology Assessment (Summary),*(43), 1–668.

Smith, C. A., Hetzel, S., Dalrymple, P., & Keselman, A. (2011). Beyond readability: Investigating coherence of clinical text for consumers. *Journal of Medical Internet Research, 13*(4), e104. doi:v13i4e104 [pii];10.2196/jmir.1842

Sudore, R. L., Landefeld, C. S., Perez-Stable, E. J., Bibbins-Domingo, K., Williams, B. A., & Schillinger, D. (2009). Unraveling the relationship between literacy, language proficiency, and patient-physician communication. *Patient Education and Counseling, 75*(3), 398–402. doi:10.1016/j.pec.2009.02.019

Svider, P. F., Agarwal, N., Choudhry, O. J., Hajart, A. F., Baredes, S., Liu, J. K., & Eloy, J. A. (2013). Readability assessment of online patient education materials from academic otolaryngology-head and neck surgery departments. *American Journal of Otolaryngology, 34*(1), 31–35. doi:10.1016/j.amjoto.2012.08.001

Tarn, D. M., Paterniti, D. A., Heritage, J., Hays, R. D., Kravitz, R. L., & Wenger, N. S. (2006). Physician communication about the cost and acquisition of newly prescribed medications. *American Journal of Managed Care, 12*(11), 657–664.

U.S. Department of Health and Human Services. (n.d.). *Plain language: A promising strategy for clearly communicating health information and improving health literacy.* Office of Disease Prevention and Promotion. Retrieved from http://www.health.gov/communication/literacy/plain language/PlainLanguage.htm

U.S. Department of Health and Human Services. (2005). *Proceedings from the 2005 White House Conference on Aging Mini-Conference on Health Literacy and Health Disparities.* Chicago, IL: American Medical Association.

Weiss, B. D., & Coyne, C. (1997). Communicating with patients who cannot read. *New England Journal of Medicine, 337*(4), 272–274. doi:10.1056/NEJM199707243370411

White, M., Garbez, R., Carroll, M., Brinker, E., & Howie-Esquivel, J. (2013). Is "teach-back" associated with knowledge retention and hospital readmission in hospitalized heart failure patients? *Journal of Cardiovascular Nursing, 28*(2), 137–146.

Wicke, D. M., Lorge, R. E., Coppin, R. J., & Jones, K. P. (1994). The effectiveness of waiting room notice-boards as a vehicle for health education. *Family Practice, 11*(3), 292–295. doi:10.1093/fampra/11.3.292

Williams, M. V., Baker, D. W., Parker, R. M., & Nurss, J. R. (1998). Relationship of functional health literacy to patients' knowledge of their chronic disease. A study of patients with hypertension and diabetes. *Archives of Internal Medicine, 158*(2), 166–172.

Woloshin, S., Schwartz, L. M., Black, W. C., & Welch, H. G. (1999). Women's perceptions of breast cancer risk: How you ask matters. *Medical Decision Making, 19*(3), 221–229.

Woloshin, S., Schwartz, L. M., Moncur, M., Gabriel, S., & Tosteson, A. (2001). Assessing values for health: Numeracy matters. *Medical Decision Making, 21*(5), 382–390. doi:10.1177/0272989X0102100505

Zraick, R. I., & Atcherson, S. R. (2012). Readability of patient-reported outcome questionnaires for use with persons with dysphonia. *Journal of Voice, 26*(5), 635–641. doi:10.1016/j.jvoice.2011.01.009

Zraick, R. I., Atcherson, S. R., & Ham, B. K. (2012). Readability of patient-reported outcome questionnaires for use with persons with swallowing disorders. *Dysphagia, 27*(3), 346–352. doi:10.1007/s00455-011-9373-x

APPENDIX A

Abbreviations

ADL	Activity of daily living
AUC	Area-under-the-curve
CAD	Coronary artery disease
COPD	Chronic obstructive pulmonary disease
CRT	Chemoradiation therapy *or* Cognitive rehabilitation treatment
CSE	Clinical swallowing evaluation
CT	Computed tomography
CXR	Chest x-ray
DHT	Dobhoff tube
DML	Direct microlaryngoscopy
EAT-10	Eating Assessment Tool
EGD	Esophagogastroduodenoscopy
EGFR	Epidermal growth factor receptor
EKG	Electrocardiogram
EUA	Examination under anesthesia
FDG PET/CT	Fluorodeoxyglucose F18 positron emission tomography
FEES	Fiberoptic endoscopic evaluation of swallowing
FNA	Fine-needle aspiration
FOIS	Functional Oral Intake Scale
FR	*Federal Register*
FU	Follow-up *or* 5-flouro-uracil (a chemotherapeutic agent)
GERD	Gastroesophageal reflux disease

Gy	Gray (a unit of radiation therapy dose)
HBO	Hyperbaric oxygen
HME	Heat moisture exchange
HNC	Head and neck cancer
HNSCC	Head and neck squamous cell carcinoma
HPV	Human papillomavirus
HTN	Hypertension
IGRT	Image-guided radiation therapy
IMRT	Intensity-modulated radiation therapy
LPR	Laryngopharyngeal reflux
M-Stages	M0: No metastasis to other organs M1: Distant metastasis present
MAR	Medication administration record device
MBS	Modified barium swallow
MBSImP	Modified Barium Swallow Impairment Profile
MBSS	Modified barium swallow study
MDADI	M.D. Anderson Dysphagia Inventory
MI	Myocardial infarction
MRI	Magnetic resonance imaging
N-Stages	NX: Regional lymph nodes cannot be assessed N0: No palpable regional nodes N1: <3 cm in a single node N2a: 3 to 6 cm in single node N2b: Two or more nodes <6 cm N2c: Contralateral or bilateral nodes <6 cm N3: Metastatic node size >6 cm
NG	Nasogastric
NGT	Nasogastric tube
NPO	Nothing by mouth
OPSCC	Oropharyngeal squamous cell carcinoma
OSA	Obstructive sleep apnea
p16	A surrogate marker for HPV-16

PAS	Penetration-Aspiration Scale
PCA	Patient-controlled analgesia
PEG	Percutaneous endoscopic gastrostomy
PET	Positron emission tomography
PET-CT	Positron emission tomography–computed tomography
PO	By mouth
QoL	Quality of life
RAD	Radiation-associated dysphagia
RT	Radiation therapy
SCC	Squamous cell carcinoma
SES	Socioeconomic status
SICU	Surgical intensive care unit
SIT	Sensory integration treatment
SLP	Speech-language pathology/pathologist
SUV	Standardized uptake value (reported in PET scans)
T-Stages	Tx: Tumor cannot be evaluated Tis: Carcinoma in situ T0: No signs of tumor T1, T2, T3, T4: Size and/or extension of the primary tumor
TE	Tracheoesphogeal
TEP	Tracheoesophageal prosthesis
TL	Total laryngectomy
TNM	Tumor, nodes, metastasis—Tumor staging system
TOLM	Transoral laser microsurgery
TORS	Transoral robotic surgery
UES	Upper esophageal sphincter
UW-QOL	University of Washington Quality of Life Questionnaire
VFSS	Videofluoroscopic swallow study
VLS	Visible light spectroscopy

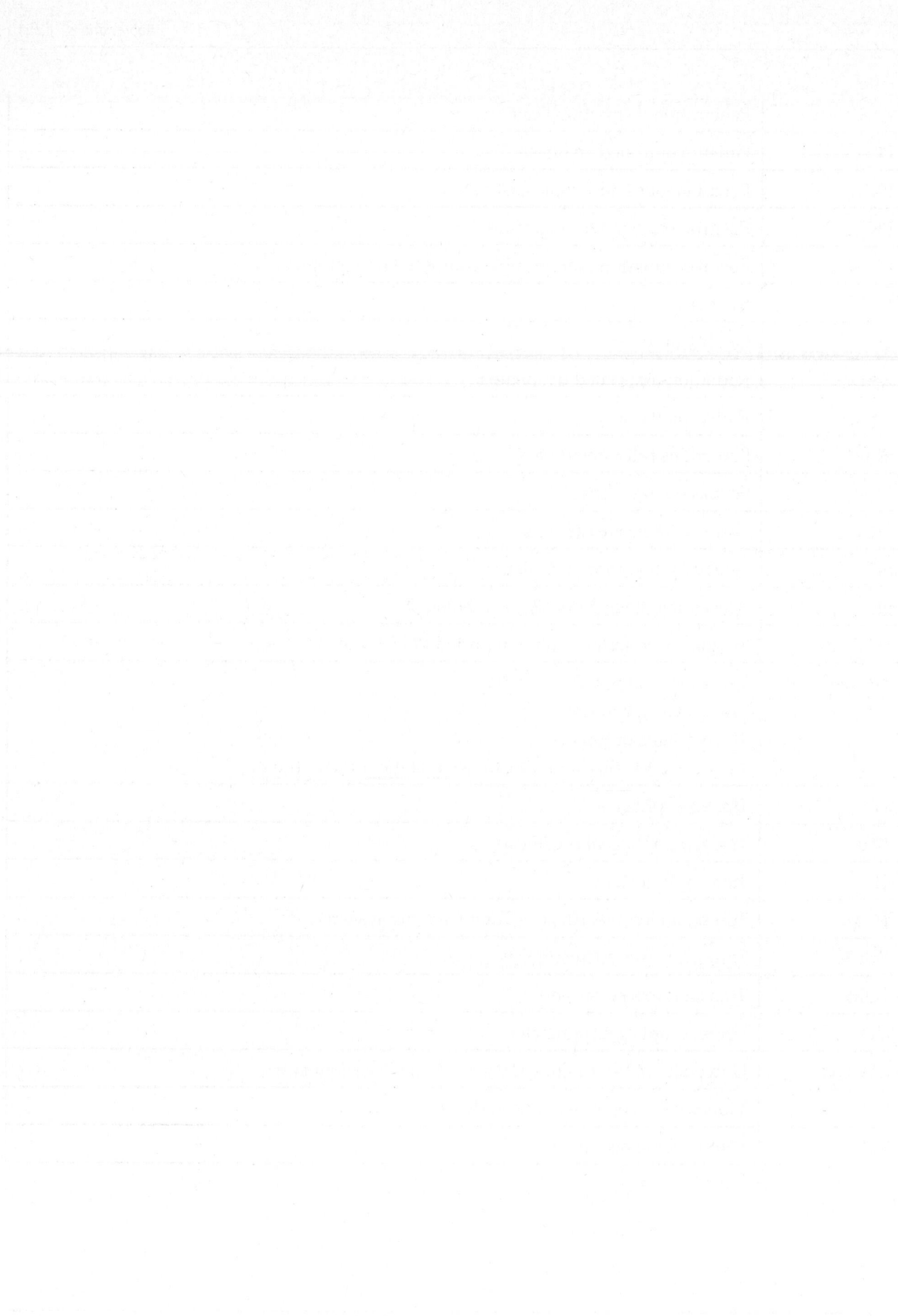

APPENDIX B

Consulted References for Glossary

http://www.asha.org

http://www.atosmedical.com/

http://www.cancernetwork.com/ars-2015/late-radiation-associated-dysphagia-late-rad-lower-cranial-neuropathy-after-oropharyngeal-imrt

http://dictionary.reference.com

http://www.electrolarynx.com/pages/catalog/SV02.html

http://www.hani-shaker.com/

http://www.practicalslpinfo.com/

http://www.hopkinsmedicine.org/

http://www.icr.ac.uk/our-research/our-research-centres/clinical-trials-and-statistics-unit/clinical-trials/parsport

Whittle, J., & Mythen, M. (2011). Anesthesiologist's manual of surgical procedures. *BJA: The British Journal of Anaesthesia, 106*(4), 611–612.

http://www.mdanderson.org/education-and-research/departments-programs-and-labs/departments-and-divisions/symptom-research/symptom-assessment-tools/MDASI_userguide.pdf

http://www.medicinenet.com

http://www.medilexicon.com

http://www.medscape.com/

http://www.merriam-webster.com/

http://www.nlm.nih.gov/

http://www.nlm.nih.gov/medlineplus/medlineplus.htm

http://path.upmc.edu/cases/case626/dx.html

http://psychiatry.duke.edu/divisions/geriatric-behavioral-health/geriatric-epidemiology/older-americans-resources-and-services-

http://www.researchgate.net/profile/James_Coyle/publication/14481478_A_penetration-aspiration_scale/links/00b7d5374ef977950b000000.pdf

http://www.researchgate.net/publication/43553645_McNeill_Dysphagia_Therapy_Program_A_Case-Control_Study

http://www.speechpathology.com/

Venes, D., & Taber, C. W. (2013). *Taber's cyclopedic medical dictionary.* Philadelphia, PA: F.A. Davis.

Uloza, V., Vegienė, A., Pribuišienė, R., & Šaferis, V. (2013). Quantitative evaluation of video laryngostroboscopy: Reliability of the basic parameters. *Journal of Voice, 27*(3), 361–368.

https://vula.uct.ac.za/access/content/group/ba5fb1bd-be95-48e5-81be-586fbaeba29d/Pectoralis%20major%20flap-1.pdf

Glossary

5-Flourouracil. A nucleoside metabolic inhibitor. The mechanism of action of fluorouracil is as a nucleic acid synthesis inhibitor.

Acneiform. Resembling acne.

Acuity. Sharpness, clearness, and distinctness of perception or vision.

Adenocarcinoma. A malignant neoplasm of epithelial cells with a glandular or glandlike pattern.

Adjuvant. In context of cancer therapy, any additional treatment modality added after the primary treatment modality. Radiation therapy can be adjuvant as well, when delivered after surgery.

Aerodigestive. Denoting that part of the respiratory and digestive tracts that course in common through the pharyngeal and cervical regions.

Alaryngeal Communicator. A method of speech used after laryngectomy.

Alloderm. Acellular dermis used for reconstruction following resection of tumor.

Alveolar Ridge. The ridgelike border of the upper and lower jaws containing the sockets of the teeth.

Alveolus. A small angular cavity or pit, such as a tooth socket or an air sac.

Anastomosis. The connection of separate parts of a branching system to form a network, especially among blood vessels, used in free-flap reconstruction after tumor resection.

Ancillary. Relating to or being auxiliary or secondary.

Angiogram. An angiographic x-ray of blood vessels used in diagnosing pathological conditions of the cardiovascular system.

Anosmia. Lack of the sense of smell.

Antiemetic. Preventing or arresting vomiting.

Aphonic. Mouthed but not spoken; noiseless; silent.

Arthritis. Inflammation of a joint or joints resulting in pain and swelling.

Articulator. A mechanical device representing the temporomandibular joints and the jaw bones, used in dentistry to obtain proper articulation of artificial teeth.

Aryepiglottic. Pertaining to or connecting the arytenoid cartilage and the epiglottis.

Arytenoid. Pertaining to either of two small cartilages on top of the cricoid cartilage at the upper, back part of the larynx.

Arytenoid Cartilage. One of a pair of small triangular pyramidal laryngeal cartilages that articulate with the lamina of the cricoid cartilage. It gives attachment at its anteriorly directed vocal process to the posterior part of the corresponding vocal ligament and to several muscles at its laterally directed muscular process. The base of the cartilage is hyaline, but the apex is elastic.

Aspiration. The act of removing a fluid, as pus or serum, from a cavity of the body, by a hollow needle or trocar connected with a suction syringe. Also, lack of airway protection from pharyngeal content. Fine-needle aspiration often results in removal of cells from a solid mass in the body.

Asymmetric. Not identical on both sides of a central line; unsymmetrical; lacking symmetry

Atelectasis. Incomplete expansion of the lungs, as from lack of breathing force.

Atherosclerosis. A form of arteriosclerosis characterized by the deposition of plaques containing cholesterol and lipids on the innermost layer of the walls of large- and medium-sized arteries.

Atraumatic Technique. Surgical technique minimizing intraoperative tissue damage, to maximize healing and minimize risk of subsequent tissue necrosis or infection.

Atrophy. A wasting or decrease in the size of an organ or tissue, as from death and reabsorption of cells, diminished cellular proliferation, pressure, ischemia, malnutrition, decreased function, or hormonal changes.

Audiology. The scientific study of hearing, often including the treatment of persons with hearing defects.

Audiometry. The testing of hearing by means of an audiometer.

Barium. Barium compounds are used in x-raying the digestive system and in making fireworks and white pigments.

Barium Contrast. A fine white powder used as a pigment and as a contrast medium in x-ray photography of the digestive tract.

Benign. Denoting the mild character of an illness or the nonmalignant character of a neoplasm.

Bilateral. Having or formed of two sides; two-sided.

Binucleated. Having two nuclei.

Biofilm. A complex structure adhering to surfaces that are regularly in contact with water, consisting of colonies of bacteria and usually other microorganisms such as yeasts, fungi, and protozoa that secrete a mucilaginous protective coating in which they are encased.

Biopsy. The removal and examination of a sample of tissue from a living body for diagnostic purposes.

Bolus. A soft, roundish mass or lump, especially of chewed food.

Bronchoscopy. An examination by means of a bronchoscope.

Buccal. Pertaining to, adjacent to, or in the direction of the cheek.

Bucco-Gingival. Relating to the cheek and the gum; more commonly referred to as gingivobuccal.

Candida. A genus of the potentially pathogenic yeastlike fungi.

Cannula. A flexible tube, usually containing a trocar at one end, that is inserted into a bodily cavity, duct, or vessel to drain fluid or administer a substance such as a medication. Can also refer to the rigid tubing of a tracheostomy.

Carboplatin. A platinum-containing anticancer agent much like cisplatin but more toxic to the myeloid elements of bone marrow while producing less nausea and neuro-, oto-, and nephrotoxicity; used in the chemotherapy of solid tumors.

Carcinoma. An invasive malignant tumor derived from epithelial tissue that tends to metastasize to other areas of the body.

Carotids. Either of two major arteries, one on each side of the neck, that carry blood to the head.

Cerebrovascular Accident. A sudden interruption of the blood supply to the brain caused by rupture of an artery in the brain (cerebral hemorrhage) or the blocking of a blood vessel, as by a clot of blood (cerebral occlusion); stroke.

Cervical. Relating to a neck, or cervix, in any sense.

Cetuximab. This drug is used alone or in combination with other agents and is effective in squamous cell carcinoma of the head and neck.

Chemoradiation. Chemotherapeutics—e.g., 5-FU, cisplatin, etoposide—followed by, or concurrently with, radiation therapy to treat cancer.

Chemotherapy. The treatment of disease by means of chemicals that have a specific toxic effect upon the disease-producing microorganisms or that selectively destroy cancerous tissue.

Chrondrosarcoma. A malignant tumor derived from cartilage cells or their precursors.

Chronic Obstructive Pulmonary Disease (COPD). Chronic lung disease, such as asthma or emphysema, in which breathing becomes slowed or forced.

Ciproflaxin. A broad-spectrum antibiotic used against Gram-negative bacteria. It is effective against anthrax.

Cisplatin. A platinum-containing chemotherapeutic drug used in the treatment of head and neck cancers.

Clinical Swallowing Evaluation (CSE). Addresses the swallowing-based activities of eating, drinking, and secretion management and, in addition, may address the activities of taking oral medications and teeth brushing.

Cochlea. A spiral-shaped cavity in the petrous portion of the temporal bone of the inner ear, containing the nerve endings essential for hearing and forming one of the divisions of the labyrinth.

Colloid. A translucent, yellowish, homogeneous material of the consistency of glue, less fluid than mucoid or mucinoid, found in the cells and tissues in a state of colloid degeneration, often in the context of thyroid cysts.

Computed Tomography (CT) Scan. Imaging anatomic information from a cross-sectional plane of the body, each image generated by a computer synthesis of x-ray transmission data obtained in many different directions in a given plane.

Concomitant. Existing or occurring with something else, often in a lesser way; accompanying; concurrent.

Conglomerate. Gathered or aggregated into a mass.

Contralateral. Taking place or originating in a corresponding part on an opposite side, as pain or paralysis in a part opposite the site of a lesion.

Coronary Artery Disease (CAD). Atherosclerosis of the coronary arteries, which can cause angina pectoris or heart attack. A positive family history, hypertension, smoking, diabetes mellitus, and elevated blood lipids increase the risk of developing coronary artery disease.

Cranial Nerves. Those nerves that emerge from, or enter, the cranium or skull, in contrast to the spinal nerves, which emerge from the spine or vertebral column. The 12 paired cranial nerves are the olfactory [CN I], optic [CN II], oculomotor [CN III], trochlear [CN IV], trigeminal [CN V], abducent [CN VI], facial [CN VII], vestibulocochlear [CN VIII], glossopharyngeal [CN IX], vagal [CN X], accessory [CN XI], and hypoglossal [CN XII] nerves.

Crico-Arytenoid. Relating to the cricoid and arytenoid cartilages.

Cricoid. The lowermost of the laryngeal cartilages; it is shaped like a signet ring, being expanded into a nearly quadrilateral plate (lamina) posteriorly; the anterior portion is called the arch (arcus).

Cricopharyngeal. Relating to the cricoid cartilage and the pharynx; a part of the inferior constrictor muscle of the pharynx.

Cricopharyngeal Myotomy. Division of the cephalad portion of the cricopharyngeus muscle, usually for treatment of Zenker esophageal diverticulum.

Crystalloid. Resembling a crystal, used in the context of intravenous fluids with dissolved electrolytes.

CT Scan. Short for *computed axial tomography scan.* An image of a body structure produced by computed axial tomography.

Cystic. Of, relating to, or having the characteristic of a cyst.

Cytokeratin. A global term for the family of intermediate filament proteins of epithelial origin; the pattern of cytokeratins (CKs) expressed may help differentiate colorectal from lung carcinomas based on low and high molecular weight types.

Débrided. To clean (a wound) by débridement.

Decannulated. The removal of a cannula or tube that may have been inserted during a surgical procedure, used in the context of tracheotomy tube removal.

Dehiscence. A bursting open or splitting along natural or sutured lines.

Delineated. To trace the outline of; sketch or trace in outline; represent pictorially.

Denervation. To deprive an organ or body part of a nerve supply, as by surgically removing or cutting a nerve or by blocking a nerve connection with drugs.

Deviated Septum. The nasal septum is a thin structure, separating the two sides of the nose. If it is not in the middle of the nose, then it is deviated.

Dexterity. Skill or adroitness in using the hands or body; agility.

Diflucan. Trademark for a broad-spectrum antifungal agent (fluconazole).

Dilation. The act of stretching or enlarging an opening or the lumen of a hollow structure.

Dobhoff Tube (DHT). A small-lumen feeding tube that can be advanced into the duodenum.

Docetaxel. An antineoplastic agent used particularly in treating carcinoma of the breast, head and neck cancer, and non small-cell lung cancer.

Dorsum. The upper, outer surface of an organ, an appendage, or a part.

Dosimetric. An instrument that measures the amount of radiation absorbed in a given period.

Dovetailed. Noting a partition line or a charge, as an ordinary, having a series of indentations suggesting dovetails.

Doxycycline. A tetracycline antibiotic used to treat conditions caused by a wide range of bacteria, including anthrax.

Dysgeusia. An impairment or dysfunction of the sense of taste.

Dysphagia/Aspiration-Related Structures (DARS). Pharyngeal constrictor muscles and the supraglottic and glottic larynx.

Dysphasia. Inability to speak or understand words because of a brain lesion.

Dysphonia. Difficulty in speaking, usually evidenced by hoarseness.

Echocardiogram. An ultrasound image of the heart that demonstrates the size, motion, and composition of cardiac structures and is used to diagnose various abnormalities of the heart, including valvular dysfunction, abnormal chamber size, congenital heart disease, and cardiomyopathy.

Eczema. An acute or chronic noncontagious inflammation of the skin, characterized chiefly by redness, itching, and the outbreak of lesions that may discharge serous matter and become encrusted and scaly.

Edematous. Effusion of serous fluid into the interstices of cells in tissue spaces or into body cavities causing swelling.

Edentulous. Having no teeth; toothless.

Electrocardiogram (EKG). A graphic recording of the electrical activity of the heart, used to evaluate cardiac function and to diagnose arrhythmias and other disorders.

Embolization. The process by which a blood vessel or organ is obstructed by an embolus or other mass. Specifically, a technique used by invasive radiologists to intentionally occlude arteries.

Emesis. The act or process of vomiting.

Emphysema. A pathological condition of the lungs marked by an abnormal increase in the size of the air spaces, resulting in labored breathing and an increased susceptibility to infection. It can be caused by irreversible expansion of the alveoli or by the destruction of alveolar walls. One of the COPDs.

Empirically. Relying on or derived from observation or experiment.

Endoscope. An instrument for examining visually the interior of a bodily canal or hollow organ such as the larynx or paranasal sinuses.

Eosinophilic. Having an affinity for eosin and other acid dyes; acidophilic.

Epidermal Growth Factor Receptor (EGFR). A protein found on the surface of cells to which epidermal growth factor (EGF) binds. When EGF attaches to EGFR, it activates the enzyme tyrosine kinase, triggering reactions that cause the cells to grow and multiply. EGFR is found at abnormally high levels on the surface of many types of cancer cells, which may divide excessively in the presence of EGF. Cetuximab is effective in blocking this mechanism.

Epistaxis. Bleeding from the nose.

Equivocal. Of doubtful nature or character; questionable; dubious; suspicious.

Erythema. Redness of the skin caused by dilatation and congestion of the capillaries, often a sign of inflammation or infection.

Esophagoscopy. Examination of the interior of the esophagus by means of an esophagoscope.

Esophagram. A series of x-ray images of the esophagus. The x-ray pictures are taken after the patient drinks a radio-opaque solution that coats and outlines the walls of the esophagus.

Esophogeal Stenosis. Stricture or a general narrowing of the esophagus.

Etiology. Cause or origin of a disease.

Eustacian Tubes. The tube that runs from the middle ear to the nasopharynx. The function of the eustachian tube is to protect, aerate, and drain the middle ear and mastoid.

Excision. The act of cutting out; the surgical removal of part or all of a structure or organ.

Exophytic. Descriptive term used for tumors that grow outward from the surface, rather than downward, deeper into the tissue.

External Beam Radiation. External radiation therapy where the energy source is outside the body, as opposed to interstitial radiation therapy (brachytherapy) or radioactive iodine therapy.

Extracapsular. Feature of tumor growth characterized by tumor extension beyond the surface of the lymph node.

Extranodal. Outside of a lymph node

Extubate. To remove a tube in the airway.

Falsetto. High-pitched voice produced by vibration of the anterior third of the vocal folds while the posterior folds are tightly adducted.

Fasciocutaneous Free Flap. Flap constructed of the deep muscle fascia with its overlying skin, and based on fasciocutaneous perforators arising from regional arteries and passing along fascial septa between adjacent muscles. The vascular anastomoses among the fasciocutaneous perforators within the deep fascial plexus are axial, therefore enabling a greater length:width ratio in the fasciocutaneous flap than in the random pattern skin flap.

Fiberoptic. An optical system in which light or an image is conveyed by a compact bundle of fine flexible glass or plastic fibers.

Fiberoptic Endoscopic Evaluation of Swallowing (FEES). A diagnostic technique for evaluation of deviant swallowing patterns, using a transnasal fiberoptic endoscope to visualize the larynx and pharynx.

Fibrosis. The formation of excessive fibrous tissue, as in a reparative or reactive process.

Fibular Flap. Transfer of tissue from the fibular area (leg) to a recipient site(s) for reconstructive purposes.

Fine-Needle Aspiration. The aspiration and removal of tissue or suspensions of cells through a small needle.

Fistula. An abnormal passage from a hollow organ to the body surface, or from one organ to another.

Flexible Fiberoptic Videonasendoscopy (FFV). A long cylindrical bronchoscope that may be placed through nose or mouth; allows visualization of upper and lower airways, as well as projection to a screen or monitor of received image. Used in tracheal intubation when indirect laryngoscopy has failed.

Friable. Readily crumbled; brittle, used to describe the gross characteristic of a tumor.

Functional Oral Intake Scale (FOIS). Diet level of safe oral intake meeting nutritional and hydration needs; contains seven levels: (1) Nothing by mouth (NPO); (2) Tube dependent with minimal attempts of food or liquid; (3) Tube dependent with consistent intake of liquid or food; (4) Total oral diet of a single consistency; (5) Total oral diet with multiple consistencies but requiring special preparation or compensations; (6) Total oral diet with multiple consistencies without special preparation, but with specific food limitations; (7) Total oral diet with no restriction.

Gait. A manner of walking, stepping, or running.

Gastroenterology. The medical specialty concerned with the function and disorders of the stomach, intestines, and related organs of the gastrointestinal tract.

Gastroesophageal. Relating to the stomach and the esophagus.

Gastroesophageal Reflux Disease (GERD). A syndrome due to structural or functional incompetence of the lower esophageal sphincter (LES), which permits retrograde flow of acidic gastric juice into the esophagus.

Gastrointestinal. Relating to the stomach and the intestines.

Gastrostomy. Surgical construction of a permanent opening from the external surface of the abdominal wall into the stomach, usually for inserting a feeding tube.

Geniculate Ganglion. A ganglion of the intermediate nerve located within the facial canal and containing sensory neurons that innervate taste buds on the front two-thirds of the tongue.

Genioglossus. One of the paired lingual muscles; origin, mental spine of the mandible; insertion, lingual fascia beneath the mucous membrane and epiglottis; action, depresses and protrudes the tongue; nerve supply, hypoglossal.

Glaucoma. Any of a group of eye diseases characterized by abnormally high intraocular fluid pressure, damaged optic disk, hardening of the eyeball, and partial to complete loss of vision.

Glissandos. A rapid slide through a series of consecutive tones in a scalelike passage.

Globus. A round or spherical body.

Globus Sensation. Commonly referred to as having a "lump in one's throat"), is the persistent sensation of having phlegm, a pill or some other sort of obstruction in the throat when there is none.

Glossectomy. Surgical removal of all or part of the tongue

Glossopharyngeal. Relating to the tongue and pharynx.

Glottic. Of or relating to the tongue.

Granulation Tissue. Tissue formed in ulcers and in early wound healing and repair, composed largely of newly growing capillaries and so called from its irregular surface in open wounds; proud flesh.

Granulomatous. A mass of inflamed granulation tissue, that is usually associated with ulcerated infections.

Granulomatous Disease. A group of diseases characterized by the formation of granulomas (e.g., tuberculosis).

Hard Palate. The anterior bony portion of the roof of the mouth, extending backward to the soft palate

Head and Neck Cancer (HNC). Head and neck cancer refers to any cancer that occurs in the head and neck, although commonly confined to the cancers of the aerodigestive tract of the head and neck.

Heat Moisture Exchange (HME). A humidifying filter that fits onto the end of the trach tube and comes in several shapes and sizes. Also known by several other terms, including Thermal humidfying filters, Swedish nose, Artificial nose, Filter, Thermovent T.

Hematologic. Pertaining to or emanating from blood cells.

Hemostasis. The stoppage of bleeding or hemorrhage.

Hepatitis. Inflammation of the liver, caused by infectious or toxic agents and characterized by jaundice, fever, liver enlargement, and abdominal pain.

Heterogeneous. Composed of parts having dissimilar characteristics or properties.

Hiatal Hernia. A hernia in which part of the stomach protrudes through the esophageal opening of the diaphragm.

Hiatus. An aperture or fissure in an organ or a body part.

Histopathologic. The study of the microscopic structure of diseased tissues

Human Papillomavirus (HPV). A large family of viruses, some of which cause genital warts; HPV can be transmitted to a fetus during birth. HPV-16 can cause cancer of the oropharynx.

Hyoglossus Muscle. Origin, body and greater horn of hyoid bone; insertion, side of the tongue; action, retracts and pulls down side of tongue; nerve supply, motor by hypoglossal, sensory by lingual.

Hyoid Bone. A U-shaped bone at the base of the tongue that supports the muscles of the tongue.

Hyolaryngeal Excursion. A movement that occurs during the normal swallowing process. The hyoid and thyroid are pulled together while both are pulled upward and forward as well as contraction of the paired thyrohyoid muscles.

Hyperbaric Oxygen (HBO). Oxygen at a pressure that is above one atmosphere used to promote nonhealing wounds.

Hypercholesterolemia. An abnormally high concentration of cholesterol in the blood.

Hyperkeratosis. Hypertrophy of the cornea or the horny layer of the skin

Hypertension (HTN). Persistent high blood pressure.

Hypertonicity. An increased level of muscle tone in laryngology.

Hypertrophy. General increase in bulk of a part or organ, not due to tumor formation. Use of the term may be restricted to denote greater bulk through increase in size, but not in number, of cells or other individual tissue elements.

Hypoglossal Nerve. Either one of the 12th pair of cranial nerves, consisting of motor fibers that innervate the muscles of the tongue.

Hypopharyngeal. Located beneath the oropharyngeal level, posterior to the larynx.

Hypothyroidism. Insufficient production of thyroid hormones by the thyroid gland.

Iatrogenic. Caused by care provider, usually referred to adverse outcome from a therapeutic intervention.

Idiopathic. Of or relating to a disease having no known cause; agnogenic.

Illicit. Not legally permitted or authorized; unlicensed; unlawful.

Immunohistochemical. Microscopic localization of specific antigens in tissues by staining with antibodies labeled with fluorescent or pigmented material.

In situ Hybridization. A technique developed in 1969 for annealing nucleic acid probes to cellular DNA for detection by autoradiography. Under proper laboratory conditions, the binding process occurs spontaneously. In situ hybridization constitutes a key step in DNA fingerprinting.

Incisors. A tooth with a chisel-shaped crown and a single conical tapering root; there are four of these teeth in the anterior part of each jaw, in both the deciduous and the permanent dentitions.

Indurated. Hardened, as a soft tissue that becomes extremely firm.

Infraglottic. Inferior to the glottis.

Intensity-Modulated Radiation Therapy (IMRT). A specialized method of delivering radiation so that the beam enters the body from many different angles to get to the tumor with pinpoint accuracy while sparing much of the surrounding healthy tissue.

Intralaryngeal. Within the larynx.

Intraoperative. Occurring during a surgical operation.

Intraoral. Within the mouth.

Invasive. Of or relating to a medical procedure in which a part of the body is entered, as by puncture or incision.

Inversion. A turning inward, inside out, or other reversal of the normal relation of a part.

Ipsilateral. Pertaining to, situated on, or affecting the same side of the body.

Isocenter. The convergence of the three axes of rotation in radiation therapy; the intersecting point of the axis of rotation of the gantry, the collimator, and the treatment couch.

Isometric. Of or exhibiting equality in dimensions or measurements.

IVA Disease. In the TNM staging for tumor classification, Stage IVA stands for advanced stage of disease, without distant metastasis.

IVC Syndrome. In the TNM staging system of tumor classification, stands for advanced stage of disease with distant metastasis.

Jugulodigastric Lymph Node. A prominent lymph node in the deep lateral cervical group, lying below the digastric muscle and anterior to the internal jugular vein; it receives lymphatic drainage from the pharynx, palatine tonsil, and tongue, usually referred to as Level IIa node.

Keratinize. To make or become horny tissue.

L-Discs. The five vertebrae situated between the thoracic vertebrae and the sacral vertebrae in the spinal column. The lumbar vertebrae are represented by the symbols L1 through L5.

Labial. Relating to the lips.

Lamictal. Trademark for an anticonvulsant drug (lamotrigine).

LaryClips. A two-piece system, consisting of a square adhesive base and a hook-and-loop clip that helps to optimize the airtight attachment of the Provox LaryButton and Provox LaryTube to the stoma.

Laryngeal. Of, relating to, affecting, or near the larynx.

Laryngeal Vestibule. The upper part of the laryngeal cavity from the superior aperture to the vestibular folds or rima vestibuli, bounded anteriorly by the epiglottis, laterally by the mucosa overlying the quadrangular membranes and posteriorly by the mucosa overlying the arytenoid cartilages and arytenoideus muscle.

Laryngologist. The branch of medicine dealing with the study and treatment of disorders of the larynx.

Laryngoscopy. Examination of the larynx by means of a laryngoscope.

Larynx. The part of the respiratory tract between the pharynx and the trachea, having walls of cartilage and muscle and containing the vocal cords enveloped in folds of mucous membrane.

Larytube. A soft laryngectomy tube.

Lateral Lisp. A speech defect or mannerism characterized by mispronunciation of the sounds /s/ and /z/ as /th/ and /th/.

Lateralization. Causing a structure to move laterally. Also referring to sidedness.

Left Main Bronchus. Primary division of the tracheobronchial tree arising as the left branch of the bifurcation of the trachea, then passing in front of the esophagus and enters the hilum of the left lung where it divides into a superior lobe bronchus and an inferior lobe bronchus. It is longer, of narrower caliber, and more nearly horizontal than the right main bronchus, and hence, aspirated objects enter it less frequently.

Lesion. A pathologic abnormality, often synonymous with tumor.

Lethargy. A state of sluggishness, inactivity, and apathy.

Leukoplakia. A condition characterized by white spots or patches on mucous membranes, especially of the mouth.

Lingual Artery. An artery with origin in the carotid artery, with distribution to the undersurface of the tongue, terminating as the deep artery of the tongue, and with branches to the suprahyoid and dorsal lingual branches and the sublingual artery.

Locoregional. Limited to a localized region or area, as contrasted with systemic or metastatic.

Lumen. The inner open space or cavity of a tubular organ, as of a blood vessel.

Lymphadenopathy. A chronic, abnormal enlargement of the lymph nodes, usually associated with disease.

Lymphoid Tissue. The part of the body's immune system that is important for the immune response and helps protect it from infection and foreign bodies. Lymphoid tissue is present throughout the body and includes the lymph nodes, spleen, tonsils, adenoids, and other structures.

Lymphovascular. Pertaining to lymphatic vessels.

M.D. Anderson Dysphagia Inventory (MDADI). A multisymptom patient-reported outcome measure for clinical and research use. The MDASI's 13 core items include symptoms found to have the highest frequency and/or severity in patients with various cancers and treatment types.

Malaise. A vague feeling of bodily discomfort, as at the beginning of an illness.

Malar. Relating to the mala, the cheek or cheek bones.

Malignancy. Usually used to describe a malignant growth, or cancer.

Mandible. The bone of the lower jaw.

Mandibular Arch. The curved structure of the mandible.

Mandibular Tori. A bony protuberance on the lingual aspect of the lower jaw in the canine-premolar region.

Mandibulectomy. Resection of the lower jaw.

Masako Maneuver. During a swallow, maintenance of the larynx for a few seconds at the highest position in the neck by voluntary muscular contraction. This laryngeal elevation results in a wider and longer esophageal opening and is a therapeutic technique for management of swallowing disorders.

Maxillary. Of or relating to the upper jaw.

McNeill Dysphagia Therapy. A systematic exercise-based rehabilitation framework for swallowing remediation.

Medication Administration Record (MAR) Device. A computer-generated schedule for administering medications to a patient for a defined period of time, including dosing, timing of administration and details about the physician's orders.

Melanoma. A dark-pigmented, malignant, frequently widely metastasizing tumor arising from a melanocyte and occurring most commonly in the skin.

Mendelsohn Maneuver. During a swallow, maintenance of the larynx for a few seconds at the highest position in the neck by voluntary muscular contraction. This laryngeal elevation results in a wider and longer esophageal opening and is a therapeutic technique for management of swallowing disorders.

Mentum. The prominence formed by the anterior projection of the mandible, or lower jaw; chin.

Metastasis. The transference of malignant or cancerous cells to other parts of the body by way of the blood or lymphatic vessels or membranous surfaces.

Metastatic. The term used to describe a secondary cancer, or one that has spread from one area of the body to another.

Microlaryngoscopy. Examination of the interior of the larynx with a laryngoscope and the binocular magnification provided by a microscope.

Microvascular. Pertaining to small blood vessels requiring magnification in order to perform surgical procedures.

Microvascular Free Radial Forearm Flap. The radial forearm consists of thin, pliable skin that can be molded in three dimensions and transferred as a sensate flap, making it ideal for most head and neck reconstructions. This requires microvascular surgery to perform blood vessel anastomoses.

MiraLax. Also known as polyethylene glycol and is an osmotic laxative. Polyethylene glycol works by retaining water in the stool, resulting in softer stools and more frequent bowel movements.

Modified Barium Swallow Impairment Profile (MBSImP). An evidence-based, standardization of the MBS study in adults. The MBSImP assesses 17 critical components of swallowing and provides an objective profile of the physiologic impairment affecting adult swallowing function.

Modified Barium Swallow Study (MBSS). Radiologic examination performed while the person swallows barium-coated substances, done to assess quality of the swallowing mechanisms of the mouth, pharynx, and esophagus.

Monoclonal. Derived from a single cell.

Mononeuropathy. Disorder involving a single nerve.

Morphologic. The patterns of word formation in a particular language, including inflection, derivation, and composition.

Mucinous/Myxoid Matrix. Permanent histologic sections reveal numerous small papillary structures surrounded by single layer of cuboidal or columnar cells. The cells have round nuclei and delicate chromatin and lack obvious cytoplasmic processes. The cores of the papillae are either completely filled up with the mucinous/myxoid matrix or have a central blood vessel surrounded by the matrix.

Mucocutaneous. Relating to mucous membrane and skin; denoting the line of junction of the two at the nasal, oral, vaginal, and anal orifices.

Mucosa. A membrane lining all body passages that communicate with the exterior, such as the respiratory, genitourinary, and alimentary tracts, and having cells and associated glands that secrete mucus.

Mucositis. Inflammation of a mucous membrane.

Multidimensional Functional Evaluation (OARS). Assesses level of functioning in five areas: social and economic resources, mental and physical health, activities of daily living (ADL).

Multinucleated. Having multiple nuclei.

Musculature. The arrangement of the muscles in a part or in the body as a whole.

Musculocutaneous. Pertaining to, composed of, or supplying both muscles and skin.

Mylohyoid. Muscle contributing to the floor of mouth.

Myocardial Infarction (MI). Heart attack; Necrosis of a region of the myocardium caused by an interruption in the supply of blood to the heart, usually as a result of occlusion of a coronary artery.

Myofascial. Of or relating to the fascia surrounding and separating muscle tissue.

Nasal Regurgitation. The nasopharynx closes through a combination of soft palate elevation and contraction of the upper pharyngeal constrictor muscles (the superior pharyngeal constrictors). Failure of this closure mechanism, pharyngeal retention, or esophagopharyngeal regurgitation can result in nasal regurgitation.

Nasogastric. Relating to or involving the nasal passages and the stomach.

Necrosis. Death of cells or tissues through injury or disease, especially in a localized area of the body.

Neopharynx. A surgically reconstructed pharynx.

Neoplastic. An abnormal new growth of tissue that grows by cellular proliferation more rapidly than normal, continues to grow after the stimuli that initiated the new growth cease, shows partial or complete lack of structural organization and functional coordination with the normal tissue, and usually forms a distinct mass of tissue which may be either benign or malignant.

Nephrectomy. Surgical removal of a kidney.

Nephrotoxic. Pertaining to nephrotoxin; toxic to renal cells.

Neurology. The branch of medical science concerned with the various nervous systems (central, peripheral, and autonomic), plus the neuromuscular junction and muscle, and their disorders.

Neuropathic. Relating in any way to neuropathy.

NID Prosthesis. A non-indwelling voice prosthesis, designed to be inserted, removed and cleaned by the patients themselves. Each prosthesis comes with a nonsterile, reusable NID Inserter.

Nodal Disease. Cancerous involvement of lymph node or nodes.

NPO Status. Abbreviation for nothing by mouth.

Nystatin. An antibiotic produced by the actinomycete *Streptomyces noursei* and used especially in the treatment of fungal infections.

Obstructive Sleep Apnea (OSA). A potentially life-threatening condition characterized by episodes of breathing cessation during sleep alternating with snoring or disordered breathing. The low levels of oxygen in the blood of patients with OSA may eventually cause heart problems or stroke.

Obturator. In head and neck surgery, pertains to a prefabricated denture-like device made by a prosthetic dentist, used to occlude palatal defects.

Occlusion. A complete closure (e.g., in the vocal tract) causing stoppage of the flow of air and accumulation of pressure.

Odynophagia. Pain on swallowing.

Oncology. The branch of medicine concerned with the study, classification, and treatment of cancer.

Opacification. Pertaining to a cloudiness on x-ray suggestive of fluid in a normally air-filled space.

Opioids. A drug containing opium or its derivatives, used in medicine for inducing sleep and relieving pain.

Oral Herpes. A disease caused by herpes simplex virus Type 1, characterized primarily by a cluster of small, transient blisters chiefly at the edge of the lip or nostril; herpes labialis.

Orifice. An opening, especially to a cavity or passage of the body; a mouth or vent.

Oropharyngeal. The pharynx located between the level of the palate and the hyoid bone.

Osteonecrosis. Necrosis of bone.

Osteoradionecrosis. Bone tissue death induced by radiation.

Osteotomies. Surgical division or sectioning of bone.

Otalgia. Pain in the ear; earache.

Otitis. Inflammation of the ear.

Ototoxic. Having a harmful effect on the organs or nerves concerned with hearing and balance.

Otolaryngologist. A physician that deals with diagnosis and treatment of diseases of the ear, larynx, and upper respiratory tract.

Otolaryngology. The branch of medicine that deals with diagnosis and treatment of diseases of the ear, nose, and throat.

Pachydermia. Abnormally thick skin or mucosa.

Palatal. Relating to the palate or the palate bone.

Palatine Tonsil. A large oval mass of lymphoid tissue embedded in the lateral wall of the oral pharynx on either side between the pillars of the fauces.

Palmaris Longus. Muscle of superficial layer of anterior (flexor) compartment of forearm; origin, medial epicondyle of humerus; insertion, flexor retinaculum of wrist and palmar fascia; action, tenses palmar fascia and flexes the hand and forearm; is absent about 20% of the time; when tensed, its tendon stands out sharply at the wrist and overlies the median nerve; nerve supply, median.

Palmaris Tendon. A superficial muscle of the forearm, arising from a humeral and an ulnar head and ending in a flat tendon that inserts into the radius. It functions to pronate the hand.

Palpable. Capable of being touched or felt; tangible.

Palpitation. Perceptible forcible pulsation of the heart, usually with an increase in frequency or force, with or without irregularity in rhythm.

Palsy. Paralysis or paresis.

Papillomatosis. Papillary projections of the epidermis forming an undulating surface; also refers to the condition of numerous papillomas associated with HPV

Paresis. Slight or partial paralysis.

Parotid Gland. Paired salivary glands situated in the cheek areas.

Parotid-Sparing IMRT Approach. Radiation technique that seeks to avoid delivering radiation dose to the parotid salivary glands.

PARSPORT Trial. A Phase III multicenter randomized controlled trial of parotid-sparing IMRT in patients with head and neck cancer. It is designed to demonstrate a difference in the proportion of patients suffering xerostomia (dry mouth) of Grade 2 or more, 1 year after treatment, in head and neck cancer patients treated with parotid-sparing intensity-modulated radiotherapy or conventional radiotherapy.

Patency. The state or quality of being open, expanded, or unblocked.

Pectoralis. Either of two muscles on each side of the upper and anterior part of the thorax, the action of the larger (pectoralis major) assisting in drawing the shoulder forward and rotating the arm inward, and the action of the smaller (pectoralis minor) assisting in drawing the shoulder downward and forward.

Pectoralis Flap. Comprises the pectoralis major muscle, with or without overlying skin, and may include the underlying ribs. It has an axial blood supply, and is based superiorly on the pectoral branch of the thoracoacromial artery. It is very useful in the head and neck, and can *inter alia* be used for the following: reconstruction of soft tissue defects of the oropharynx, oral cavity, hypopharynx, and skin of the neck; to augment pharyngeal repairs following salvage laryngectomy following previous chemoradiotherapy, and to cover carotid or jugular vein blowouts, and so on. Rib may be included to bridge mandibular defects.

Penetration-Aspiration Scale (PAS). The development and use of an 8-point, equal-appearing interval scale to describe penetration and aspiration events are described. Scores are determined primarily by the depth to which material passes in the airway and by whether or not material entering the airway is expelled. (1) Material does not enter the airway. (2) Material enters the airway, remains above the vocal folds, and is ejected from the airway. (3) Material enters the airway, remains above the vocal folds, and is not ejected from the airway. (4) Material enters the airway, contacts the vocal folds, and is ejected from the airway. (5) Material enters the airway, contacts the vocal folds, and is not ejected from the airway. (6) Material enters the airway, passes below the vocal folds and is ejected into the larynx or out of the airway. (7) Material enters the airway, passes below the vocal folds, and is not ejected from the trachea despite effort. (8) Material enters the airway, passes below the vocal folds, and no effort is made to eject.

Pentoxifylline. A bitter-tasting compound that decreases blood viscosity and improves blood flow, used in the treatment of intermittent claudication.

Percutaneous Endoscopic Gastrostomy (PEG). A gastrostomy performed without opening the abdominal cavity; usually involves gastroscopy, insufflation of the stomach, and puncture of stomach and abdominal wall, followed by placement of a special tube.

Piriform Sinus. A recess in the anterolateral wall of the nasopharynx on each side of the vestibule of the larynx separated from it by the aryepiglottic folds.

Perinural Invasion. Surgical pathology term describing extension of epithelial cells around nerves which, while typical of malignancy, may be seen in sclerosing adenosis–breast, and is not per se an indication of malignancy.

Pharyngocutaneous Fistula. The most common nonfatal complication following total laryngectomy. It creates a communication between the pharynx and cervical skin around the surgical incision or, less frequently, the stoma of the tracheostomy.

Pharyngotomy. Surgical incision into the pharynx.

Phonation. Rapid, periodic opening and closing of the glottis through separation and apposition of the vocal cords that, accompanied by breath under lung pressure, constitutes a source of vocal sound.

Phonotraumatic. Any abuse or misuse of the vocal cords (folds), more commonly seen in those with professional voices, which gives rises to various lesions (e.g., polyps, nodules, degenerative polyps, cysts, varices) and other benign conditions.

Pneumonia. An acute or chronic disease marked by inflammation of the lungs and caused by viruses, bacteria, or other microorganisms and sometimes by physical and chemical irritants.

Polyneuropathies. A nontraumatic generalized disorder of peripheral nerves, affecting the distal fibers most severely, with proximal shading (the feet are affected sooner or more severely than the hands), and typically symmetrically; most often affects motor and sensory fibers almost equally, but can involve either one, either solely or very disproportionately; classified as axon degenerating (axonal), or demyelinating; many causes, particularly metabolic and toxic; familial or sporadic.

Positive Margins. When the cut edges of the cancer specimen is involved with cancer on histopathology.

Prevacid Solutabs. A proton pump inhibitor used to inhibit gastric acid secretion for the treatment of duodenal or gastric ulcer, gastroesophageal reflux disease, and hyperchlorhydria.

Prognosis. A forecasting of the probable course and outcome of a disease, especially of the chances of recovery.

Prophylactic. Defending or protecting from disease or infection, as a drug.

Prophylaxis. The preventing of disease.

Propulsion. A driving or propelling force.

Prosthodontist. A professional in the branch of dentistry that deals with the restoration and maintenance of oral function by the replacement of missing teeth and other oral structures by artificial devices (see obturator).

Proton Therapy. A type of particle therapy which uses a beam of protons to irradiate diseased tissue, most often in the treatment of cancer. The chief advantage of proton therapy is the ability to more precisely localize the radiation dosage when compared with other types of external beam radiotherapy.

Protonix. Trade name for a proton pump inhibitor used for short-term treatment of erosion and ulceration of the esophagus caused by gastroesophageal reflux disease.

Proton Pump Inhibitor (PPI). Agents that block the transport of hydrogen ions into the stomach and hence are useful in the treatment of gastric hyperacidity.

Protrusion. To project or cause to project from or as if from a surface.

Pterygoid Muscle. Head of origin from the infratemporal surface and crest of the greater wing of the sphenoid; this part of the muscle attaches to the discocapsular system (fibrous layer of the joint capsule and articular disc) of the temporomandibular joint and has been determined by electromyography to be active during both protrusion and retrusion of the mandible serving in both to ensure that the disc moves in concert with the excursion of the head of the mandible.

Pterygopalatine Fossa. A small pyramidal space, housing the pterygopalatine ganglion and third part of the maxillary artery, between the pterygoid process, the maxilla, and the palatine bone.

Pulmonary Pleural Disease. Inflammation of the pleura covering the lungs.

Pulsed-Dye Laser (PDL). Extremely short bursts of focused yellow light absorbed by hemoglobin, used to treat hemangiomas without anesthesia in young children.

Piriform. Pear shaped. Refers to the funnel shaped portion of the hypopharynx on either side of the larynx that drains into the esophageal inlet.

Queried. To question as doubtful or obscure.

Radiation-Associated Dysphagia (RAD). A debilitating, delayed toxicity of nonsurgical organ preservation for head and neck cancers.

Radiation-Oncology. The medical specialty concerned with the use of ionizing radiation in the treatment of disease.

Randomized Phase III Trial. Clinical trials are conducted in a series of steps, called phases—each phase is designed to answer a separate research question. **Phase I:** Researchers test a new drug or treatment in a small group of people for the first time to evaluate its safety, determine a safe dosage range, and identify side effects. **Phase II:** The drug or treatment is given to a larger group of people to see if it is effective and to further evaluate its safety. **Phase III:** The drug or treatment is given to large groups of people to confirm its effectiveness, monitor side effects, compare it to commonly used treatments, and collect information that will allow the drug or treatment to be used safely. **Phase IV:** Studies are done after the drug or treatment has been marketed to gather information on the drug's effect in various populations and any side effects associated with long-term use.

Recurrent. Occurring or appearing again or repeatedly.

Reflux. A flowing back.

Renal. Of or relating to the kidneys or the surrounding regions.

Resection. Surgical removal of part of an organ or a structure.

Retropharyngeal Lymph Nodes. The three groups of lymph nodes (one median and two lateral) located between the pharynx and the prevertebral layer of cervical fascia; they receive lymph from the nasopharynx, the auditory tube, and the atlantooccipital and atlantoaxial joints.

Rhinolalia. A nasal tone in speech.

Right Main Bronchus. Primary division of the tracheobronchial tree arising as the right of branch at the bifurcation of the trachea; it enters the hilum of the right lung, giving off the superior lobe bronchus and continuing downward to give off the middle and inferior lobe bronchi. It is shorter, of larger caliber, and more nearly vertical than the left main bronchus; thus, aspirated objects more frequently lodge on the right side.

Rinne. A hearing test in which a vibrating tuning fork is held against the mastoid process until the sound is lost and then brought close to the auditory orifice.

Ritalin. Trademark preparation of methylphenidate, a drug related to amphetamine, used to treat attention-deficit disorder in children

Robotic Surgery. Pertains to use of a surgical robotic system which employs multiple arms controlled by the surgeon at an actuator console. These arms are designed to hold and position a three-dimensional camera system as well as to manipulate specialized instruments.

S-Discs. There are five sacral vertebral bones. They are represented by the symbols S1 through S5 and are situated between the lumbar vertebrae and the coccyx (the lowest segment of the vertebral column). The sacral vertebrae are normally fused to form the sacrum.

Sclerosis. The hardening of a tissue or part due to chronic inflammation.

Segmental Composite Resection. Full thickness of a segment of mandibular bone is resected, often along with the floor of mouth and a part of the tongue, generally for advanced squamous cell carcinoma, though occasionally for osteoradionecrosis following complications of prior irradiation or for other malignancies such as osteosarcoma.

Sensate. Perceived by a sense or the senses.

Sequelae. A pathological condition resulting from a disease.

Serous Middle Ear Effusion. Fluid behind the eardrum in the middle ear. It occurs without an ear infection.

Servox Electrolarynx. The only speech aid that offers the possibility of programming both buttons with different volume and frequency settings.

Shaker Exercise. The patient lies flat and, keeping the shoulders on the bed/mat, raises the head to look at the toes. The patient maintains this position (the goal is 60 s) and then repeats this two more times. The second part of the exercise is a repetitive movement. In the same starting position, the patient raises the head to look at the chin, lowers the head back to the bed and then repeats this 30 times. Three sets of 30 are the goal.

Sham-Controlled. A treatment or procedure that is performed as a control and that is similar to but omits a key therapeutic element of the treatment or procedure under investigation.

Skelaxin. A centrally acting muscle relaxant.

Snuff. A preparation of finely pulverized tobacco that can be drawn up into the nostrils by inhaling; people also put this in the gingivolabial sulcus.

Soft Palate. The posterior fleshy portion of the roof of the mouth. It forms a movable muscular flap that seals off the nasopharynx during swallowing and speech.

Sphenopalatine. Pertaining to the sphenoid and palatine bones.

Squamous Cell. A flat, scalelike epithelial cell.

Stasis. Stoppage of the normal flow of a body substance, as of blood through an artery or of intestinal contents through the bowels.

Stent. A device that is used to maintain a bodily orifice or cavity after skin grafting or other surgical manipulation, or to immobilize a skin graft following placement.

Sternocleidomastoid Muscle. A muscle with origin from the anterior surface of the episternum and from the sternal end of the clavicle, with insertion into the mastoid process and the superior nuchal line, with nerve supply from the accessory nerve, and whose action turns the head obliquely to the opposite side and flexes the neck and extends the head when both sides act together.

Stomal. A temporary or permanent opening in a body surface, especially the abdomen or throat, that is created by a surgical procedure, such as a colostomy or laryngectomy.

Stricture. A constriction of airflow within a passage.

Stridor. A harsh, high-pitched sound in inhalation or exhalation.

Stroboscopic. Pertaining to an instrument producing a flashing light, the frequency of which can be synchronized with some multiple of the frequency of rotation, vibration, or operation of an object, and so on, making it appear stationary. It is used to determine speeds of rotation or vibration, or to adjust objects or parts.

Stroboscopy. Endoscopy performed with an intermittent light at a frequency that approximates the frequency of movement of the object visualized so that it appears to be motionless; useful in analyzing vocal fold structure and motion.

Stromal. Relating to the background tissue on histopathology or the connective/structural tissue of an organ or other structure.

Submandibular. Beneath the mandible or lower jaw.

Sulcus. Any of the grooves on the brain surface, bounding the gyri; a fissure.

Supraglottic. Above the glottis.

Supraglottic Swallow Technique. It is also called the voluntary airway closure technique. (1) Take a deep breath and hold it tightly. (2) Take a bite of food or a sip of liquid. (3) Swallow while holding your breath until it is completed. (4) Cough immediately after the swallow. (5) Swallow again. (6) Breathe.

Surgical Robot. A device that seeks to improve surgical outcomes by reducing or eliminating most of the disadvantages of traditional (manual) surgery. The surgeon is seated near the patient and controls the device, which contains high-resolution cameras and microsurgical instruments; the robot scales, filters, and translates the surgeon's gestures into precise movement in the operative field, resulting in improved outcomes, faster recuperation, and fewer complications.

Sutured. The surgical method used to close a wound or join tissues.

Symptomatology. The medical science of symptoms.

Synergistically. Acting together

Taxol. Trademark for drug developed from the toxin of specific types of yew trees and bushes and used to kill dividing cells, especially tumor cells.

The Eating Assessment Tool (EAT-10). A 10-item self-administered questionnaire developed to evaluate dysphagia symptoms in persons with a wide variety of causes of dysphagia and in different clinical settings.

Therabite. A portable system specifically designed to treat trismus and mandibular hypomobility.

Thyroidectomy. Surgical removal of thyroid gland.

Tinnitus. A sound in one ear or both ears, such as buzzing, ringing, or whistling, occurring without an external stimulus and usually caused by a specific condition, such as an ear infection, the use of certain drugs, a blocked auditory tube or canal, or a head injury.

Tomography. Any of several techniques for making detailed x-rays of a plane section of a solid object, such as the body, while blurring out the images of other planes.

Tonsil. Intramucosal collection of lymphocytes or aggregated lymphoid tissue closely associated with the overlying epithelium, commonly referred to as the palatine tonsil.

Tonsillar Fossae. The depression between the palatoglossal and palatopharyngeal arches occupied by the palatine tonsil.

Tonsillar Pillars. Synonymous with the palatoglossal and palatopharyngeal arches; Folds of mucous membrane in the palatine arch that correspond to the underlying palatoglossus and palatopharyngeus muscles.

TORS. Transoral robotic surgery. This is a specific application of robotic surgical technology to address tumors of the oropharynx, hypopharynx, tongue base, and upper larynx. The improved visualization and the capability for wristed action of the instruments can allow for an en bloc resection of tumors without having to resort to open exposure techniques.

Tracheoesophageal Voice Prosthesis (TEP). A tracheoesophageal voice prosthesis is a device made of medical-grade silicone, which is positioned within the "party wall" which is the shared wall between the trachea and the esophagus. The voice prosthesis itself does not produce a voice. The purpose of the prosthesis is to allow air to be delivered from the lungs into the esophagus where it is expelled through the mouth. The passage of air as it travels from the esophagus to the mouth, results in vibration of tissues in the lower pharynx, or throat, producing sound which serves as the new voice for laryngectomy patients.

Tramadol HCI. An analgesic drug with a mechanism of action that is unusual in that one optic isomer exerts typical opioid-type effects and the other isomer interacts with the reuptake and/or release of norepinephrine and serotonin in nerve terminals.

Transurethral. Performed through the urethra.

Transoral Robotic Surgery (TORS). The surgical approach that allows for a guided endoscope to provide a high-resolution, 3D image of the back of the mouth and throat that is a difficult area to reach with conventional tools. With two robotically guided instruments that act as a surgeon's arms, tumors are able to be dissected free from surrounding tissue safely.

Trapezius. A broad, flat muscle on each side of the upper and back part of the neck, shoulders, and back, the action of which raises, or rotates, or draws back the shoulders, and pulls the head backward or to one side.

Trismus. A firm closing of the jaw due to tonic spasm of the muscles of mastication from disease of the motor branch of the trigeminal nerve. It is usually associated with general tetanus.

True Vocal Fold. The sharp-edged fold of mucous membrane overlying and incorporating the vocal ligament and the thyroarytenoid muscle and stretching along either wall of the larynx from the angle between the laminae of the thyroid cartilage to the vocal process of the arytenoid cartilage; airflow causes the vocal folds to vibrate in production of the voice.

Tuberculosis. An infectious disease of humans and animals caused by the tubercle bacillus and characterized by the formation of tubercles on the lungs and other tissues of the body, often developing long after the initial infection (a granulomatous disease).

Tuning Fork. A steel instrument consisting of a stem with two prongs, producing a musical tone of definite, constant pitch when struck, and serving as a standard for tuning musical instruments, making acoustical experiments, and the like.

Tympanogram. The printout of immittance showing the stiffness or the compliance of the middle ear structures as it varies with changes in pressure within the external auditory canal.

Ulcerative. Causing ulceration.

Ultrasonography. Diagnostic imaging in which ultrasound is used to visualize an internal body structure or a developing fetus.

Unasyn. An intravenous antibiotic combination of ampicillin and sulbactam with broad-spectrum antibacterial activity.

University of Washington Quality of Life Questionnaire (UW-QoL). An English-language survey instrument used worldwide to assess the quality of life of patients with head and neck cancer.

Uvula. The small, fleshy, conical body projecting downward from the middle of the soft palate.

Vallecula. An anatomical crevice or depression on any surface, such as the deep hollow on the inferior surface of the cerebellum, between the hemispheres, in which the medulla oblongata rests.

Vallecula Epiglottica. A depression immediately posterior to the root of the tongue between the median and lateral glossoepiglottic folds on either side.

Valtrex. A trademark for the drug valacyclovir hydrochloride; Rapidly converts to acyclovir, which interferes with viral DNA synthesis and replication.

Vancomycin. An antibiotic that is produced by the actinomycete *Streptomyces orientalis,* and is effective against staphylococci and spirochetes.

Varibar. A contrast agent tailor made for oropharyngeal examination, it is not uncommon to find clinicians using other imaging products in videofluoroscopy; these products may be mixed in ways that differ from the manufacturer guidelines for intended use.

Velar. Concerning or using the soft palate.

Velopharyngeal. Of or relating to the soft palate and the posterior nasopharyngeal wall.

Viable. Capable of living, developing, or germinating under favorable conditions.

Videofluoroscopy. Fluoroscopy using an image intensifier and television camera for image detection and a video monitor for display.

Video Laryngeal Stroboscopy (VLS). Allows early detection of infiltrative processes of the vocal folds, thus increasing potential possibilities of early diagnostics of laryngeal carcinoma; can also be used in diagnosing and treating benign vocal disease.

Vidian Nerve. The nerve constituting the parasympathetic and sympathetic root of the pterygopalatine ganglion; it is formed in the region of the foramen lacerum by the union of the greater and deep petrosal nerves and runs through the pterygoid canal to the pterygopalatine fossa.

Volitional. The act or an instance of making a conscious choice or decision.

Waldeyer's Ring. The broken ring of lymphoid tissue, formed of the lingual, faucial, and pharyngeal tonsils.

Weber. The standard unit of magnetic flux and magnetic pole strength in the International System of Units (SI), equal to a flux that produces an electromotive force of 1 volt in a single turn of wire when the flux is uniformly reduced to zero in a period of 1 s; 10^8 maxwells

Wellbutrin. The trademark for the antidepressant bupropion.

Xerostomia. Dryness of the mouth caused by diminished function of the salivary glands due to aging, disease, drug reaction, and so on.

Zegerid Powder. A proton pump inhibitor used in the treatment of dyspepsia, peptic ulcer disease (PUD), and gastroesophageal reflux disease (GERD).

Zosyn. Zosyn is an injectable combination of two antibiotics, piperacillin and tazobactam, with broad-spectrum activity against an extended range of bacterial species.

Index

Note: Page numbers in **bold** refer to illustrations and tables.